Beyond the Bottom Line:
Management in Government

Beyond the Bottom Line: Management in Government

by

Timothy W. Plumptre

The Institute for Research on Public Policy
L'Institut de recherches politiques

Printed in Canada

Legal Deposit Second Quarter
Bibliothèque nationale du Québec

Canadian Cataloguing in Publication Data

Plumptre, Timothy W. (Timothy Wynne)

Beyond the bottom line

Prefatory material in English and French.
ISBN 0-88645-069-1

1. Public administration. 2. Civil service —
Personnel management. 3. Canada — Officials and
employees. 4. Great Britain — Officials and
employees. I. Institute for Research on Public
Policy. II. Title.

JF1351.P58 1988   351.007   C88-098550-X

The camera-ready copy for this publication was created
on a Xerox 6085 Desktop Publishing System.

The Institute for Research on Public Policy/
L'Institut de recherches politiques
P.O. Box 3670 South
Halifax, Nova Scotia B3J 3K6

To my mother, Beryl Plumptre,
and to the memory of my father, Wynne Plumptre,
for whom public service was a way of life.

Contents

CONTENTS

CONTENTS

Foreword

Some of the most fundamental issues of public policy at the end of the twentieth century relate not to the substance of specific policy fields, but to the underlying philosophical foundations and principles governing the conduct and management of the public service itself. Principles of responsible behaviour, mechanisms for establishing accountability, structures for public participation all go to the heart of our social organization and determine the prospects for meeting successfully the challenges of government in a complex federal structure in an increasingly competitive international economy. Structural limitations to the governability of parliamentary democracies run through contemporary dilemmas of public policy in a pervasive manner.

It was for these reasons that the subject of public management was introduced as a central part of this Institute's program of work on problems of governability and institutions of governance. There are many dimensions to this program of work, including for example, public service employment, compensation, collective bargaining, and a concern for civilized procedures in the exercise of restraint and "downsizing". In addition, questions of structure and process in the management of evaluation, crisis management and planning have been addressed. The structures of public enterprise, crown corporations, and regulatory mechanisms have been reviewed in the context of growing pressures for privatization and deregulation. More generally, avenues of public participation, in the social policy process, in business-government relations, or through other interest groups have been a central concern. Constitutional rules and structures of federalism provide the context for public sector management, though that is obviously not the basis on which they will be judged. But underlying all these aspects of rules, structure, and process are the psychological issues of morale and motivation within the public service, and general public confidence in the institutions of government, along with the philosophical principles of responsible behaviour, and ethical guidelines in the proper exercise of administrative discretion.

Spanning several of these subjects is the present study of management in the public service by Timothy Plumptre.

Some consider the expression "management in the public service" self-contradictory, an oxymoron; some consider it an impossibly difficult objective; and some, perhaps, think it is happening but needs a better press.

For some decades there has been an interplay between public and private sector traditions of management, a shifting balance as the separated disciplines of public administration and private sector management have passed through distinct cycles. Attempts have sometimes been made to offer a synthesis which would recognize business administration and public administration as disciplines sharing a common interest in the organization and management of complex enterprises, even though operating in different social environments under differing accountability regimes or agency rules. Nevertheless, successive waves of enthusiasm for more formal systems of planning and analysis seem to have washed over the two communities at different times, leaving the business schools now propounding as conventional practice a much more organic approach to management responsibilities while cadres of public managers continue to contend with the legacy of overarching concerns for efficiency and value for money, as recorded in the systems imposed at the behest of successive recent Auditors General.

FOREWORD

Not intended as a text in the well-travelled fields of public administration, nor an authoritative review of the existing public administration literature, this book is primarily directed instead toward the management community. From the perspective of the literature on management, it explores whether and how management principles can be deployed in mobilizing and managing resources in the public sector, while recognizing the institutional structures and conventions developed to provide a framework for conflict resolution and accountability in the exercise of the powers delegated to government by voters.

It thus is designed to interpret the particular setting and features of the public service to a professional community generally familiar with management principles and applications in the private sector.

The message of this book is that solutions to the fundamental problems of management in the public service do not lie in sophisticated systems or elaborate equipment. Rather they lie in fundamental principles and values, in the exercise of leadership to motivate and channel individual effort in large organizations, and in sustained efforts to communicate objectives and promote understanding of management's purposes throughout the organization.

The present volume provides a survey of some principles of broad applicability in public sector organization, and an overall framework into which more detailed work on structure, systems and values can be fitted.

It suggests that business critics of management in government too readily urge autonomy for managers and delegation of authority in a manner not consistent with the political setting Plumptre describes. At the same time it suggests that government managers too readily accept controls that are not consistent with personal performance and individual initiative. Both groups, however, appear to have rejected the more extreme versions of a formal planning apparatus; it remains to be seen whether the public sector can escape from under the burden of formal monitoring to unleash the individual performance of managers below the most senior levels. (A forthcoming Institute monograph by Prof. David Zussman pursues the comparison of management attitudes and motivation in public and private organizations reported in his recent Institute working paper and employed in the concluding sections of the present book.)

The Institute is pleased to have had the opportunity, with the financial support of the Public Service Commission and William M. Mercer Limited, gratefully acknowledged, to undertake this study and make it generally available as a backdrop and framework for further work in this critically important area.

A.R. Dobell
President

March 1988

Avant-propos

Certaines des questions les plus fondamentales de la fin du vingtième siècle, en matière de politique générale, ont moins à voir avec les problèmes particuliers à des domaines politiques spécifiques qu'avec les principes philosophiques de base sur lesquels reposent la conduite et l'administration du service public lui-même. Les raisons d'un comportement responsable, les mécanismes permettant à l'Administration de rendre compte de ses activités, les procédures de participation du public, tous ces éléments sont au coeur de notre organisation sociale et influencent les chances que nous avons de relever avec succès les défis posés par le fait de gouverner dans un système fédéral complexe et à une époque où la situation économique internationale s'avère de plus en plus concurrentielle. Les limitations structurelles à la capacité de gouverner rencontrées par les démocraties parlementaires sont à la base même des problèmes de politique générale contemporains.

C'est pour ces raisons qu'il a été décidé de faire de la gestion du secteur public l'un des sujets principaux du programme de recherche de l'Institut sur la capacité de gouverner et sur les institutions de gouvernement. Ce champ d'étude comporte d'ailleurs plusieurs dimensions, notamment : le problème de l'emploi dans la fonction publique, la question de la compensation, les négociations collectives et le besoin de prévoir des procédures raisonnables permettant la mise en pratique des mesures de modération et restrictives particulières à ce secteur. En outre, on a tenu compte des questions de structure et de procédure dans l'évaluation de la gestion du secteur public, dans le traitement des crises et dans la planification. Les structures de l'entreprise publique et des compagnies de la Couronne, ainsi que les mécanismes régulateurs, ont été examinés dans le contexte des pressions croissantes qui s'exercent en faveur de la privatisation et de la déréglementation. Et plus généralement, la recherche s'est orientée vers les moyens de faire participer le public aux questions de politique sociale, aux relations entre le gouvernement et les milieux d'affaires ou par l'entremise d'autres groupes d'intérêts. L'exercice de la gestion du secteur public s'effectue à partir des règles constitutionnelles et des structures fédérales, sans pourtant servir de critère pour juger ces institutions. En fait, derrière tout cet appareil de réglementation, de structures et de procédure, il y a les problèmes psychologiques du moral et de la motivation dans la fonction publique, celui de la confiance témoignée par le public à l'égard des institutions gouvernementales, ainsi que d'autres considérations touchant à la justification philosophique d'un comportement responsable et à des règles de conduite conformes à une éthique professionnelle dans l'exercice discrétionnaire de la fonction administrative.

Dans la présente étude sur le problème de la gestion dans la fonction publique, l'auteur Timothy Plumptre considère plusieurs de ces questions.

Pour certains, l'expression "gestion à l'intérieur de la fonction publique" renferme des termes contradictoires et constitue un oxymoron; pour d'autres, c'est un objectif presque impossible à atteindre; d'autres encore pensent peut-être que le processus est en cours de réalisation et qu'il y a lieu de l'encourager.

Pendant des décennies, les traditions administratives des secteurs public et privé se sont mutuellement influencées, dans un rapport qui n'a cessé de fluctuer au gré des vicissitudes propres à chacun de ces secteurs. On a quelquefois tenté d'intégrer les deux disciplines, celle de l'administration et celle des affaires, dans une synthèse reposant sur un commun intérêt dans l'organisation et l'administration d'entreprises complexes, sans tenir compte du fait que les deux secteurs opèrent dans des contextes sociaux différents et suivant des régimes de responsabilité ou des codes divergents. Des vagues successives d'enthousiasme pour des systèmes de planification et d'analyse plus formels semblent néanmoins avoir déferlé à plusieurs reprises sur les deux secteurs. Le résultat, c'est que les écoles d'administration des affaires préconisent maintenant une approche conventionnelle beaucoup plus systématique à l'égard des responsabilités de gestion, tandis que les cadres de l'administration publique continuent à se débattre avec l'héritage de préoccupations dépassées, relativement à l'efficacité et au rendement de l'argent dépensé, comme l'illustrent les mesures imposées à la demande réitérée des derniers vérificateurs généraux.

Cet ouvrage ne prétend ni être un nouveau manuel dans le domaine déjà très étudié de l'administration publique, ni une recension officielle des écrits consacrés à ce sujet; il vise avant tout à informer la communauté des gestionnaires. Du point de vue théorique, il explore les conditions d'exercice des principes de gestion dans la fonction publique et les manières dont ces principes peuvent être mis en oeuvre, à partir de l'emploi et de la gestion des ressources existantes, tout en tenant compte des structures institutionnelles et des conventions élaborées en vue de fournir un cadre propice à la résolution des conflits et à l'exercice de la responsabilité budgétaire, dans les limites des pouvoirs délégués au gouvernement par les électeurs.

Il est donc conçu pour faire comprendre les caractéristiques et le contexte particulier de la fonction publique à une communauté de professionnels généralement familiarisés avec les principes de la gestion et leurs applications dans le secteur privé.

La leçon à retirer de ce livre, c'est que ce n'est pas grâce à des systèmes sophistiqués ni à un équipement dernier cri que l'on trouvera les solutions aux problèmes fondamentaux qui se posent au sujet de la gestion dans la fonction publique. Ces solutions dépendent plutôt de valeurs et de principes fondamentaux, d'un leadership capable de motiver et de canaliser les efforts individuels au sein des grandes organisations, et d'une activité soutenue pour communiquer les objectifs à tous les niveaux de l'organisation et faire connaître et accepter les intentions de la direction.

BEYOND THE BOTTOM LINE

Le présent volume passe en revue certains des principes largement applicables à l'organisation du secteur public, et il fournit un cadre général dans lequel peuvent s'inscrire et s'adapter des sous-structures, des systèmes et des valeurs plus particuliers.

Il laisse entendre que les critiques professionnels de la gestion dans la fonction publique recommandent trop facilement l'autonomie des administrateurs et la délégation des pouvoirs, sans tenir suffisamment compte du contexte politique que M. Plumptre décrit. Il indique par ailleurs que les administrateurs du gouvernement sont trop disposés à accepter des contrôles qui ne tiennent pas compte du travail et de l'initiative individuels. Les deux groupes, cependant, paraissent avoir écarté les versions les plus extrêmes d'une planification trop rigide; toutefois, il reste à voir si le secteur public saura se libérer du fardeau d'une stricte surveillance, pour être en mesure de stimuler les initiatives individuelles des gestionnaires n'appartenant pas aux échelons les plus élevés des cadres supérieurs. (Une monographie en cours de préparation, due au professeur David Zussman, s'attache à poursuivre la comparaison des attitudes et de la motivation des administrateurs des secteurs public et privé, dont il a déjà fait état dans un récent document de travail pour l'Institut et dont les données ont été utilisées dans la conclusion du présent ouvrage.)

L'Institut désire exprimer ici sa gratitude envers la Commission de la Fonction publique et envers la compagnie William M. Mercer Limited, dont l'aide financière a permis de mener à bien cette étude et de lui donner le plaisir de la mettre à la disposition du public, dans l'espoir qu'elle servira de point de départ et de cadre de travail à de futurs travaux dans ce domaine d'une importance cruciale.

A.R. Dobell
Président

Mars 1988

Introduction

"You're writing a book about government management? Why!?"

"Well, that'll be a very short book!"

"On that subject, you'll have to write a veritable tome!"

"I guess that'll be a book with a lot of blank pages!"

"Management in government. Isn't that a contradiction in terms?"

Many friends and acquaintances reacted with sentiments ranging from disinterest to incredulity when they learned of my intention to write this book. Why would *anyone* want to write on such a topic?

Why a Book on Management in Government?

Why, indeed? There are several answers. First, government is here to stay. Some may wish it were somewhat bigger, some smaller; but few persons would suggest that we can do without any government whatsoever. Since, for better or for worse, we have governments, we ought to manage them properly.

Government is big business. The Canadian federal government, including government corporations and enterprises where the government owns more than half the shares, employs well over 500,000 persons.[1] It spends in the order of $100 billion annually. It is larger and more complex than the top 20 Canadian companies combined.[2]

If one takes into account the different levels of government in society, including the municipal level, it becomes apparent that a very large proportion of the labour force works for government. Total government employment in 1986 in Canada was 2.1 million persons – almost 20 per cent of the total employed labour force of 11.7 million. (This includes 580,000 teachers, hospital workers and other employees working for local governments who are not normally counted by Statistics Canada.)[3] In most developed countries, a lot of resources are administered by governments, and a lot of persons' working lives run their course in government institutions. In light of this, it is perhaps surprising how few publications exist on the subject of management in government, by comparison with business administration.

In my view, there is a need for more study and writing in this area. When it comes to management, governments do not enjoy the best of reputations. Scarcely a day goes by that some conference speaker is not lamenting the spread of red tape, government overspending, the unresponsiveness of the public service, or the inefficiency of government bureaucracies. Why, we are asked, do civil servants refuse to follow practices tested in the tough competitive environment of business? Why can't we get good management in government?

There is, of course, no shortage of books about management. Many such books purport to apply to all organizations, large or small, new or old, private or public sector. However, books which intimate that they are universally applicable should be approached with caution. It is becoming more and more accepted that even in the world of business there are few universal truths, that there is no single "best" way to manage, and that due account must be taken of the differences between organizations. Managing a multinational is acknowledged to be different from directing a small entrepreneurial company; a professional firm cannot be run like a manufacturing organization; a research and development operation requires different methods of management from an industrial plant; a hospital or a theatre company cannot be directed as if it were a railway or an airline. Each type of organization has its special characteristics; and, increasingly, each has its own literature on management and its own techniques.

Yet, despite the size of the public sector, one finds little about management in this sphere. In conducting the research for this book, I was able to find only half a dozen books specifically on the topic of management in government. Most of what was available was in Royal Commission reports and special studies which were often directed to a particular problem or context.

There was, of course, no lack of books on public administration; but the preoccupations of this discipline, certainly until recently, have tended to be somewhat different from those of "management". Where the literature on management has been concerned with institutional and individual productivity, public administration seems to have been more focused upon constitutional traditions and conventions; where management was interested in the performance and productivity of individual organizations, public administration tended to be more interested in the structure of government as a whole, in the legitimacy of government institutions, or in policy questions; where management was seeking methods for effective delegation, public administration was worried about accountability; where management tried to determine how to motivate employees, public administration asked how to control them or protect them from political interference. Moreover, much of the literature on public administration seemed weighted more toward theory and principle than day-to-day practice.

Of course, there are exceptions to these generalizations. But, on the whole, my impression is that the bulk of the intellectual effort which has been invested in government administration has, at least until the last 10 or 20 years, been concerned with questions which are different in subtle but important ways from the classic preoccupations of management theory. As we shall see, there is cause to believe that, in the public sector, the concept of management has itself been quite widely misunderstood. Hence this book, whose objective is to help fill the gap in the literature about management in the public sector, to try to eradicate some of the misunderstandings and to contribute to the blending of management theory and experience with the traditions of public administration.

The Scope of Management

Many persons, particularly those in government, have limited ideas about the scope of management. They consider it to be concerned with such matters as procedural manuals, accounting systems, routine administrative functions, and the like. In this interpretation, management is, indeed, not very interesting or challenging; a book on the subject would hardly be of very broad appeal.

There is, however, more to management than this. Management is not just concerned with administrivia. Fundamentally, management has to do with organizational performance. When elections are called, we hold elected governments to account for the policies they have devised and the way they have "managed" the affairs of state. We expect governments to serve us efficiently. We expect them not to waste our money, and to be effective in the functions which they discharge. We also expect governments to operate with due regard for prevailing standards in such areas as ethics, morality and equity. We want them to respect the legitimacy of constitutional conventions. We require them to be responsive to different interests, and even-handed in their approach to policy questions. All these concepts: "efficiency", "effectiveness", "waste", "equity" and "legitimacy" have a bearing upon the concept of management as it applies in the public sector.

Our ideas about what constitutes good management thus play a significant role in establishing our expectations in a democracy. They set some of the standards which help us to hold both our elected representatives and our public servants to account. They provide a frame of reference for the work of officials such as auditors general who are responsible for monitoring the state of administration in government organizations. In addition, ideas about management influence a great deal of what goes on inside government. They affect critical relationships between powerful institutions, who gets promoted, how much people get paid, what programs get funded, how resources get allocated, and who gets blamed when things go wrong.

In summary, there is more to management than meets the eye; and, in the public sector, there are problems associated with management which are quite different from (and some would say, more intractable than) those which one encounters in most private sector organizations. Managing to the bottom line, the task of the private sector is difficult enough. In the public sector, the problem is to manage in an environment where there is no "bottom line", where uncertainties are more prevalent than in business, relationships more complex, problems more difficult, and mistakes more exposed to the possibility of public criticism. As we shall see, "success" is itself often harder to define than in the private sector. Officials in government have to learn to cope with a context in which the very concept of "good management" is susceptible to different, and potentially incompatible, interpretations. The challenge of managing in this situation — "beyond the bottom line" — is the subject of this book.

Defining the Public Sector

This book originally began as a study of management in the public sector. One of the difficulties in writing on this topic is to decide how broadly to cast one's net. What is the "public sector"? Should it include government-owned corporations? What about organizations funded by government but at arm's length from government control? What about voluntary and not-for-profit entities, dependent upon public support? I ultimately decided that the book needed a more specific focus than "the public sector" at large, and resolved to focus my attention upon the heart or core of government: that is, departments and agencies whose institutional environment is too specialized to be encompassed successfully in the same volume with other types of "public sector" organizations.

The next conundrum was: which government should be the focus of this study? Many books in the field of public administration and political science condemn themselves to early obsolescence by narrowing their scope to one jurisdiction at one particular time. Governments evolve constantly. By the time such jurisdictionally specific books have made their way from the authors' desks to the booksellers, they are already partially out of date. Moreover, my interest was in identifying broader principles and themes, and in highlighting parallels among the efforts to improve management in different jurisdictions, not just to discuss one-of-a-kind concerns of a specific government. I therefore wished to preserve a certain generic perspective by dealing with more than one government, and by using specific examples as illustrations of more general issues.

Conversely, it soon became evident that there were limits to how general a book on management in government could be. To try to write about management while referring simultaneously to other systems of government, such as the congressional system in the U.S., or to several different levels, such as the federal, provincial and municipal levels, promised to involve too many conceptual and institutional complications. I decided that the main focus of this book was to be management within parliamentary democracies. I chose the Canadian federal government as my principal frame of reference, but a certain amount of the discussion also relates to the British government, the original model for most parliamentary democracies. In passing, I refer to other jurisdictions such as Ontario and other Canadian provinces. Occasionally, where the parallel is appropriate, references to the United States are included. However, throughout, parliamentary democracy remains the principal model.

In view of this orientation, I would hope that the governments of parliamentary democracies, most notably those of Commonwealth countries modelled on Westminster, will find something of value in these pages. Despite differences in context, I believe that much of this book will also find application at the municipal and provincial levels. Many of its topics may also have a general application to the American situation – and perhaps to other governments as well – although the arguments would clearly have to be transposed to fit each institutional context.

Even with the limited focus on parliamentary government, my approach has entailed certain problems of terminology. For example, in Canada the official head of a department is known as the deputy minister, while in Britain the title is permanent secretary; Canada has a Department of Finance while Britain has a Treasury which is similar in some, but not all, respects; Canada has a Public Service Commission while Britain has a (somewhat different) Civil Service Commission; for many years, a Chief Executive Officer was a lower- to middle-level management grade in the British civil service, whereas in North America this term is commonly used to designate the head of a business enterprise; people who work for government in Canada are called public servants, whereas in Britain they are called civil servants.

Insofar as possible I have tried either to use terminology such as "department head", which is institutionally neutral, or to make my meaning clear through the context. If, occasionally, the terminology is a trifle loose, I hope the sense will nonetheless be clear; my principal concern has been to write a book which is readable and accessible, and there comes a point at which concern for the niceties of vocabulary creates a text which is correct but pedestrian.

Improving Management in Canada and Britain, 1960-1985

Although the academic and research literature on what might be called public management is not as yet very extensive, a lot of people inside governments have been concerned with management issues. In appendix 1 and appendix 2, an overview of the efforts to improve management in Canada and Britain over the last 25 years may be found. A brief summary appears below.

The history of each jurisdiction is somewhat different. In Canada, the story begins in the early 1960s with the publication of the report of a Royal Commission on Government Organization, known as the Glassco Commission, which urged greater delegation of responsibility to managers within the bureaucracy and which recommended various other changes to the structure of government. There were a number of major developments during the 1960s in addition to the implementation of Glassco recommendations. It was in this decade that collective bargaining was introduced in Ottawa. A major program to render the public service bilingual was launched. The government also decided during this period to implement a new budgeting and expenditure management system known as PPBS (Program Planning and Budgeting System). This system greatly increased the number of staff specialists in the federal government involved in planning and policy development work, and this change, combined with the others mentioned above, made the process of government a good deal more formal and bureaucratic than it had been previously.

The pace of change did not abate in the 1970s. New efforts were mounted to develop other types of government-wide planning systems, as a sort of overlay to PPBS. Several new ministries and agencies with responsibilities for planning and policy coordination were set up, in such fields as urban affairs, science and technology, economic policy and social policy. Systems for performance measurement were introduced. A great fascination with "accountability" developed and, with a view to "increasing" accountability, the mandate of the federal Auditor General was expanded, new units responsible for evaluating government programs were set up in the bureaucracy, and a new central agency known as the Office of the Comptroller General was established. A Royal Commission on Financial Management and Accountability, better known as the Lambert Commission, was struck, in 1976. It conducted a wide-ranging review of government planning, the roles of top officials, financial and personnel management practices, and a variety of related issues. By the end of the decade, the government was awash in auditors, assessors and evaluators, and increasingly one heard the plea from officials, "Why can't they leave us alone and let us get on with our jobs?"

Nonetheless, the changes continued through the late 1970s and into the 1980s. It began to become evident during this period that several of the new management initiatives and organizations that had been launched with fanfare a few years previously were working less successfully than their proponents had predicted. For example, PPBS, which had been touted as the tool to bring government expenditures under control and to make the process of planning much more systematic and rational, had relatively little impact on the substance of expenditure policy or on the federal deficit, which continued to climb; meanwhile it added enormously to the workload of the bureaucracy. By the late 1970s, in fact, the Auditor General was suggesting that government spending was virtually out of control. For these and other reasons, PPBS was substantially amended, eventually turning into a policy planning and budgeting methodology known as PEMS (Policy and Expenditure Management System).

In addition, it became apparent that the various coordinating agencies created during the 1970s were overburdening and confusing policy development. There was, perhaps, better coordination; but the decision-making process became so byzantine, informed observers were no longer able to discern who was responsible for key spheres of government policy. Accountability, in whose name many changes in government structures and procedures had been made, became diffused among a raft of departments and agencies with overlapping mandates. As a result, in the early 1980s the government disassembled much of the machinery which had been created only a few years earlier, and most of the coordinating agencies disappeared from the scene. Planning systems developed for the Cabinet were allowed to slip into obscurity. Similarly, a request that departments prepare annual strategic plans was quietly dropped.

The most recent significant development, at time of writing, was the development of a new approach to delegation of authority within the public service. This initiative, known as IMAA (Increased Ministerial Authority and Accountability), returned to the fundamental preoccupation of the Glassco Commission 25 years earlier, that is: how to provide departments with adequate managerial flexibility while maintaining sufficient control over the system of government. The IMAA initiative, described in more detail in chapter 7, represents an attempt to approach this difficult issue from a fresh perspective; it was necessary because the philosophy urged upon the federal government by the Glassco Commission had, in the opinion of many informed observers, never been properly implemented.

If one takes the long view of Canadian experience over the last 25 years, what one sees amid all the complexity is a government wrestling with the fundamental issue of how, on the one hand, to keep control over government expenditures while, on the other, allowing large complicated bureaucracies to function efficiently and effectively and with due regard for special government priorities such as the "bilingualization" of the public service. The story is essentially that of the familiar struggle between centralization and decentralization of authority, and between the desire to secure autonomy for working units of a big organization, while maintaining an appropriate measure of coordination . . . all this set in an environment of great complexity.

The Canadian approach during the period 1960-1985 might be described as "systems-oriented", that is, the belief seems to have persisted that the "solution" to problems of management in government lay in the development of procedures and structures.

What one witnesses over the period is a continual process of experimentation with different procedures and structures. There has, in my view, been considerable progress made during the period. On the other hand, there have certainly been more false starts and misconceived initiatives than desirable. Rather a lot of time and energy have been wasted correcting problems that might have been avoided had there been a little more forethought, a little less enthusiasm for untried approaches among some officials at the centre of government and, perhaps, a slightly better understanding of some of the basics of management.

Turning to Britain, we see various attempts to wrestle with what were, fundamentally, the same sorts of problems. Whitehall (as the centre of government in Britain is sometimes called, after a large avenue in London where key government departments are located) has traditionally been rather less interested in management issues than the Canadian government. This fact in part reflects its greater distance from the United States, where so much thinking on management has originated. Class traditions may also have something to do with this attitude. Management has traditionally been seen as something faintly below the salt in Britain. Senior officials, according to the U.K. tradition, were responsible for policy development; management was the province of subordinate officials. To a considerable degree as a result of this disinterest, the pace of management change, at least up to the 1980s, was much less intense than it was in Canada.

Nonetheless, during the 1960s and 1970s a few developments of note did occur. One was the institution of a new method of expenditure management which became known in Whitehall as PESC, after the Public Expenditure Survey Committee. The PESC process involved a very considerable increase in the complexity and workload associated with planning and budget preparation; like PPBS, it set in place a whole new technology of procedures for expenditure management which had then to interact with the political process which overlaid them. Its overriding objective was to make planning and budgeting more rational and systematic, and to ensure that, through the operation of the new system, expenditure decisions got taken in the context of some appreciation of available resources and competing priorities, rather than in a vacuum, as had tended to be the case prior to 1960.

Broadly speaking, PESC was intended to address some of the same issues as was PPBS in other jurisdictions, but the system was directed primarily to the overall containment and control of public expenditures; the PESC process was much less ambitious in its goals with respect to the management of individual programs within departments than was PPBS. Originally instituted in the early 1960s, PESC has been progressively modified and adapted over the subsequent decades and, like the PEMS system in Canada which superceded PPBS, it lies at the heart of the present expenditure management process in the U.K.

Another important development in the 1960s was the publication of a report on the British civil service called the Fulton Report, which proposed a number of changes to personnel management practices, including the establishment of a new Civil Service Department and a Civil Service College, and more attention to management training. The report generally was poorly received by the senior bureaucracy due in particular to its ill-chosen decision to chastise civil servants as "amateurs" and also to a contentious recommendation concerning the establishment of new policy units in government reporting directly to ministers. Although the Civil Service College proposed by Fulton was established, the report's broader recommendations were not well received and, ultimately, the study did not have a major impact on the operations of the civil service. (Some have suggested that a recalcitrant bureaucracy sandbagged its implementation — see appendix 2.)

A few years after Fulton, the election of Prime Minister Edward Heath brought with it a fresh interest in new techniques of planning and analysis. A development which received a lot of attention in the early 1970s was the institution of a new system for reviewing and analyzing blocks of government expenditure known as PAR (Programme Analysis and Review). As in Canada, the expectation was that, through new centrally operated structures and systems, the beast of government could be tamed and made more orderly. However, PAR did not endure; it had little general impact on expenditures and gradually lost its profile. It ultimately disappeared from view in the late 1970s.

In short, with the exception of the ongoing elaboration of the PESC process from year to year, efforts to improve management practices in the U.K. over the period from 1960 to the mid-1970s were somewhat sporadic and discontinuous. Margaret Thatcher changed that, as she did so many other aspects of Britain. Under Thatcher, a number of important initiatives were set in motion. Among these was an ongoing program of examinations of portions of the Whitehall bureaucracy under the direction of Lord Rayner, which were designed to promote efficiencies and which soon became known as Rayner Scrutinies. Another initiative involved a process that became known as the FMI (Financial Management Initiative), which constituted a general review of accountability, objective-setting, management information and financial procedures in all British government departments. The FMI led to changes in many structures and procedures, and had the general effect of raising the profile of management in a bureaucracy that had, on the whole, been relatively uninterested in better management. Concurrently with FMI, a limited amount of attention was directed to the question of how to delegate more authority to departments, but changes in this area had tended, at time of writing, to remain somewhat exploratory.

As in Canada, there has been a continuing tendency for the British to continue tinkering with the structure and division of management-related responsibilities among the central departments of government. While Canada was making and unmaking its coordinating ministries, the British were establishing a Civil Service Department (in the wake of Fulton), then unmaking it (under Thatcher) and transferring most of its responsibilities to a new office called the Management and Personnel Office. This Office was amalgamated with the Cabinet Office in the early 1980s; then, in another episode in the continuing jousts for power one sees among central departments of governments, in 1986 most of the MPO responsibilities were taken over by the Treasury Department. (A new, much-reduced entity called the Office of the Minister of the Civil Service (OMSC) was established in the Cabinet Office.) This has left the Treasury (a department which until very recently has not displayed a great interest in, or a very broad understanding of, management issues other than those directly related to expenditure control) largely in control of management policies affecting the

INTRODUCTION

British civil service. Just what this unification of ex-MPO responsibilities with the Treasury will mean in practice remains to be seen.

In summary, as discussed in detail in Appendices 1 and 2, what we see in both Canada and Britain over the period 1960 to 1985 is a continuing attempt to develop and improve systems to facilitate the planning and control of expenditures. We witness a process of experiment with a variety of structures which were set up and then dismantled, the purpose of which was to improve coordination or institute new approaches to management in government. We also observe a see-saw battle between the forces of centralization and decentralization, as governments tried to find the right balance between autonomy and control.

The preoccupations in both countries (as in other jurisdictions) during the 1960s and 1970s was with better methods for planning and control and with accountability for public funds. There appears to have been belief underlying developments in both countries that the key to making government "work" was to get the right procedures and structures in place. While procedures and structures play an important role in management, there is more to management than this.

Indeed, in my view, if one looks closely at all the different approaches that were tried and the experiments that went off the rails, what one sees are the consequences of some significant misunderstandings of management, in both jurisdictions. In the case of Canada, the concept of accountability was confused with another related but different concept, that of control. In Britain, there has been a persistent tendency to think of management in terms of the implementation of routine work procedures, and there seems to have been a lack of appreciation of the broader dimensions of the discipline. Certainly until recently, there seems to have been a tendency in both jurisdictions (particularly in Britain) to make decisions on advancement on the basis of individuals' policy advisory skills, and there has been a good deal less emphasis than one might wish on those qualities of leadership which motivate others. In addition, both countries have tended to think of management in terms of systems, structures and financial procedures to too great an extent. While significant progress has been made in both countries in these areas, the consequence of this orientation has been insufficient emphasis on the human or "people" aspects of management. Similarly, there has been too great a tendency to believe that management can be "delegated" by senior officials to lower levels of government organizations.

If these problems are to be avoided in future, it will be necessary to ensure that senior government officials, particularly those in central departments, have a firm grasp of what management entails, and of how management principles should — and should not — be applied to different types of organizations. There will, in my view, have to be a greater recognition of the unique features of government, as compared with business, more awareness within government of the diversity of government institutions, and a greater willingness to give effect to this in management policies and practices.

Objectives and Organization of the Book

This is a book, first and foremost, for senior officials, or for those who aspire to become senior officials in government. In much of the book, I have adopted a top-management perspective. This is for two reasons. First, nowhere is the perspective on internal relationships within an organization clearer than from the top. Second, my experience has again and again brought home to me the pervasive impact of top officials, and in particular the chief executive, on the character and the performance of the organization, whether it be in a government department or a private corporation. Systems, structures and procedures are not unimportant. Above all, however, what makes organizations work is people; and what makes people work, first and foremost, is the leadership they receive from the top. As a former Chairman of the Board of Dupont has written:

> In Ralph Waldo Emerson's time, it was accurate for him to say that an institution was the lengthened shadow of a man. That is less true today.... Emerson is not entirely out of date, though. Each modern corporation, for all its diversification and decentralization, despite chains of command and shared authority, is still the lengthened shadow of a few people. Those who are board members and senior managers establish the climate within, and casting the shadow is their main work.[4]

INTRODUCTION

If this book helps those at senior levels in government organizations to achieve a better understanding of how to exercise their influence, one of its main purposes will have been attained.

However, the book is not addressed exclusively to top officials. It has also been designed to be useful to other readers. Among these are students of public administration, who may be seeking a better understanding of how government actually works and of the key issues and dilemmas with which officials must cope in trying to make the institutions of government work. Others who may find something of value here are business executives (and students of business administration) baffled by the behaviour of government officials and perplexed by the institutional structure of the bureaucracy. Governments are a fact of life for businesses today, and a business of any size usually has to deal with governments for a number of different purposes.

Business executives may not want to explore some of the more specialized chapters of this book, such as those dealing with planning and control systems (see below); but they may find other parts useful in gaining an appreciation of the roles of the different players, the kinds of pressures to which public servants have to respond, and the way the different pieces of the institutional puzzle that is government fit together. (It is not as illogical as it may appear from the outside!)

The book is divided into four parts. Part 1 sets the context. It explores the meaning of management with a view to eradicating misunderstandings surrounding the concept which, as I have suggested above, tend to prevail in the public sector. It also sketches the institutional and psychological landscape within which public servants have to work. Some of them understand this landscape; others, particularly those who have not had occasion to work at the centre of government, may not. Many government officials are principally concerned with the affairs of their own organization, and are not very familiar with the larger institutional environment or the constitutional traditions of the public service. For such readers, and for those from a business background, chapters 2 and 3 may provide some helpful perspective. Other readers, however, may prefer to skip these chapters and move directly into parts 2 and 3 of the book.

There were several choices to make in deciding how much material to cover in part 1. I had originally thought to include chapters tracing the history of management thought, and discussing in some depth the efforts of the Canadian and British governments in improving management practices during the past 25 years or so. However, this seemed to impede the flow of the book so, apart from the brief overview of Canada and Britain which appears above, the historical material on management and on Canada and Britain, as noted previously, now appears in three appendices.

Part 2 discusses the major players and institutions of government by moving progressively from the centre toward the margins of the public service. Thus, the first chapter in part 2 deals with the role of a minister of the Crown. The next two deal with the job of the department head and the problem of the multiple accountabilities with which the head must cope. The following chapter, 7, reviews the role of what are known in Canada as the central agencies of government (they are referred to as central departments in the U.K., but the term central agencies will be used for convenience in this book). It examines their relationship to departments which deliver most of the programs and develop most of the policies. As the discussion of Canada and Britain earlier in this chapter may have suggested, getting this relationship "right" is one of the most critical and difficult challenges in public management.

Part 3 moves a further step out from the centre of government. It is concerned with management at the level of the individual department. The section opens with a short chapter entitled "The Architecture of Effective Organizations", which discusses management theory about how organizations should be designed in order to perform well. In order to keep this book to manageable proportions, only key areas of management in government are then dealt with: the planning and control of expenditures and departmental operations; the function of policy development; and the management of people.

While the first three parts of the book are occasionally prescriptive, they are mainly intended to describe how the process of management works and how the elements fit together. In part 4, however, the orientation changes somewhat, and the tone becomes more normative. Government is so complex that it is not easy to suggest what kinds of changes might improve performance. However, after several years of pondering the subject, I have formed some views on the subject which are contained in the final two chapters. Chapter

12 deals with the question of relationships and accountabilities of the public service, while chapter 13 considers the issue of people and performance.

The Basis for this Book

This book is based upon a combination of experience, observation, management theory and political science. My association with government began with eight years as a Canadian public servant, which included line experience in both policy and administrative departments, as well as service in both the office of a minister and of a deputy minister. In 1972 I was fortunate to receive a Canadian government scholarship to study at Oxford University in England. During this year I was also associated with the now-defunct Civil Service Department in London, which provided an opportunity to observe the workings of the British civil service from the inside. My work on a paper on planning in government brought me face-to-face with the complexity of the whole subject, and I resolved that, if I could broaden my exposure to the different aspects of government, I would one day expand my preliminary thoughts into a book.

For the past 17 years, with the exception of the year at Oxford, I have worked as a management consultant. Much of my activity during this period has been in the public sector. Specifically, I have had the opportunity to work for some 30 departments of the Canadian government, and I have conducted studies of organization and planning for several deputy ministers and heads of agencies, as well as many other officials at subordinate levels. I have also carried out engagements for a number of Crown corporations and agencies, provincial government departments, municipal governments and voluntary agencies, in addition, of course, to business enterprises. This work has involved a wide range of subjects: general management reviews, the development of planning and budgeting systems, strategic planning, evaluations of government programs, studies of the machinery of government, policy development, the analysis of management information systems, the management of computer technology, examinations of the roles of policy groups as well as several economic studies.

The chance to write this book came in 1984 with a two-year partial leave of absence from consulting, made possible by support from the Institute for Research on Public Policy, the Public Service Commission of the Government of Canada, and the generosity of my own consulting firm, William M. Mercer Limited. This half-sabbatical permitted me to arrange a program of interviews in Britain to supplement my earlier experience in that country in 1972/73. These interviews, made possible through the assistance of the British Cabinet Office, included two ministers from different parties, half a dozen permanent secretaries, some departmental managers, and senior officials in both the Cabinet Office and the Treasury associated with efforts to improve administrative practices in Whitehall and with the management of public expenditures. I conducted subsequent interviews with a number of officials in Ottawa, including several deputy ministers whose views were particularly valuable in connection with part 2. These interviews were supplemented by research in both recent and past literature on politics, public administration and management, as well as the opportunity to teach a class in organization behaviour at the University of Ottawa, where some of my ideas about motivation were refined.

However, the main foundation for this book lies not in academic theory but in day-to-day contact with the many officials with whom I have had the privilege of working during the last 20-odd years, as well as those whom I interviewed specifically for this book. Discussions of their work, ambitions, frustrations, problems and ideas for the improvement of their organizations have contributed immeasurably to my own thinking; they have helped me to create a book which, I hope, has the strong flavour of the practical world. Without the patience and co-operation of all these public servants, this book would not have been possible, and although they must remain anonymous, they should know that I am most grateful for their help.

Acknowledgements

A number of individuals, however, can and should be identified. Very special thanks are due to Gordon Robertson, formerly Secretary to the Cabinet in Ottawa and latterly President of the Institute for Research on Public Policy. Gordon took this project under the wing of the

INTRODUCTION

Institute with the promise of publication and support that made the idea of a book a reality rather than a doubtful dream. Rod Dobell, Gordon's able successor as President of the Institute, provided his own enthusiastic backing over a period of three years, and Jeffrey Holmes, responsible for communications at the IRPP, guided the process of promotion with more zeal and imagination than an author could hope for. Another key supporter for the project has been Edgar Gallant, former Chairman of the Public Service Commission, who shared Gordon's initial optimism about the book and who was able to provide much-needed financial assistance, which was continued by his successor at the Commission, Huguette Labelle. Edgar has been a continuing source of encouragement throughout the writing and, following his retirement from government, he provided valuable comments at key stages in the development of the manuscript.

Particular recognition is also due to my employer, the consulting firm of William M. Mercer Limited, and especially to my friends and colleagues Robert Brochu, Jean-Louis Bourbeau and Jack Marshall. All supported the project from the start, and the firm's decision to contribute financially and also to agree to a partial leave of absence for me constituted a vote of confidence that was heartening at the early stages of research. Moreover, my colleagues' patience as the manuscript made its uneven progress toward completion greatly facilitated the task of writing! I have certainly appreciated their understanding and forbearance.

I was most fortunate to receive the help of the British Cabinet Office in arranging interviews. Colin Peterson, formerly of the Cabinet Office (MPO), in his courteous, low-key and effective way, went far beyond the call of duty, opening doors that might otherwise have remained firmly shut and helping out in many other ways. John Chilcot, also formerly of the Cabinet Office, spent hours in a critical analysis of an early draft, and provided insights into subtleties of British bureaucracy at several stages of writing that were exceptionally useful.

A number of individuals have been kind enough to review individual chapters, or larger portions of the text, as the book progressed, as the result of which major revisions were often made, as they will see. Among these I wish to thank David Brown, Robert Bryce, Ron Corbeil, Alan Darling, Richard Paton, Beryl Plumptre,

Mitchell Sharp, and Sharon Sutherland. John Langford was particularly perceptive on issues related to the overall organization of the book; David Zussman was especially helpful in connection with the research into people in the public service, as related in part 3.

Despite all this help, and despite my efforts to excise them, I expect that this book contains its share of errors and omissions. For these, as well as the opinions and conclusions in the following chapters, the responsibility rests with me.

Finally, I cheerfully acknowledge my many debts to four individuals who provided the most immediate and personal support. First, Ken Huffman, my undefatigable research assistant, saved me hours of work, showing a singular capacity for ferreting out one useful and relevant book after another. Ken never complained about unreasonable requests and had a remarkable capacity for tracking down obscure references. Second, Penelope Williams, my editor, somehow managed to get me to organize my ideas and repeatedly saved me from myself by helping me to prune and weed first-draft text into more direct prose. She did this with a combination of boundless good humour, goodwill and professional acuity that made her a pleasure to work with. Loranne Gauthier's dependable assistance with the typing of editorial revisions was a great help to both Penny and me.

Last, my wife Barbara has given unswerving support to this venture. From the microcomputer which she gave me in 1983 (along with the challenge to "get started!"), to the title she conceived toward the end of writing, she has been a continuing source of encouragement and intelligent criticism. Her assumption of many domestic chores in addition to her own taxing professional responsibilities provided me with much-needed time to write; her moral support carried me through periods of uncertainty; her belief that the book could and would be done meant that, ultimately, it was.

Tim Plumptre
Ottawa

March 1988

INTRODUCTION

Footnotes:

1. *Federal Government Employment,* Oct. - Dec. 1986, Statistics Canada Catalogue 72-004, (Ottawa: Supply and Services Canada, 1987), table 1, p. 20.

2. Gordon Osbaldeston, "Dear Minister, Letter to and Old Friend on Being a Successful Minister," remarks to the Association of Professional Executives (Ottawa: January 22, 1988).

3. See footnote 1 above; also *Provincial and Territorial Government Employment,* Oct. - Dec. 1986, Statistics Canada Catalogue 72-007, table 1, p. 20; *Local Government Employment,* Oct. - Dec. 1986, Statistics Canada Catalogue 72-009, and likewise the Jan. - March issue, tables 2 and 7, pp. 21-22 and 30. On the growth of government generally, see Richard Bird, Meyer Bucovetsky and David Foot (eds.), *The Growth of Public Employment in Canada,* (Ottawa: Institute for Research on Public Policy, 1979) and Sharon L. Sutherland and G. Bruce Doern, *Bureaucracy in Canada: Control and Reform,* (Toronto: University of Toronto Press in cooperation with the Royal Commission on the Economic Union and Development Prospects for Canada and the Canadian Government Publishing Centre, Supply and Services Canada, 1985.)

4. Irving S. Shapiro, *America's Third Revolution: Public Interest and the Private Role,* (New York: Harper & Row, 1984), p. 68.

Part One:

Management in a Government Context

Introduction to Part One

To address the complex issues associated with management in a government setting, one must understand the meaning of management and the environment of the public sector. These provide the intellectual or conceptual cornerstones for public management.

As noted in the previous chapter, my own experience has been that many persons in government have somewhat limited, and even distorted, ideas about the scope and purpose of management. Therefore, the first chapter in this part of the book deals with the definition of management and the scope of the discipline. It suggests that, in the terminology of the economist, management is one of the key factors of production, and that "productivity improvement" is simply a synonym for sound management.

It then considers the difficulties associated with defining what constitutes "good management" in an environment where there is no bottom line, where conflicting values constantly must be reconciled, and where objectives are often unclear. It examines two alternative approaches to defining "good management" and concludes that, while both approaches have their merits, in the final analysis what constitutes "good management" will often be a matter of judgment in a government setting.

The two subsequent chapters describe the institutional environment of government. Chapter 2 describes the different types of organizations and agencies and provides an overview of their relationships. Chapter 3 looks at the "softer" aspects of government. It considers norms, values and conventions which affect the behaviour of public servants. Many of these define what it is to be a public servant in a parliamentary democracy; unless one understands them, one cannot appreciate why people who work in government think and act as they do.

Some public servants will find little new in these chapters. However, readers who are not familiar with such matters as the role of central agencies, the different types of departments, the relationship between departments and their ministers and the impact of interdepartmental meetings on the business of government may find these chapters helpful in orienting their impressions.

In short, part 1 sets the context. It points out that there are no universal rules in management, and that it is a "situational" discipline which has to take into account the kind of institutions to which it is applied and the environment within which those institutions function. The explanation of the structure and culture of government in chapters 2 and 3 differentiates government from the private sector, and sets the stage for the remainder of the book.

Chapter One:
Management in the Public Sector

No broad consensus exists about what constitutes good management in the
Federal context . . . *

This chapter addresses the meaning of management with particular
reference to the public sector. It sets forth a number of the more
common misbeliefs about management, and explains where the real
focus of the discipline resides. It then poses the question, what
constitutes good management? What are the standards by which we
should hold managers in government to account? It suggests that the
answers to these questions are often ambiguous and susceptible to
quite different interpretations. The story which follows illustrates
this point nicely. The chapter concludes with a discussion of the
relationship between business administration and public
management.

---

* Opening statement in a U.S. study on management in government. See U.S.
General Accounting Office staff study, "Selected Government-Wide Management
Improvement Efforts – 1970 to 1980," G.A.O. Catalogue GGD-83-69, (Washington,
D.C.: 8 August, 1983), pp. i and 39.

The Story of the Spence Bay Craft Shop

In 1976, I was requested by the Department of Indian Affairs and Northern Development to help resolve a problem in connection with a craft shop in Spence Bay, a tiny community located about 200 miles from the magnetic north pole, on Canada's most northerly coast. It is one of a number of little communities that have sprung up in the Arctic as the Inuit people have come off the land, abandoning their previous nomadic existence to cluster around schools, the local Hudson Bay stores and government facilities.

What income there is, in these isolated settlements, is typically derived from the sale of furs, of crafts such as soapstone carvings in some villages, or prints in others, and from a handful of jobs associated with the local store and municipal offices.[1] To a great extent, people continue to subsist on a diet of fish, caribou and seal: there are few other resources. In Spence Bay, the average annual income in 1976 was under $4,000: there were 35 jobs in a community of about 435 persons, of whom 160 were over 16 years old — an unemployment rate of around 70 per cent.

The fact that most people are dependent on welfare and other government grants reinforces a sense of dependency among a proud and independent people. Social problems such as alcoholism and wife-beating, previously rare, have become more common. An already difficult situation is made worse by friction between some members of the transient white population (many of whom are there principally to save money for a few years) and the local Inuit, who have an understandably different attitude to the land and who consider the area to be home.

In these circumstances, any economic activity that promises some employment for local people, particularly for Inuit women who have virtually no chance at a job, is an opportunity to be nurtured. The community of Spence Bay was fortunate to have just such an opportunity. Two independent and plucky women from southern Canada had collaborated with an able Inuit woman, Anaoyok Alookee, to create a craft shop which developed hand-made parkas for the southern market, based on original Inuit designs but modified for southern tastes. The founder of the project, Judy McGrath, had taught the Inuit women how to use local material such as lichens from rocks to make dyes in beautiful, soft colours. Eva Strickler, a Swiss-trained weaver, helped to organize the shop and showed the women how to maintain the high standards of quality expected in the fashion-conscious South. The local women had been encouraged to explore their own ideas about design, and as a result the parkas and other products from this unique enterprise had won design awards and had been featured in a national magazine.

Spence Bay products had a cachet among knowledgeable southern stores and consumers. The shop itself occupied a special place in the local community, offering partial or full employment for about two dozen women, affording them a sense of personal purpose and achievement, as well as providing the local women with a social setting in which to enjoy each other's company. A long-term resident of Spence Bay commented at the time of the study, "It would be a calamity for the community if the craft shop was ever closed."

The shop had received financial support from two sources: a federal government program intended to create employment opportunities, and the Government of the Northwest Territories' economic development program. Both programs required that periodic evaluations be undertaken. One of the key criteria upon which the continuation of funding was to be based was the quality of management. It was to conduct such an evaluation that I was retained.

The federal government took the view that local circumstances, as well as non-economic contributions of the project, had to be taken into account in assessing the quality of management. The territorial government, however, took good management to mean that the shop had to be "economically viable". The Spence Bay project was expected to make money, although it was thousands of miles from southern markets, it had to function in a drafty, government-owned building, and to pay heating costs in a land where the temperature fell to -60 degrees Celsius. The workers had never worked in a business enterprise, most spoke no English, and all supplies and products had to be shipped in and out by air (except for the brief hiatus when the sea was not frozen). In addition, the project was dependent upon problematic and inexpert services of the territorial government itself for purchasing and shipping its supplies, for marketing its product, and for maintaining its accounts.

The women managing this project were in an impossible situation. The federal government's definition of good management encompassed the achievement of social as well as economic goals. Aware that the local women, if not employed at the craft shop, would increase the drain on the local social welfare system, federal officials wanted to continue subsidizing the project, and felt that the managers were doing a responsible job. Officials of the territorial government of the day defined good management in commercial terms. Good managers earned a profit. Good managers followed prescribed procedures, no matter what the external variables. Since the shop was not earning a profit, territorial officials were constantly threatening to close it down. An enterprise requiring a subsidy was by definition badly managed, in their estimation.

The continuation of funding for this project, and the livelihood and well-being of some 30 to 40 Inuit women and their families, hung on the outcome of the evaluation, which in turn hung on the definition of "good management".*

Misconceptions of Management

Clearly, different beliefs about what constitutes good management can lead to very different expectations and standards for the performance of government programs. It is therefore important that government officials, both elected and appointed, avoid some of the misconceptions about management which are quite prevalent in the public sector. Such misconceptions have contributed to many of the difficulties associated with attempts to improve management practices in government. In Whitehall, for example, as discussed in the previous chapter (see also appendix 2), officials have tended to equate management with "controlling and supervising routine functions", with "programmed implementation of predetermined policies" or "techniques of control".[2] I have encountered similar

---

* The evaluation supported the federal government's interpretation of good management; territorial officials remained unconvinced. Nonetheless, the shop managed to struggle on for a decade or so after the evaluation; ultimately, it was shut in December 1986.

beliefs in other jurisdictions. Some government officials do not see themselves as managers at all. (One former senior public servant has written, "[P]ublic servants are not managers: they are policy advisers and/or emissaries (negotiators) and/or administrators."[3])

One especially tenacious misconception about management is the notion that financial administration constitutes its core; all other aspects are secondary. This view sees management as little more than minding the money: if one gets the financial policies right, any other management problems will more or less look after themselves. (It leads to a related misconception: that financial auditors are qualified to resolve almost any management problem.) Another misbelief equates "sound management" with adherence to official policies regarding the control of money and personnel. The bureaucrat who follows these policies and procedures (or ensures that others are following them) must by definition be managing well. This belief obviously has to rest upon the assumption that official policies and procedures in such areas as personnel, administration and finance provide managers with a reliable cookbook of management recipes which can be applied in all circumstances — an assumption of questionable merit, in my experience.

A related perversion is the belief that management consists of a set of universal principles or rules, equally relevant to every organization. Good managers know these rules and apply them, whatever the setting. Yet another misconstruction, still particularly prevalent in the U.K., is that management is something done by subordinate officials within the framework of policies conceived by their superiors. This is the "all management is administration, and administration is implementation" fallacy. It gives rise to the view of the civil servant as a rather passive custodian, interpreting legislation and applying rules. It rests on the idea that policy and management occupy two different worlds, roughly corresponding to the upper and lower levels of the management hierarchy in a department. Policy types occupy the senior levels, managers the subordinate ones. A variation on this theme is the belief that management is something that heads of departments delegate to their chief financial (and/or personnel) officers, so that they can get on with the "real" work of the department.

Then there is the belief that management is business administration. That is, management is primarily, if not exclusively, concerned with marketing, production and similar business-specific functions. This idea leads straight to the conclusion that, since government does not involve most of these functions, government officials do not need to know about "management". (Some business people go to the opposite extreme, and argue that government's problems arise from its failure to behave like a business; if it did, it would be "well-managed", and its inefficiencies would disappear.)

Related to this view is the idea that management is a collection of prescriptions designed to help people engaged in routine, repetitive work, such as loading boxcars or assembling automobiles. Management then is not really relevant to organizations engaged in more intellectual or creative tasks such as, say, policy analysis or scientific research. Management is for doers and drones.

Many members of Parliament seem to harbour the belief that "applying management principles" means reducing the size of the public service. They are conveniently blind to the relationship between the growth of the service and the programs approved by Parliament, or the resources voted in annual appropriations. Public servants (read "bad managers") have somehow slipped a lot of extra money past Parliament. The public service is "too big", according to some undefined standard. Good management thus involves "downsizing"; it leads also to what the British have called "hiving off", to "privatization" of government services, or to slashing budgets and staff. While there are certainly circumstances in which cost reductions are desirable in government organizations not subject to the discipline of the "bottom line", the idea that "good management" involves little more than cross-the-board reductions in budgets and personnel is simple-minded. Good management requires that the volume of work and the demands placed upon an organization be correlated with the resources at its disposition. Wholesale cost reductions may well lead to a situation where a responsible job can simply no longer be done by the people employed in the organization. Cuts in these circumstances are demoralizing and contribute nothing to better management.

Each of the foregoing interpretations of management carries different implications for how top officials should carry out their roles;

for relationships between important institutions of government; for policies affecting appointments and promotions in the public service; for working relationships within the bureaucracy; and for determining which procedures and practices should be imported from business to government. Defining management is not just an exercise in semantics: it establishes a foundation upon which to build other ideas about the functioning of the public service and the institutional environment of government.

The Language of Management

One of the reasons why there is confusion over the meaning of management lies in the absence of any well-defined terminology for management concepts. A necessary step in the evolution of any new discipline is the development of a specialized vocabulary to describe its concepts and ideas. The mark of an established discipline is a lexicon of terms understood by persons who are expert in the field, terms which facilitate the analysis of problems and which permit communication among specialists. The more recent the discipline, the more inconsistency there tends to be in the use of technical terms.

This is certainly true of management, and it is a major impediment to the manager or student interested in a broader knowledge of the field. There are, for example, few concepts as fundamental to the study of management as objectives. Organizations exist to achieve certain purposes; it is generally recognized that there is a hierarchy of such purposes, with broad statements of intent providing an overall framework for organizational activity. Within this, there are more detailed and specific ends which relate to the activities of subordinate units within the organization. One might have thought that, after three generations of evolution, management would have agreed on the terminology to be used to describe different sorts of objectives. The broad statement of purpose at the top of the hierarchy might be referred to as an aim, subordinate statements might be called objectives, and the most specific and detailed statements might be called goals. With agreement on these terms, managers could more readily communicate on matters related to the determination of organizational purposes.

However, even on a matter as basic as this, there is no consistency in terminology. I have often heard managers debating what the words "goal" or "objective" mean, not realizing that there is no standard meaning, and it is simply up to them to agree on one. Management literature is littered with different terms used to describe ends and intentions: mandates, aims, goals, normative goals, objectives, strategies, priorities, policies, missions, vision...all used in ways that are inconsistent.

Similar problems arise with other management concepts. "System", an important idea in management, is used variously to mean a procedure, a method of operation, a strategy for achieving an end, a computerized method of handling information, a performance requirement, an entity comprising a number of related parts, and an organism that interacts with its environment. Concepts such as decision analysis, planning, human resource management, financial management, control, information system, accountability, operational audit, performance management or evaluation have no standard meaning. Even persons working in the same organization often have quite varied understandings of what key management terms mean. I have known these misunderstandings to interfere seriously with organizational performance, by causing conflict among managers as to the scope of their responsibilities. Such conflicts have arisen simply from the fact that each individual understood a certain term to mean something different.[4]

Financial management provides a good illustration. In a number of government departments, I have known senior financial officials who believed that their "financial management" role invested them with a substantive authority over resource allocation decisions. Colleagues with line responsibilities hotly contested what they perceived as meddling in line authority. Planning affords another example: the many different meanings that may be assigned to this concept can easily lead to battles over organizational turf. Control is a classic source of conflict: assigning a manager a "control" responsibility may create more problems than it solves, for control may be interpreted to mean "monitoring" or it may be understood to mean "decision-making".

The Evolution of Management Thought

What, then, is management concerned with? The idea that management is interested primarily in routine sorts of tasks, or in business functions, is quite understandable. A good deal of thinking about management originated with the work of an American, Frederick Taylor. Taylor, who published his major works soon after the turn of this century, was convinced that there had to be one best way of carrying out many routine manual jobs (such as loading boxcars). His efforts to find more "scientific" approaches to such tasks led to the development of a school known as "scientific management" (see appendix 3). Although the notion that there is "one best way" to carry out most tasks is now largely discredited, the idea that management consists of a set of rules or principles that are generally applicable to all situations became adopted by what became known as the "classical school" of management. It still holds remarkable sway, and colours many persons' ideas about what management is.

Management has in fact gone far beyond its roots in industrial engineering and the rather limited ideas of the classical school. It has spread through all the remaining functions of the business organization — marketing, finance, personnel — and into the executive suite. Whereas in its early days, management was principally concerned with the internal operations of companies, it has expanded to address the external relationships of the organization. When management was mainly directed at subordinate occupations within business enterprises, the line between planning or business strategy and management was relatively easy to maintain. Management was concerned with "implementation", and such activities as determining the global objectives of the corporation lay outside its sphere. However, management's progress into such fields as business strategy and corporate finance has put an end to the notion that management is directed solely to routine sorts of tasks: it now embraces all the functions of the corporation and all its relationships, both internal and external.

In addition, management has moved beyond the field of business. It has also extended its concerns well outside the "hard" aspects of productivity — technology, time-saving, the layout of production facilities, etc. — and become engaged in studies of motivation and morale, in recognition of the key role played by people in making institutions work. Indeed, it is a fallacy to think that the discipline has traditionally been concerned only with shop floor productivity or with business problems. For example, one of the earliest and most influential writers on management, Max Weber, dealt with questions of organization design and the need to establish more formal systems and structures within institutions, without restricting himself to business enterprises. His concern was to develop a general model or a set of principles of administration that would be applicable to any type of organization, public or private. Similarly Chester Barnard, one of the early giants of management thinking, was greatly interested in such "soft" questions as leadership and motivation.

Today, it is useful to think of management as being broadly concerned with the problem of organizational productivity or performance. Indeed, to use the language of the economist, management might be described as the fifth factor of production. According to economic theory, productivity is achieved by appropriately blending together the three "classical" factors of production (land, labour and capital) with technology. This view of the productive process ignores the fact that these four factors do not unite of their own free will. Productivity will be attained only when they are consciously assembled in a purposeful, well-managed organization where tasks are divided among different persons and then co-ordinated. Productivity can no more be achieved without sound management than it can without land or labour.

Management provides guidance, in the form of concepts, principles and standards, to determine organizational goals and to implement agreed strategies. Management is not limited to business organizations: it is a discipline which should be appropriately applied in different institutional settings (business, government departments, municipalities, not-for-profit organizations, hospitals, etc.) with due regard for the particular objectives and character of each type of organization. Business practices constitute one source of ideas and precedents about how to manage, but they are not necessarily applicable, or even relevant, in other organizations and contexts.

Management has aptly been called a situational discipline — one where a wide variety of tools or "answers" exist, and where the challenge is to determine what tool is best suited to a particular situation or context. Jay Lorsch, a prominent contemporary management theorist, has written, "[W]hat is effective management behaviour and action depends on the specifics in each situation.... What the behavioural sciences can, and should, provide are ... 'walking sticks' to guide the managers along decision-making paths about human affairs."[5] Peter Drucker asserts that we must abandon "the belief of traditional organization theory that there must be 'one best principle' which alone is 'right'.... There must be one final answer."[6]

How then are we to determine when an organization is well managed? What standards should be employed in assessing managerial performance?

Good Management = Means and Processes

A good manager is often thought to be one who plans ahead, is organized, motivates others and follows up. That is, he or she follows the plan-organize-motivate-control precepts with which many managers will be familiar (see appendix 3). This is, of course, a procedural, or instrumental, view of management. It says nothing about results: the good manager is not the one who gets things done, but the one who follows the rules.

The management auditor reviewing organizational performance under these criteria looks for evidence of procedural rectitude, preferably documented. Do you plan? How can I tell unless it is written down? Where is the manual? What process do you use? There should be a flow chart. What about organization? The well-organized institution is the one where there are up-to-date, clear job descriptions. Let me see them. How do you control? There has to be a system, and it should be documented. Some of the territorial government officials monitoring Spence Bay clearly believed that management should be assessed in this manner.

Defining management in procedural terms makes life in a bureaucracy a lot simpler, and requires less judgment or discretion on the part of managers (or auditors monitoring departments' activities). Since they only have to apply defined standards and rules, auditors can be more junior and lower paid. When surrounded by a hedge of procedures, government officials are less likely to stray outside and take an initiative that might embarrass a minister.

BEYOND THE BOTTOM LINE

There is nothing intrinsically wrong with documented plans, formalized control systems and the like; but to conclude that management is sound on the basis of such evidence is akin to concluding that good soldiers are the ones who polish their shoes, arrive on time at drills and salute smartly. It can lead to disproportionate attention to means rather than ends. In practice, it often seems to create a bias toward a document-dependent, procedure-bound approach to administration, which, in turn, may generate an atmosphere that poisons initiative, imagination and flexibility. It enshrines the "one best way" of doing things in manuals and guidelines that become difficult and time-consuming to alter. People working in the organization tend to develop vested interests in the existing procedures and systems, regardless of whether these procedures actually work.

Another problem is that the "means" definition of management conjures up a vision of the managerial situation that is at odds with most managers' reality. It suggests that management occurs in an environment of relative serenity and predictability, and that the functions of management can proceed in a measured and linear fashion, moving from planning through to implementation. For individuals who manage projects where there is a clear beginning and a process of building, or who are starting up new ventures, the plan-organize-motivate-control model may offer a certain relevance. For managers caught up in the day-to-day turbulence of running a program, the model is less helpful.

When there are unexpected changes in priorities and workload arising from, for example, a Cabinet shuffle, a question in the House, a political crisis or a change in minister, planning tends to be a matter of grabbing whatever time can be salvaged amid the pressures of responding to the latest crisis. Organizing is not the cool design of organization charts to respond to a previously-articulated plan, but rather the on-the-run adjustment and adaptation of people and functions to the exigencies of the relentless flow of daily tasks. In such an environment, the good manager may be the one who spends little or no time planning and organizing and carrying out the other recommended functions in textbook fashion; rather, the good manager may simply be the one who is able, by using the resources and imagination at his or her command, to get a Cabinet document to the minister before the proroguing of the House, or a batch of welfare cheques delivered to pensioners during a postal strike. A good formula for demoralizing such managers is to criticize them for failing to have a documented planning system.

Procedural definitions of good management raise the danger that management performance will be judged, not on its true merits, but on the basis of what can be conveniently observed, documented or counted. The need to record transactions is important in certain functions, the field of accounting and large information systems being two good examples. However, systematic documentation of procedures, transactions and decisions in other realms of management may simply result in paper for paper's sake. In personnel management, for example, and particularly in the field of performance appraisal, it may be counterproductive to commit certain matters to paper. Some decision-making situations move too quickly to be conveniently recorded and often, in the context of the organization's own internal requirements, there is no need to record why a particular decision was reached. Documentation for documentation's sake is a danger that is especially acute in government, because of the increasing prevalence of external, publicly reported auditing. If we are to avoid cluttering government records with reams of "memoranda to the file" written for potential auditors afflicted with a narrow interpretation of what constitutes sound administration, we must be wary of procedural definitions of management.

In the development and application of procedural standards, due allowance must also be made for the nature of the organization and the circumstances of the moment. Only rarely will one set of standards fit every situation. (In Spence Bay, certain methods of accounting or inventory control devised in some southern metropolis were an affront to common sense.) Furthermore, it is clear that a degree in accounting and experience in financial auditing are not sufficient training for this type of analysis. A broader understanding of management and the functioning of organizations is required.

An official who was deeply involved in Britain's FMI (Financial Management Initiative) program spoke of the dangers of a process-oriented approach to management:

You're in a difficult area of judgment here about the reality of management, as opposed to the cosmetics and process. The great temptation is to rely on process, because it's easier, and because it's the only thing a drowning man can grip. . . . You say, "Ah yes ! On the third Thursday of the second month, they sit around a table and set objectives, so they're all right, and they also have a return that comes in every month...which reviews how those objectives are going. . . ." It becomes a caricature of management.

[F]ormulating this kind of criticism is like taking confectionery off children. . . . The problem is unique to government, because you've got proxies in business, and you can . . . know when something is going wrong more quickly and more assuredly. You take a short cut and you say, I don't know exactly what's wrong . . . at the moment; but I can tell the systems are wrong because we're not making any money.

[In government], the problem is identifying what the deficiency is before you can even get on to it. The trouble with the external auditor is that unless he is prepared to do very laborious legwork, like a whole succession of test bores, he is reduced to a mechanistic, process sort of thing. "Have they got this, have they got that?" and so forth. And you're left at the end saying, "Well, they have got all that. But is it well managed, or is it not?"[7]

Furthermore, the "good management = means and processes" view does not pay enough attention to the motivational dimensions of management. To date, in Canada and Britain, government management-improvement initiatives seem to have focused mainly on procedures and systems. It is, after all, relatively simple to tell departments, "You shall have a commitment control system," and then to go out and inspect to see if such a system has been installed. To say to departments, "You shall have a well-motivated work force" is an injunction that is much less precise and much less susceptible to measurement. Yet the issue is surely of equal, if not greater, importance.

In summary, the definition of good management in terms of the observance of certain processes or practices raises a lot of problems. Procedural standards have their place, but they must be sufficiently general to allow flexibility in their application and interpretation.

Overuse or misapplication of such standards may lead to a confusion of means with ends. Certainly they should not be devised without allowance for the context of the particular organization. Excessive use of such standards will continue to force government officials to produce paper for its own sake and to create a document- and procedure-bound bureaucracy. The cost of government will rise, and overall performance will almost certainly deteriorate.

Moreover, reliance on means and methods encourages officials to focus on the "harder" procedural or analytic aspects of administration, while ignoring the "softer" motivational issues, presumably because the latter are too intangible. Yet employees' attitudes and motivation clearly exercise a major impact on organizational productivity, particularly in white-collar environments such as government departments.

Managing for Results: An Alternative View

"The good manager gets results!" It seems difficult to argue with this. The notion appears particularly suited to the world of business, where, it is well known, good management generates profits. The good manager makes money. With such a clear goal, surely there can be no difficulty identifying the good manager in business. But does assessing management according to profits really provide an unequivocal yardstick for judging performance?

An American study of the process of determining corporate goals and strategies in 12 major industrial firms shows how business results can be subject to different interpretations. The study documents the conflicting pressures on such corporations. It identifies three principal "constituencies" to whom a big corporation is accountable (in the sense that these groups have legitimate claims, enforceable through law, politics or economics, upon the company): those who provide capital, including both shareholders and debtors; the "product market" constituency, including suppliers and customers; and the organizational constituency of managers and career employees. (A more general "constituency" which is identified but which receives little attention because of its amorphous nature is "society at large".) The study notes how the satisfaction of one constituency usually involves trading off against competing objectives sought by another.

"[M]anagers cannot afford to overlook the legitimate demands placed on them by the capital market, the product market, and the organization of which they too are a part. Yet these demands are not easily reconciled."[8]

Some shareholders may be looking for dividends, others for capital appreciation; debtors are interested in secure returns and the preservation of their principal; communities where the firms are located look for tax revenues, for minimal environmental damage and for employment opportunities; suppliers want high prices, unions high wages and job security; management wants freedom from constraints (whether imposed by unions or outside owners), a stable, secure organizational environment and attractive compensation; customers want low prices. These are not mutually consistent goals. Yet managers must not overlook the legitimate demands of all the constituencies.

The conventional view is that a business has only one accountability, that is, to the shareholders, a view which suggests that "success" or "good results" can be easily defined in terms of shareholders' interests. The reality is more complicated, especially in a large concern. What seems good management to one constituency may appear as a serious error in judgment to another. To say that good management is merely a matter of achieving results begs the question: which results? Serving whose interests? Is a manager who is more effective at serving the interests of one constituency "better" than the manager who is more successful at meeting the demands of another? Donaldson and Lorsch, the study authors, propose that top executives' responsibility is to maintain a strategic equilibrium among competing interests; but such an equilibrium may assume many forms. Even in the world of business, values and context enter into one's definition of "success" or of good management.

If a business needs a major change in labour relations strategy, then the good manager will be the individual with the right mix of skills to bring about that change. On the other hand, if a new product is needed, or perhaps new international markets have to be developed for the firm, the good manager may have to possess quite different skills. The entrepreneurial company will have very different requirements from the mature organization. The "good" top manager is the one with the capacity to cope with the strategic demands of the moment. Rather than speaking of "good management", it might be better to speak of "appropriate management skills" – that mix of abilities and aptitudes which is suited to the context.

Defining good management in a business environment also requires a judgment concerning the conflict between short-run and longer-term performance. Thornton Bradshaw, Chief Executive Officer of RCA, says that one of the toughest challenges facing top executives is the need to "walk the tightrope" between "short-term results and the absolute necessity for a long-term positioning . . . . It's very, very hard to do."[9] We have all heard of the high flier who moves from one job to another so quickly that mistakes never catch up, who engineers impressive short-run results while leaving long-term problems for others to resolve. Without knowing the context, who is to say whether it is more prudent to manage for shorter-term performance or for sustained results over the longer-term?

Brilliant short-run results may lead to great difficulties in the longer term; conversely, too much emphasis on the long term may cause short-run cash flow problems. Apparently astute investments in developing countries may generate profits but may entail human costs that are unacceptable. Ignoring pollution regulations may initially increase revenues but lead to troubled community relations and damaging fines. Closing a marginally productive plant in a small community may simplify the job of top management, but throw several hundred persons out of work. The "bottom line" may be more sound – but is this "good management"? Is this corporate success? Clearly, different interpretations of success are possible, even in the supposedly simple world of business.

The previous discussion has been directed to the business environment because it is often thought that success is easier to define in this context. However, there are still difficulties: to assess management in business, one must take into account a company's competitive environment, its stage of evolution, its organizational traditions and its responsibilities to different stakeholders. Moreover, if good management is defined as the attainment of results, then the assessment of management performance must be linked to an assessment of what goals the company should be pursuing.

Defining success is a good deal more difficult and complex in the public sector. The multiplicity of objectives and clients served by most government programs leads to the possibility of many more views as to what constitutes "results". Business has three main constituencies; government has dozens. What constitutes a signal achievement in one constituency's eyes – say, placing tariffs on foreign imports or imposing censorship on certain publications – may be a disaster to others.

It is often difficult to tell what the results of government initiatives have been, either because a program's impact cannot be measured or because its effects are not easily distinguishable from other events. If results cannot be readily observed or quantified (and this is in the nature of the work itself), it is that much more difficult to judge managerial performance.

A good example of this problem is provided by an international development project, in which a rich "donor" country provides assistance to a poorer, "recipient" nation. Would a "well-managed" aid project be one that got funds quickly into the recipient country, so that they were spent abroad, or one that resulted in the highest expenditures on domestic goods and services in the donor country? What if the goods in question were more costly than comparable items available to the recipient from other donor nations: could procurement at home be called "economical" under these circumstances? What if an audit of the project revealed that, because of the extensive involvement of nationals of the recipient country, the project advanced more slowly than it would have, had "trained professionals" been running it? Is that waste, or an inexpensive price to pay to give a recipient nation greater experience in administration? Clearly, assessing "success" in these circumstances involves some difficult judgments.

Management in the public sector is vastly complicated by the problem of incommensurability: the apples-and-oranges difficulties one encounters in trying to assess the merits of one public program relative to another. In business, costs and revenues provide a convenient common yardstick for considering alternative investment possibilities or comparing the performance of different divisions or products. In government, there are many different yardsticks. "Fairness" is the one which is commonly used to compare the advantages and disadvantages of, say, opening a new customs office, giving a grant to a voluntary organization, increasing the staff of a regulatory agency or purchasing a new piece of military equipment. Fairness, and the related standard of the politician, "Will it sell back home?" are crude measurement tools at best, certainly open to many interpretations.[10] But few other tools are available to assist with judgements where competing values are involved.

A final problem is resource reallocation in government. Many groups in society will agree that government should be smaller and less costly, but never at the expense of a program in which they have a vested interest. Cutting programs can be bad politics. Therefore, in light of the intransigence of voters, ministers may try to make existing programs run on a shoestring so that funds can be extracted for a new priority. This creates an invidious, but not uncommon, situation in the public service. "Good management" in this context may mean keeping a number of different client groups within the limits of tolerable discontent, as resource shortages gradually compromise the efficiency of existing programs. Officials caught in this vise will feel understandably aggrieved if a news story or a question in the House criticizes the quality of their service to the public, or if an audit cites them for inefficiency.

The Impact of Context on Management Concepts

Judgments about what constitutes good management cannot be taken in isolation from the context. What appears to be prudent, responsible, efficient or economical in one set of circumstances may appear quite different when viewed from another perspective or in other circumstances. In short, these are relative, not absolute, concepts.

Take executive jets as an example. Are expensive private jets for corporate executives or government ministers efficient? When viewed in the narrow context of the costs involved in getting from one place to another, the answer is, "No." Commercial airlines are cheaper. Clearly executive jets are inefficient. The use of private jets is the kind of extravagance upon which auditors love to pounce.

Considering the costs in a wider context leads to a different interpretation of what constitutes "efficiency". If a private jet permits top executives to use their time more productively on behalf of the organization, then the jet becomes a sound business investment, not a luxury.

The theme of executive jets turns up in the biography of Lee Iacocca: the business leader who made history while he was busy pulling Chrysler back from the brink of bankruptcy, thereby saving half a million jobs. While Chrysler was struggling back to its feet, Iacocca's judgment came under fire from Washington. Good managers, the officials knew, don't waste money on jets. Iacocca relates the episode:

> Then we ran into a problem that could only have come from the fertile mind of a real bureaucrat. The board ordered us to sell our Gulfstream jet. To the minds in Washington, the Chrysler jet was a symbol of the profligate spending of a big corporation. . . . Nobody blinks when you spend $100 million for new robots, but when you send one of your top guys around to the factories to teach the workers how to use those new robots, that's OK — but only if he flies commercial. . . .
>
> Some of our plants can't be reached very easily by commercial aircraft. And if I'm paying a guy two hundred grand a year, I don't want him spending his time in airports.
>
> Private planes save a lot of wear and tear on our employees. People outside the business world often have the impression that most executives goof off. Not the ones I know. They work twelve and fourteen hours a day, and their time is valuable.
>
> The corporate jet is not a perk. It's a necessity. . . . [T]he company jet is a great time-saver — and a stress-saver as well.[11]

An illustration from the public sector shows how an apparently objective concept such as productivity can be open to different interpretations. During the late 1960s and early 1970s, an increasingly tense relationship developed in Canada between the then Auditor General, Max Henderson, and the Government of Prime Minister Pierre Trudeau. They could not agree on the areas suitable for scrutiny by the auditor general, or what constituted the responsible spending of public funds. A case in point was the matter of government disbursements on the approaches for a proposed new causeway to connect Prince Edward Island to the mainland (an issue that has recently returned to the news). After incurring some $64 million in costs (thereby creating a number of jobs in an economically depressed area of the country), the federal government decided to abandon the project.[12]

The auditor general criticized the government for wasting taxpayers' money, arguing that no return had been secured for the expenditures and that they were, therefore, "unproductive". The government took a broader view, asserting that it was a general manager 's prerogative, indeed duty, to review priorities from time to time. This had been done in the case of the causeway; the government had prudently decided not to pursue the project but to divert resources to a more pressing need. Thus the abandonment was not wasteful but a sound management decision adopted in the light of new information.

It is easy to see how the same decision can be interpreted quite differently depending on the context within which it is viewed. Within the scope of the project, the decision was clearly a bad one, as no causeway was built, and the resources that had been employed in preparing the approaches were wasted. In a larger context, that is, if the cost of continuing the project is weighed against other funding requirements that may have emerged, then the decision to abandon the causeway may have been legitimate. Presumably the negative consequences of such a decision were considered and rejected by Cabinet. Was the decision an example of waste or good management? Although in this particular case, the Government's decision to start and then terminate the project was somewhat difficult to defend, it is clear that a wider context makes possible a different interpretation of the concept of good management, just as it did in the case of the executive jet.

Should Government Emulate Business?

As noted above, much early work on management was concerned with business problems, and even today, students who wish to learn about management are often advised to go to universities that offer courses in business administration. In our day-to-day conversation, we speak of people acting in a "business-like manner", using this term as a synonym for efficient, responsible behaviour. To learn business' way of doing things, according to this view, is to learn how to manage well.

Business practices do not provide a guaranteed recipe for success in non-commercial organizations, an important point to understand if governments are to be prevented from importing practices unsuited to the government environment. The private sector is not infrequently viewed through rose-coloured glasses. The fact that an enterprise is in the private sector provides no assurance that it is well managed. How many business leaders would claim that a published external appraisal of their management practices, of the kind conducted by auditors general of government departments, would yield a clean bill of health? Four authors who have examined managerial competence in the private sector in America have written,

- "One is continually surprised by the number of obvious mistakes made by otherwise sophisticated organizations."

- "[A] clear majority of businesses, even in the most sophisticated economy in the world, are mismanaged in some obvious and preventable ways."

- "There is clear evidence of widespread managerial weakness."

- "[C]orporate top management does not deserve its reputation for marvelous efficiency and decisiveness."[13]

The conventional wisdom about business is that the goad of competition prevents wasteful behaviour. In some companies, this certainly applies. However, there are circumstances where business success may have little to do with managerial skill or the elimination of wasteful practices. Good luck helps. (Napoleon is reputed to have said, "If I had to choose between the skillful general and the lucky general, I'd take the lucky one.") Being in the right place with the right product at the right time, not as a result of planning but simply because the breaks went your company's way, may be the main reason for profitability.

If a business is able to charge comfortable prices without fear of serious competition, there may be even less incentive to eliminate extravagance or waste than there is in government. Long-standing customer loyalties, inertia, monopoly, government subsidy, technological dominance, tariff barriers, exchange-rate fluctuations, political influence can all contribute to business success. Some companies – perhaps more than many people believe – are profitable almost in spite of their management. It is time we laid to rest the naive belief that an institution must be well run because it is in the private sector. And since the work of business is different from the work of government, we should not assume that business practices consistently provide a model worthy of emulation in the public sector.

As efforts have been made to develop useful principles and precepts for management in non-business organizations, it has become apparent that management in government is harder than in the private sector. There are many reasons for this: less clarity of direction, less control over resources, more relationships to maintain, fewer indicators of success, less privacy, more influences to take into account in decision-making, less flexibility to motivate and reward subordinates. Business executives who have worked in government will often acknowledge this.[14] Lord Bancroft, former head of the U.K. Home Civil Service, has made this comment:

> Much has been said about the analogy between running a business and running a government. This is a sloppy analogy for a start. If one simply substitutes "running a business" on the one hand and "governing a parliamentary democracy" on the other the falsity of the conceit is obvious.... [In government] there is immense concern to see that individuals and groups, large and small, are treated fairly and equally, and receive all the benefits that may be open to them.... [T]he pursuit of even handedness in the treatment of the enormously varied individual circumstances of the millions whose affairs become the business of government... makes for highly complex administration....[15]

Too much emphasis on the adoption of business practices in government institutions may obscure why they were situated in the public sector in the first instance. For many, perhaps most, government organizations, to suggest that the formula for better management is to run them like a business is somewhat akin to saying that if only elephants were monkeys, they could climb trees better. Wallace Sayre's oft-cited observation provides an apt summary of the degree of similarity between the two sectors: "Business and government administration are alike in all unimportant respects."[16] If government is to adopt models from the world of business, it should ensure that it is importing practices that are tried and proven, not myths; and it should ensure that the practices are suited to the public sector environment.

Once Again, What is Good Management?

The preceding discussion reinforces the idea that management is a situational discipline, not a set of absolute rules. There are real problems associated with defining good management in terms of means, processes and procedures rather than ends; there are equally serious difficulties with defining good management as the achievement of results, or as the pursuit of business practices.

In short, there is no simple formula for assessing good management in the public sector. Part of the assessment may hinge upon the degree to which program officials have conformed to certain rules, procedures or standards. However, those assessing performance have a responsibility not only to determine to what extent conformity has prevailed, but also to what extent the rules and procedures are appropriate to the context. It is my impression that governments have tended to be overly zealous in developing general rules and regulations for departments, without making sufficient allowance for institutional differences. In such circumstances, "following the book" may have little to do with good management (see chapter 7).

Any reasonable assessment of good management will involve a good deal of judgment and must take into account a combination of factors. Some of these will relate to how the work is being done (process or procedural considerations); some may relate to employees' engagement and commitment (motivational considerations); some will relate to the attainment of results, appropriately defined.

In view of this, it is clear that any general assessment or review of performance of a government program will have to call upon particular kinds of aptitudes. Because government has no bottom line, audits and examinations of performance are becoming increasingly common in many jurisdictions. Both external reviews and internal audits must be staffed by people with the breadth of knowledge and experience appropriate to the mandate. A procedural review of management practices clearly requires different competence from a general assessment of organizational performance and management.

This leads to a final conclusion. Care and balance are due in assessing performance in the public sector. Numerous factors must be taken into account in judging the quality of management of a project or program, a more costly approach than that of simply applying formulae. Governments, which tend to try to do things on the cheap, will have to be careful not to be penny-wise and pound-foolish in this sphere. It is tempting to draw facile conclusions about the performance of government officials and institutions, and unfortunately the media and politicians often do so. As noted earlier in this chapter, this is not difficult — it is "like taking confectionery off children." However, quick judgments are often biased and erroneous, and they will almost certainly be unfair to the officials concerned.

Footnotes

1. A profile of a typical community's employment is as follows: in a village of 430 persons (roughly the size of Spence), there might be 30 to 40 whites. Of these, about half would be employed, in the following capacities: administration (2), education (7), nursing (2), Hudson's Bay Company (2), RCMP (1), missions (2), social welfare (1), local co-operative (1). There would be very few jobs — perhaps half a dozen — for the 400-odd Inuit residents. See Hugh Brody, *The People's Land*, (Harmondsworth: Penguin, 1975), pp. 32-50.

2. Les Metcalfe, and Sue Richards, "The Impact of the Efficiency Strategy," *Public Administration*, 62, (Winter 1983), pp. 439-454.

3. D.G. Hartle, "Techniques and processes of administration," *Canadian Public Administration*, 20th anniversary ed. (1978) pp.127-138. Originally published in CPA, vol. 19 no. 1, (Spring 1976), pp. 21-33.

4. The noted American management professor, Jay Lorsch, has stated, "One difficulty with today's . . . [management] tools is that each scholar (or group of scholars) has developed his or her own language and methods. . . . Understandably, communication among behavioural scientists and their communication with managers is confused. Different scholars use different labels to mean the same thing. . . . Managers and scholars alike find it difficult to understand what one label means in one model as compared to another or how the ideas developed by one group relate to those developed elsewhere." See "Making Behavioural Science More Useful," *Harvard Business Review*, (March - April 1979), pp.171-181.

5. *Ibid.*, pp. 171-181.

6. Peter F. Drucker, *Management — Tasks, Responsibilities, Practices*, (New York: Harper and Row, 1973), ch. 41, pp. 518ff.

7. Author's interview, May 1985.

8. Gordon Donaldson and Jay W. Lorsch, *Decision Making At The Top — The Shaping of Strategic Direction*, (New York: Basic Books, Inc., 1983).

9. Interview with Harold Bradshaw, "The CEO Today: His Master's Steadier Voice," *Across The Board* magazine, (February 1985), pp. 38-43.

10. See Irving S. Shapiro, *America's Third Revolution: Public Interest and the Private Role*. (New York: Harper & Row, 1984), pp. 82-85. " 'Fairness' is a universal touchstone in politics, one of the few."

11. Lee Iacocca, with William Novak, *Iacocca: An Autobiography*, (New York: Bantam Books, 1984), p. 256.

12. Auditor General of Canada, *Annual Report, 1968-69*, pp.107-108; *Annual Report, 1971-72*, p. 150.

13. Leonard R. Sayles, Kenneth R. Andrews, Robert B. Buchele and David Finn, as cited in Lawrence E. Lynn, Jr., *Managing the Public's Business: The Job of the Government Executive*, (New York: Basic Books Inc., 1981), p. 112.

14. Lynn, *op. cit.*, pp. 120-121.

15. Lord Bancroft, "Whitehall: Some Personal Reflections," Suntory-Toyota Lecture, delivered at the London School of Economics, 1 December 1983. (Available from the library, Royal Institute of Public Administration, London.)

16. Cited in Lynn, *op. cit.*, p. 136.

Chapter Two:
The Institutions of Government

Government is like an onion. To understand it, you have to peel through many different layers. Most outsiders never get beyond the first or second layer.[1]

The political institutions which provide overall direction and hold the key levers of power — Cabinet, Parliament, the prime minister — occupy the centre of the onion, surrounded by a variety of central departments or agencies responsible for managing government as a collectivity, and for co-ordination of policy. The "line" or operating departments, occupying the next layer to central agencies, are responsible for policy advice to their minister, for drafting and administering legislation and regulations, and for delivering programs and services to the public (or each other, in some cases). Departments are staffed by officials known in some jurisdictions as public servants (e.g. Canada), and in others (e.g. Britain) as civil servants.*

---

* A second group of organizations, often also called "central agencies", are those which play a cross-governmental co-ordinating role. They may be important in certain areas of government policy but are not usually involved in overall managerial matters. In Canada's federal government at time of writing, this group includes the Department of Finance and the Ministry of State for Science and Technology, created to co-ordinate scientific policy, and External Affairs, which co-ordinates Canadian foreign policy. Sometimes an organization such as the office of the auditor general or an ombudsman may be referred to as a central agency; however, such organizations report directly to the legislature and are not part of the central machinery of the executive, which is the sense in which the term "central agency" is used in this book.

The outer rim of the onion, furthest from the centre, is composed of a mixture of agencies known colloquially as "quangos" and nationalized industries in Britain and collectively as "Crown corporations" in Canada. These organizations, which operate at varying degrees of "arm's length" from the centre of government, are distinguished from departments by their somewhat greater degree of autonomy and managerial flexibility. (Their employees are not known as public servants, although many are government employees in the sense that most or all of their pay comes from government revenues.) Exhibit 1-1 illustrates these relationships.

The "Collectivity" and the Departments of Government

To understand both the subtleties and the difficulties of managing in government, it is important to appreciate the chameleon nature of government organizations. A government department often appears to be a self-contained entity, responsible for defining its mandate and operating policies under general direction from Cabinet and its committees. On other occasions, a government department assumes a much less clearly defined identity, presenting itself as a small component of a larger organization—the government as a whole. Superficially, a department might seem to be like a major subsidiary of a large corporation. However, such an analogy hardly captures the complexity of the subtle and mobile relationship between the centre and departments. Institutional relationships in a large government are determined to a considerable degree by a web of conventions rooted in the traditions of parliamentary democracy. In addition, they ebb and flow in response to the character of the elected Government* and the personalities of senior officials. At the departmental level, this creates an environment for management that is, in certain respects, very different from that of the private sector.

In any large public service, such as that of Canada (about 240,000 staff)[2] or even Ontario (70,000),[3] a department does function

---

* Government, capitalized, is used in this book to refer to the elected Government under the leadership of the prime minister; government (lower case) refers to the institution of government.

EXHIBIT 1 - 1
THE INSTITUTIONAL STRUCTURE OF GOVERNMENT

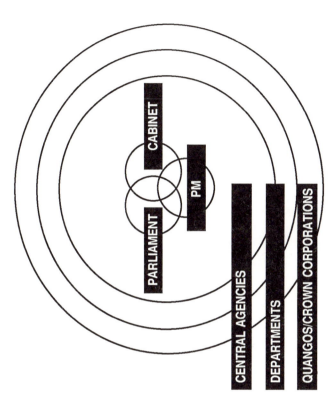

PARLIAMENT

CABINET

PM

CENTRAL AGENCIES

DEPARTMENTS

QUANGOS/CROWN CORPORATIONS

BEYOND THE BOTTOM LINE
(1988)

for many purposes as if it were a reasonably autonomous agency under the general supervision of a board of directors (Cabinet). A large department will exercise a strong influence over how its resources should be deployed; it will select staff and develop working methods and traditions that, over the years, will come to distinguish it from other departments of the same government. For example, in Ottawa, a department such as Indian Affairs and Northern Development tends to attract people with different values and modes of behaviour from, say, those of employees in a department such as Energy, Mines and Resources or National Defence.

It might be thought that people working in these departments would identify themselves as employees of their department. After all, some of these employees spend a good deal of their time vigorously promoting their department's interests. But despite this, it seems that many departmental employees think of themselves first and foremost as public servants, and secondarily as departmental employees.[4] They are recognizing a constitutional reality of parliamentary democracies, namely that government is a single entity. All government activity is undertaken on behalf of, and in the name of, the monarch or the "Crown". This is why one government organization cannot sue another: the Crown cannot sue itself. All public servants are employees of the Crown; in Canada, they are technically the employees of the Treasury Board (which acts on behalf of the Crown), not of their own department, even though their department may have made the hiring decision.

One practical consequence of this tradition is that governments tend to operate as more or less unified financial entities, with common financial policies and procedures (the degree of commonality varies somewhat from one jurisdiction to another). Obligations are assumed in the name of the monarch, i.e., on behalf of the collectivity. Many policies governing remuneration, benefits, superannuation, collective bargaining, senior staffing and other aspects of personnel management will be handled by one or more central agencies on behalf of the government as a whole. As well, certain spheres of administrative policy, such as land management and accommodation, travel, and major capital expenditures (notably computers), will often be centrally determined. (Britain is less centralized than Canada in some of these respects.)

The collectivity-departmental duality infuses the public service with a certain schizophrenia. Public servants' jobs and their individual rates of pay are determined by their departments, and their day-to-day priorities are very closely tied to those of the minister responsible for their department. This encourages strong identification with departmental objectives. However, public servants must also recognize the wider context of the collectivity and think about the implications of their actions on other spheres of government responsibility and other government institutions. This underlines the importance of consultation with colleagues in other departments, a subject about which more will be said below.

Since modern government has many responsibilities and institutions, this need to "consider the broader implications" (a classic civil service phrase) of a proposed initiative can turn into a formula for indecision and paralysis. Yet it is an intrinsic component of the government world. Part of the art of being an effective manager in the public service is to be able to work within this duality and to judge when action should take precedence over consultation, and vice versa.

The Political Centre

The single most important difference between public- and private-sector management lies in the political character of the body that controls the executive of government, the Cabinet. There is a superficial resemblance between the Cabinet, comprising the prime minister and ministers, and a corporate board of directors. However, Cabinet differs from the business board of directors in several ways. First, its composition: Cabinet typically is made up of individuals from widely divergent backgrounds and regions, who, although members of a common political party, usually hold differing views on questions of economic or social policy. Whereas the members of boards of directors are selected for their ability to contribute to the management of the enterprise, Cabinet members are chosen on the basis of many criteria, and ability to provide direction to the administrative machinery of government tends to be less important than other, more political considerations (see chapter 4).

Second, its size: particularly in Canada, where recent Cabinets have been very large, Cabinet is an unwieldy body, and the results of its deliberations can be unpredictable. (Britain gets around this problem to some degree by distinguishing between the Ministry – all ministers – and the Cabinet – a smaller, inner group of about 20 key ministers.) One former deputy minister, in an irreverent moment, told me,

> I sometimes used to refer to Cabinet as the Funny Farm. You and your staff would work hard to try to suggest a sound, sensible course of action and then you'd send your proposal to the political level. But you never knew what was going to come out. Often the decision just didn't seem to make any sense at all, and you couldn't determine how they'd reached the conclusion they did.

A third and more fundamental difference between the business board and Cabinet lies, of course, in the area of mandate. The objective of the business board of directors is to pursue the financial well-being of the corporation in a competitive market environment. Much of the language of business is competitive, even military, in nature: strategy, tactics, aggressive stances, exploitation of advantage, overcoming the competition, positioning, consolidation of position. In government, the motivation is not financial advantage, and the context is not the competitive world of the marketplace. Cabinet's mandate is the attainment of that elusive goal, "good government" (and the more immediate goal of "re-election"!). The ends of good government have to do with such abstract matters as social and economic well-being, personal freedom, equality under the law or cultural enhancement. The possibility of so many different interpretations of these objectives makes the task of government a good deal more contentious than that of business.

Civil servants tend to define "good government" in terms of policies that promote the long-term interests of the country. Politicians lean more to Keynes' observation that "in the long run, we are all dead", an attitude reinforced by the requirement that they seek re-election every four or five years. Cabinet must therefore strive to find a balance between policies with long- and short-term benefits, between policies that promote the general welfare as compared with that of specific interest groups, and between different, often unrelated policy fields, such as economic growth and social well-being, both of which make claims on the public purse.

Politicians must function in a web of traditions and conventions, some designed to circumscribe their power and limit their scope for action. These conventions are cornerstones of parliamentary democracy; many are the result of constitutional evolution that occurred over a period of centuries. Where business consciously focuses power and channels accountability to facilitate action, government will diffuse power and split accountability so that all legitimate points of view may be brought to bear in the process of decision-making, and also so that power is not abused in ways that might diminish personal freedom. Personal freedom is a privilege which most citizens in Western democracies take for granted. People forget that the conventions which impede government's ability to take prompt executive action may sometimes be making it work *well* – that is, as government is supposed to work – not *badly*.

A fourth difference between Cabinet and a board of directors lies in one of the most important conventions of parliamentary government, that of Cabinet solidarity. This convention dictates that ministers must stand or fall as an elected Government collectively.

> The members of the Cabinet are responsible to one another, and particularly to the Prime Minister. It is an essential Cabinet convention . . . that all members must openly agree on all important public questions. . . .
>
> It follows that all members of a Cabinet must consider the views of one another in making any important announcement or in taking a decision that might be considered as involving Government policy; and this leads in practice to prior consultation and discussion in Cabinet, or at least, with the Prime Minister. This done, if the Minister secures agreement on his proposal, the Cabinet will support it to a man; failing such agreement, the dissenting member must acquiesce in the rejection of his ideas or tender his resignation.[5]

A related convention is that of ministerial responsibility, requiring that ministers be personally accountable for the policies and activities of their departments, and answerable for these in the House of Commons as well as to the public. Both these conventions create profound differences between the managerial environment in government departments and that in the private sector. Two other traditions affecting ministerial responsibility, those of the neutrality and anonymity of public servants, are discussed in more depth in chapter 3.

No discussion of the political centre in Canada would be complete without reference to the role of the Prime Minister's Office (PMO). In the context of constitutional evolution, the PMO is a new arrival on the scene. Until the election of Prime Minister Lester Pearson in 1963, the staff of the office had not exceeded 30, and even under Pearson, it was only increased to 40. During the Pearson years (1963 to 1968) the PMO was almost indistinguishable from the Privy Council Office (PCO), sharing a joint telephone number and offices in the old East Block on Parliament Hill.[6]

When Prime Minister Trudeau succeeded Pearson in 1968, he greatly expanded the size and role of the PMO, clearly establishing its identity, and more than doubling the staff to 91. The publicly proclaimed rationale for this related to the growth of government and Trudeau's desire for expert assistance in developing the Government's programs and policies, in making appointments, in scheduling his time, in keeping in touch with Cabinet, colleagues, MPs, public servants, constituents, the officials of the Liberal Party, the media and the public, in answering questions in the House, in preparing speeches, in making travel arrangements and in related responsibilities. (Greater political control over the bureaucracy was undoubtedly another reason for the expansion of the office.) The PMO also assumed a key role in designing the machinery of government, a role it shared with the PCO. By 1971, the budget of the Office had reached $1 million; its budget for 1986/87 stood at $6.3 million.[7]

During the 1970s and 1980s, the PMO appears to have drawn some power away from the PCO as well as from party officials; it now plays a very significant role in the elected Government's political strategy, in appointments, and it intervenes selectively in many matters of policy. The PMO also seems to play a co-ordinating and shepherding role in relation to ministers. With all this additional clout, some believe that the non-elected officials of the PMO have more power than is appropriate in a parliamentary democracy.[8]

Central Agencies

Central departments or agencies are the units of government most closely associated with the Cabinet as a collective institution. Closest to the political heart of government in Ottawa lies the Privy Council Office, its rough equivalent being the Cabinet Office in Britain, and the Office of the Premier or the Executive Council in many provincial governments in Canada. The top official in this office (and, usually, the most senior official in the public service) is the Secretary to the Cabinet (in the Canadian provinces the incumbent is often known as the Deputy Minister to the Premier).

The PCO, or its equivalent in other jurisdictions, is usually responsible for briefing the prime minister, organizing and recording the results of Cabinet and Cabinet committee meetings, and advising on appointments to top positions.[9] It is often responsible for planning and priority-setting on behalf of the government as a whole. (In Canada, the PCO provides support of this nature to the Priorities and Planning Committee of Cabinet.) Frequently it makes recommendations to the prime minister concerning the deployment of functions among departments – the "machinery of government" role alluded to above. Because it affects the distribution of power among departments, this little-known activity has a direct impact on the authority, status and prerogatives not only of public servants, but also of ministers. It is a function of considerable importance.

Closely associated with this office are other departments with responsibilities for the formulation of government economic policy, and for the management of government as a collectivity. They develop proposals related to fiscal policy and to overall spending limits in each fiscal year. At the national level, they deal with such international economic issues as exchange rates and certain aspects of domestic and international monetary policy. In Canada, these responsibilities reside in the Department of Finance, while in Britain they are handled by Her Majesty's Treasury (H.M. Treasury or simply "Treasury").

Their responsibilities related to government as a collectivity comprise a blend of functions in financial management, personnel management and administration. These include: the operation of the system that aggregates departmental expenditure plans; negotiations with departments on proposed increases in spending; preparation of the annual Estimates for tabling in the legislature; negotiating collective agreements; determining terms and conditions of employment; hiring civil servants and supervising the methods of promotion and appointment within the service; establishing the framework for the classification of public servants' positions and the determination of pay scales; formulating government-wide policies on accounting practices, contracting procedures, and other aspects of administration, including, usually, the approval of major contracts and the establishment of public service accommodation policies. In principle, most if not all these responsibilities reside with the central agencies; in practice, some may be delegated to departments subject to monitoring from the centre. How much is delegated, and under what terms, varies from jurisdiction to jurisdiction.

In Ottawa, the Treasury Board Secretariat is largely responsible for the management of the public service as a collectivity. However, its responsibilities were shared with an organization called the Office of the Comptroller General whose mandate at time of writing overlapped that of the Treasury Board Secretariat to some degree (see chapter 7). Certain executive responsibilities in personnel management are shared with the Public Service Commission (a politically independent agency whose main role is to protect the principle of appointment and promotion on merit within the public service). In Ontario, central management responsibilities have, by and large, been assigned to a Management Board Secretariat, which supports a Cabinet committee called Management Board. Management Board works in co-operation with Ontario's Civil Service Commission.

In Britain, responsibilities for the central management of the civil service have been shifting. Before 1968, responsibilities in finance and personnel were shared primarily between the Treasury and the Civil Service Commission (CSC). In 1968, in response to the Fulton Report, an inquiry into government management, a new Civil Service Department (CSD) was created to complement the CSC, with responsibilities for personnel management and, to some degree, for the improvement of efficiency in the civil service. In 1982, however, as noted previously, Prime Minister Thatcher abolished the CSD and subsequently transferred many of its responsibilities to a new agency known as MPO (Management and Personnel Office). A subsequent reorganization linked MPO with the Cabinet Office; in 1986, MPO's responsibilities were realigned between the Treasury and a new Office of the Minister for the Civil Service (OMCS) located in the Cabinet Office. (Responsibility for improving management generally in the civil service, at time of writing, appeared to reside primarily in the Treasury.)

To grasp how the internal machinery of government works, one must understand the network of relationships that prevail between central agencies and departments. It is complicated. In policy development, departments not only must convince their minister what should be done, they must also submit any major policy proposal by Cabinet memorandum, signed by their minister, to Cabinet. Departments must submit their annual expenditure plans to Treasury Board or its equivalent. Major expenditures, even those within the approved budget, must often be resubmitted to Treasury Board or its equivalent for more detailed scrutiny. On the classification of positions, central agency rules must be observed. Appointments to positions may be recommended by the department but, subject to delegation, final decisions on staffing and other important personnel-related issues may rest with central agencies, particularly for the top posts. Thus, size of complement and any significant change in departmental organization must often be centrally approved.

The division of responsibilities for management policies among several central agencies often leads to a difficulty peculiar to the public sector – an inconsistent management context or "accountability framework" for departments. This arises when the philosophy of delegation differs from one central agency to another, resulting in uneven levels of decentralization in different functions. (This is an issue to which we return in chapter 7.) In general, inter-agency collaboration at the centre of government is a continuing problem, and differences of view among central officials on matters of management philosophy are not uncommon.

Departments

Outside the circle of central agencies lies a large cluster of organizations sometimes referred to as operating, or line, departments. These departments perform three types of activity:

(1)   They provide policy advice to the elected Government and develop draft legislation on issues of current public concern (acid rain, foreign imports, economic subsidies, etc.); on relations with other levels of government or other jurisdictions; on the workings of existing programs and policies, and what new policies or programs might usefully be implemented. Departments primarily engaged in work of this type are known colloquially as policy departments.

(2)   They administer legislation and manage "programs". This term is a convenient peg upon which almost any meaning may be (and is) hung. In Canada and the United States, a program is typically a group of activities that involves spending government money. These may range from the financing of the operations of administrative tribunals through the funding of research, regulatory activities, inspection services, incentives, income transfers, or the operation of facilities on behalf of the public such as hospitals, parks, wharves, and so forth. "Program departments" are sometimes distinguished colloquially from "service departments", in that the former undertake activities involving direct assistance to the public, whereas the latter (see below) provide support to other departments.*

(3)   A third category of departments provides services to other government organizations. Departments such as Canada's Public Works or Supply and Services, which provide a centralized service to other departments and agencies, are often alluded to as "common service departments".

Few, if any, departments are exclusively engaged in policy development or program delivery, or indeed in the delivery of common services. When governments were smaller, the distinctions between policy and operational departments were clearer. Today, most have a mix of responsibilities.** The need for management skills is obviously

---

* In the context of the preparation of departments' budgets, the word "program" is sometimes used in a more rigorously defined manner, as described in chapter 9.

** In the late 1970s, 27 Canadian deputy ministers were asked to indicate the orientation of their department — policy or operations. Seven thought of their

greater in departments with a large operational role, which tend to be the program or service departments. These also tend to be the larger departments of government, such as Canada's National Defence with a civilian staff of 33,300, National Revenue (26,900), Employment and Immigration (23,500), or Transport (20,300). However, even departments such as Canada's Department of External Affairs, classically viewed as a "policy department", now has important management tasks to discharge, employing over 4,100 staff in Ottawa and in missions around the world.[10]

Size alone does not determine a department's proximity to the political centre. A department such as Finance in Canada has a small staff relative to other departments (under 900 at time of writing), and few program responsibilities. Nonetheless its involvement in a wide range of important macro-economic, fiscal and monetary policy issues ensures that it commands political attention and ministerial involvement. By contrast, big departments such as Customs and Excise have a much greater range of managerial responsibilities and a lower proportion of policy work. The major decisions on tariffs and trade policy are the result of international negotiations in which officials from departments responsible for macro-economic policy and trade assume the key roles. While Customs and Excise would usually contribute to these discussions, its top officials would be mainly employed in developing systems and procedures to ensure that border posts are properly run and that existing legislation is enforced. With its many staff and border points, Customs has a major managerial job in training and deploying personnel.

Unless there erupts some political crisis over the way a department is administered, ministers collectively take rather less interest in the activities of departments with routine program administration or service responsibilities than they do in ones with a high policy content. (There is, in fact, rather less for ministers to do in departments with large administrative responsibilities, especially when the nature of these responsibilities is prescribed by law. A

---

department as "mostly policy" or "more policy than operations"; eight reported an "even split" between policy and operations; the remaining 12 indicated a preponderance of operational responsibilities. See the Royal Commission on Financial Management and Accountability, *Final Report*, (Ottawa: Supply and Services Canada, March 1979), p. 475.

former deputy minister of Customs and Excise noted that in his department, ministers often wondered what their own role really was.)[11]

Service departments often administer large contracts with the private sector, which may attract political attention from time to time, although not necessarily for the right reasons. Departments concerned with construction and public land must often deal with the problem of pork-barrelling as politicians seek to have contracts placed with party favourites or in their own constituencies. However, since the policy activities of such departments tend to attract little political attention, they can be viewed as somewhat distanced from the political centre.

In summary, departments operate in a tangle of overlapping, indefinite and fluid relationships, overlaid with constitutional conventions and traditions that evolved for political rather than administrative ends. Particularly at the senior levels, a government department is no place for a manager with a low tolerance for ambiguity. Effective top officials must be able to navigate with confidence in this uncertain environment, and to do that, they have to understand the institutional framework — not just its formal dimensions, but, perhaps more important, the many informal networks and ways of doing business that make it possible to function in a big bureaucracy.

The Fringes of Government

Beyond policy and administrative departments, there lies a whole other realm of government: Crown corporations, special advisory institutions set up by governments, companies in which the government owns a partial interest, commissions, regulatory agencies and tribunals, quasi-commercial enterprises, nationalized industries and independent bodies funded by government. It is the existence of these institutions on the fringe of government that makes it so difficult to define the size of government. If an organization is financed entirely by government but established according to the "arm's-length principle" to be independent of political pressure, is it part of government? (British ingenuity has coined the acronym QUANGO — Quasi Autonomous Non-Governmental Organization —

to describe some of these institutions, a phrase that has caught the fancy of Whitehall bureaucrats despite the fact that purists have pointed out that it ought, in fact, to be QUAGO.)* What about government-owned corporations, or corporations where government owns some (but not all) the shares?

Governments establish quangos and Crown corporations in order to constitute an organization which is less directly susceptible to political control and able to operate with greater autonomy. Since such institutions are closer to the private sector model of management, they are less relevant to the subject of this book. However, they present an interesting alternative to the departmental form of organization and are considered in that connection later in this book.

Interdepartmental Committees

> Nothing is ever accomplished by a committee unless it consists of three members, one of whom happens to be sick and the other absent.

> A committee is a cul-de-sac down which ideas are lured, and then quietly strangled.[12]

Part of what contributes to the chameleon nature of departments — now seemingly discrete entities, now part of an amorphous collectivity — is the accepted convention that each department should, to some extent, be responsible for the objectives of

---

* Quasi Autonomous *Governmental* Organization, the point being that these agencies are *not* non-governmental, but part of government (at least in some loose sense). Despite the fallacy of logic in the notion of an organization that is both non-governmental and quasi-autonomous, the fact remains that no one likes the sound of quago, so quango sticks in informal usage in Whitehall. Because quango has a slightly irreverent quality (and perhaps because some central agency officials are made nervous by the prospect of autonomy — or even quasi-autonomy), official Whitehall frowns upon its use. The official and unmemorable designation for these organizations is NDPB: non-departmental public bodies. Canadian government officials, more prosaically, describe these organizations as Crown corporations, an unsatisfactory term since Crown corporation has a specific meaning in law and some of these organizations do not fall within the legal definition.

other departments. A cardinal sin in government is to allow activities to go on in one organization that are inconsistent with (or worse, contrary to) the goals of another. Nothing is likely to infuriate the voter more than to discover that taxes are being used to fund activities of one government organization that are in conflict with those of another.

"Co-ordination" has, therefore, become enshrined as a special virtue in government circles. Governments co-ordinate to a fault, often incurring considerable costs and compounding red tape in the pursuit of doubtful economies. Many central agency officials seem to have a better understanding of cost analysis than they do of management; given a choice between consolidation (to realize economies) and decentralization (to create "divisional integrity" and afford line managers authority to get on with their job), they lean toward consolidation. Consolidation, as Peters and Waterman point out in *In Search of Excellence*, is often a false economy, resulting in complicated organizational structures and convoluted lines of authority.[13] They argue that successful companies display "simple form, lean staff". However, the costs arising from duplication, or lack of co-ordination, are highly visible, whereas the costs arising from organizational convolution and complexity tend to be hidden. So consolidation and co-ordination usually win out.

One of the key vehicles of co-ordination in government is the interdepartmental committee. At interdepartmental meetings, public servants from different departments convene to reconcile differences of view concerning proposals advanced by one of the institutions represented around the table, or to co-ordinate related work in separate departments. Here, bureaucrats hone their skills analyzing every aspect of a proposal. The thrust of the discussion tends to be, not "How can we make this idea work?" but "What's likely to go wrong?"

Take, as a hypothetical example, an international development project of the type alluded to in chapter 1, to provide agricultural assistance to a foreign country. To meet its objective of using development funds as efficiently as possible on behalf of the recipient nation, the Agency originating the project (e.g. Canada's International Development Agency or Britain's Overseas Development Agency) might advocate untied procurement for the project, meaning that procurement would not be "tied" to domestic firms; any country's commercial interests could bid. "Value for money" would be realized through acceptance of the most competitive bid.

If the project involved substantial expenditures, officials from the Department of Finance (or Treasury) might review the proposed financing arrangements to prevent any adverse consequences for balance of payments. Officials from the Department of Agriculture might want to ensure that the project was technically sound and that the development of an indigenous industry abroad would not damage export markets. Officials from other departments would doubtless be interested in helping domestic companies to participate in the project, and might well oppose the Agency's proposal for untied procurement. Public servants from External Affairs (or the Foreign Office) would want to ensure that the project did not jeopardize other relationships with the recipient or surrounding countries, and that project objectives were consistent with the donor's general foreign policy interests.

By the time the interdepartmental consultation was complete, months or even years might have passed. The project's original proponents may have moved on to jobs in other parts of the Agency or in other departments – as, indeed, may its proponents in the recipient country.* The project itself may bear little resemblance to the one originally advanced. With luck it may have emerged as a logical, well-planned initiative that effectively met all the interests of the departments around the table. "Value for money" would be achieved, but it would now represent not simply the greatest "bang for the buck" in development impact. Rather, it would spread the "bang" around so that the investment in the project served the multiple objectives of promoting exports, creating domestic jobs, supporting the donor's foreign policy interests, improving relations with other countries in

---

* Public servants are expected to represent the views of their departments at these meetings. An interesting illustration of the maxim, "where you stand depends on where you sit" is provided by the following anecdote. The head of a government agency in Ottawa wrote a letter to a department complaining of that department's policy toward his agency. While the letter was in transit, its author was appointed deputy minister of the department to which he had written. Upon receiving his letter, he wrote back to the agency taking issue with the letter and restating the arguments in support of the department's original position.

the area, and enhancing domestic expertise in tropical agriculture. All laudable objectives in themselves, but not always comfortable bedfellows in the context of one overseas aid project!

Interdepartmental meetings are the bureaucratic consequence of the doctrine of Cabinet solidarity and are a key aspect of government. Officials invest considerable effort to represent their minister's position accurately and effectively. Ministers count on their officials to protect their interests, a responsibility that, by and large, officials take very seriously.

The objective of the process is to ensure a homogenization of policy before its arrival at the Cabinet table – an appetizing political dish containing a subtle blend of ingredients. However, many public servants believe that what usually emerges from the kitchens of interdepartmental consultation is a sort of overcooked and unpalatable gruel. Possibly when governments were smaller and more collegial, this process worked better than it does now. One former senior official reminisced about how, during the 1940s and early 1950s in the Canadian federal government, interdepartmental meetings were informed by a common concern to identify the collective national interest.

> I recall vividly the first time I was at such a meeting when [a senior official from another department] said, "The position of my department on this issue is so and so." I remember how taken aback I was. I had never heard that phrase before at an interdepartmental meeting. Previously, everyone had tried to find common ground that reconciled the different views; but we were working together. The arrival of that kind of vocabulary, which soon became common, signaled to me an important – and very regrettable – change in officials' conceptions of their role as public servants. It turned the meetings into sessions where departments negotiated with each other and jockeyed for position, rather than trying collectively to solve a problem of government policy.[14]

Today, because the number of actors is so much larger, and also because there is perhaps less consistency of view among top government officials about what constitutes appropriate policy than there was 30 or 40 years ago (and less consistency of interest in society), the process of consultation is often exhausting and frustrating, generating a patchwork of compromises that meets no department's objectives well. One official suggested to me that interdepartmental committees are victims of what he termed the Law of Inverse Synergy: "The whole is less than the sum of its parts."

There is another problem arising from interdepartmental committees, namely, the obscuring of accountability for decision-making and results. A Canadian official has offered this perspective on the practical consequences of the tradition of interdepartmental consultation.

> Since the top of the inter-agency hierarchy is the Prime Minister, and since he is obviously beyond reach as the arbiter of departmental disagreements on powers and processes, the result is perpetual squabbling without an accessible referee. . . . As a veteran of dozens of inter-departmental committee meetings, I can attest to how good ideas can be ground down to pedestrian programs, and to how everyone is given a little piece of the action as a tribute for letting proposals go forward.[15]

This sounds not dissimilar to the British agency head who spoke of how in government departments:

> You spend your life submitting recommendations to [the minister] which are very cautiously received, which are kicked around in an endless process of consultation . . . it goes on and on and on. . . . Consultation is so much a part of the bureaucratic scene, people do feel very genuinely aggrieved when they are not consulted. . . .[16]

The solution to this problem would seem, at first exposure, to be to set up organizations whose mandates are specific, and to try to keep overlap between departments to a minimum. The need for consultation would diminish as a result.

This is what private sector practices would seem to suggest. When businesses think that an organization is getting too large to manage, they try to focus accountability and diminish bureaucracy in several ways. One option is to sell off a portion of the company that fits less well into the plans of the firm. Another is to establish a subsidiary. Yet another is to establish an organizational configuration sometimes called a divisional structure, where separate divisions develop and sell products or services of a similar character.[17]

A fourth, not dissimilar option is to set up "strategic business units" – creating a focus within the firm for the achievement of strategic objectives. Within the SBU, the company places enough authority and resources to allow the manager to get on with the job, without being unnecessarily hampered by head office procedures or policies. An SBU is thus more or less self-contained, able within broad parameters to develop and prosecute its own strategy, with bottom-line accountability for performance. Both the divisional concept and the SBU are vehicles for focussing accountability, and they involve not greater control but greater delegation of authority within a framework where the overall results expected are clearly understood.[18]

Efforts to focus accountability in government through clearer delegation of authority and a more "bottom line" approach to management in lieu of detailed controls would certainly be helpful, but they will not resolve the problem. The issues confronting government change from month to month, and departments set up to deal with one limited set of issues would in the nature of things soon find themselves involved in other questions that affected the mandates of other departments. The fundamental problem is the complexity of modern society, not the structure of departments. Education affects employment, employment affects industry, industry affects health, health affects employment, foreign affairs affects defence, taxes affect almost everything, almost everything affects women, and so it goes.

Concerning the problem of overlapping mandates among government agencies, it must be recalled that to some degree, government is designed to be inefficient on purpose. Irving Shapiro, the former head of Dupont, has commented on the reasons why government functions as it does.

> Whether government even ought to look for optimal solutions in a technical sense is moot. It is not going to happen. Efficiency, as the private sector uses the word, ranks too low in the government's priorities. There is a sensible reason for this, going back to the fundamental risks associated with unchecked power. . . . In democracies,

one might say, it is necessary to trade away some efficiency for security....

On the question of the division of powers among agencies, he observed:

> [S]uch a structure can be expensive, inconsistent, and maddeningly bureaucratic.... It is wrong, though, to take any of this as justification for reforms that would press government operations into the mold of a private corporation. The difference in accountability has not yet been factored in.... Thus we lean over backwards in government, applying checks and balances and dividing authority in ways that would never make sense for the private sector.[19]

Diffusion of executive power and participative decision-making may be political necessities. However, they have serious administrative consequences. What they create is a swamp-like environment where to take even one step toward policy development or program implementation, a department must carefully plant its foot to ensure that the ground of interdepartmental support is firm. To lift a foot for the next step, the department must pull free of the clinging ooze of overlapping mandates and competing interests of other departments and agencies, each of which is vigorously pressing the real or supposed interests of its minister(s). Those who assume, as the media often do, that civil servants are inefficient managers might be surprised at how effective they sometimes are at moving a proposal forward and achieving results in the quagmire of interdepartmental restraints.

Not only is participative decision-making as practised interdepartmentally time-consuming and inconvenient, but, worse, there is evidence to suggest that it is damaging to program performance. It may even cause needed initiatives to collapse entirely. A study of the reasons why programs fail in the United States concluded that one of the major causes of failure was the complexity of government and the problem of too many cooks in the kitchen. "[A]s a rule of thumb, the greater the number of actors and agencies involved in a program, the less likely it is to succeed...."[20]

The larger the government, the more time-consuming and frustrating is the process of consultation, the longer it takes to reach decisions, and the more susceptible the government is to accusations of unresponsiveness. However, as indicated above, interdepartmental consultation is tied to the tradition of Cabinet solidarity. It is difficult to see how the interdepartmental committee can be dispensed with as long as the concept of a collectivity exists; but it must be recognized that the need for such consultations dampens the zeal of many public servants and drags out the process of implementation. In addition, as discussed in the next chapter, it can stifle innovation and imagination.

Summary

With Cabinet at the centre, "line" departments carrying out the main tasks and "staff" central agencies co-ordinating functions such as personnel and finance, government may look a lot like a big private company. However, there are so many differences, so many inaccuracies in this analogy that it probably obscures and confuses more than it clarifies. Conventions unique to the public sector, such as ministerial responsibility, Cabinet solidarity and public service neutrality, colour everything that happens. Departments, ministers, the prime minister and central agencies function in a maze of complex, shifting relationships quite unlike the relationships at the top of most business corporations, which are by comparison far less complicated. The interdepartmental community is a forest in which officials must learn to play the games of inter-agency politics while moving forward those proposals they believe to be in the public interest.

In short, the institutional framework of government is that of . . . government. It is not an adaptation of a business model, nor is it some sort of ill-designed copy. Where business seeks to focus power and accountability, government may, for legitimate and important reasons, seek to diffuse them. This creates not only a unique institutional environment, but also a rather different organizational culture, which is the subject of the following chapter.

Footnotes:

1. Author's interview with a deputy minister, Canadian government, July 1985.

2. Federal statistics from Public Service Commission *Annual Report*, (Ottawa: Supply and Services Canada, 1986), tables 1 and 2, pp. 68-69.

3. Ontario statistics from Price Waterhouse Associates/The Canada Consulting Group, "A Study of Management and Accountability in the Government of Ontario," (Toronto: January 1985), p. 95.

4. According to an interview with a senior British civil servant, an attitude survey of prison staff in the U.K. — employees where one might anticipate a high degree of identification with the immediate employer — revealed that some 70 per cent of the staff viewed themselves in the first instance as public servants of the Crown.

5. Robert MacGregor Dawson, *The Government of Canada*, 3rd ed., (Toronto: University of Toronto Press, 1957).

6. Thomas D'Aquino, "The Prime Minister's Office: Catalyst or Cabal? Aspects of the development of the Office in Canada and some thoughts about its future," *Canadian Public Administration*, vol. 17 no. 1, (Spring 1974), pp. 55-79. See also Denis Smith's "Comments," pp. 80-84.

7. *Estimates, 1970-1971*, pp. 18-6; Privy Council Office, *Estimates, 1986-1987, Part III, Expenditure Plan*, p. 17.

8. See, for example, Donald Johnston, "The Trouble with Trudeau," *Saturday Night*, (April 1986), pp. 17ff.

9. The British Cabinet Office maintains what has become known as the list of "The Great and the Good" to assist with many prime ministerial appointments.

10. Figures from Public Service Commission as of September 1987.

11. Author's interview, February 1987.

12. Quotations attributed respectively to Hendrick van Loon and to Sir Bernard Cocks in Michael Jackman, ed., *The Macmillan*

Book of Business and Economic Quotations, (New York: Macmillan Publishing Company, 1984), p. 47.

13. Thomas J. Peters and Robert H. Waterman Jr., *In Search of Excellence*, (New York: Harper and Row, 1982), pp. 310-311.

14. Recollection of a discussion with A.F.W. Plumptre, former Assistant Deputy Minister of Finance, about 1975.

15. H.L. Laframboise, "The future of public administration in Canada," *Canadian Public Administration*, vol. 25 no. 4, (Winter 1982), p. 519.

16. Author's interview, May 1985.

17. For a classic description of the establishment of a divisional structure, see Alfred P. Sloan, *My Years With General Motors*, (New York: Doubleday and Company, 1972), especially ch. 3, "Concept of the Organization."

18. A subsidiary is not necessarily an SBU, as the reasons for creating a subsidiary are not always the same as those for establishing an SBU. A subsidiary may be established simply for legal reasons, to set up a separate corporate entity in a particular jurisdiction. The subsidiary may or may not be allocated the authority and resources that would permit it to function as an SBU within the parent corporation.

19. Irving S. Shapiro, *America's Third Revolution: Public Interest and the Private Role*, (New York: Harper & Row, 1984), pp. 84-86.

20. James Larson, *Why Government Programs Fail: Improving Policy Implementation*, (New York: Praeger, 1980). See especially pp. 1-16 and pp. 108-120.

Chapter Three:
The Environment and Culture
of Government

Organizational culture consists of beliefs, values and norms that influence the way people behave. As part of the collectivity of government, departments are influenced by a number of such beliefs and values which, in large measure, define what it means to be a public servant. Many of these are based upon traditions and conventions that are part of the fabric of parliamentary government. In the world of business, organizational culture may derive in part from the values of some key figure in corporate history, such as the founder of a company, who has sought to institutionalize certain values or patterns of behaviour. In government, individuals who have played a major role in the evolution of the public service may have made a contribution to organizational culture but, on the whole, individual contributions tend to be much less important than history, constitutional convention and, to some extent, legislation which places the force of law behind certain values.

Consultation, Risk-taking and Innovation

A key value in the public service is that of coordination among departments, a value reflecting the collective character of government described in the previous chapter. However, it can also have a significant detrimental impact on government's ability to act and to innovate. A commission reviewing productivity in the Ontario government in 1973 found, "A major complaint of managers was that implementation of decisions was often delayed or decisions were altered by other departments."[1]

The habit of consultation can become so engrained that some public servants lose sight of how it drags out the process of implementing policy or responding to concerns voiced by members of the public. Some people who have spent their life in government seem to be so inured to the public service environment that they take it for granted that work should always proceed in a measured, careful way and that no action should be taken until all viewpoints have been considered. This method of working becomes a norm; any other method of proceeding would be considered irresponsible.

Business tends to be more aware of the costs and delays involved in such consultations, and more sensitive to the need to move promptly in response to a specific client request rather than worrying about its implications for other clients. Businesses are under no obligation to treat all their clients equally, nor are they bound, as government tends to be, by precedent. This allows them to adopt a single-mindedness which government organizations, especially those in the interdepartmental community, cannot afford.

Peter Drucker has stressed the importance of maintaining an entrepreneurial flavour in business, and subsequent authors have written about the importance of preserving drive and focus in increasingly complex commercial organizations. Drucker suggests that the role of business is to "make the future happen" through the power of an idea: not a balanced reconciliation of multiple ideas or interests, but a single, dynamic, focused idea of commercial potential.

> It need not be a big idea; but it must be one that differs from the norm of today. The idea has to be an entrepreneurial one—an idea of wealth-producing potential and capacity, expressed in a going, working, producing business.... It does not emerge from the question, "What should future society look like?"—the question of the social reformer, revolutionary or philosopher....

The very fact that an entrepreneurial idea does not encompass all of society or all of knowledge but just one narrow area makes it more viable. The people who have this idea may be wrong about everything else in the future economy or society. But that does not matter as long as they are approximately right in respect of their own business focus.[2]

Ideas in business are ultimately tested in the marketplace. Successful businesses tend to be those which create an internal environment where creativity can flourish and new ideas can make their way on to the street to be assessed by the consumer rather than becoming entrapped in an endless round of internal meetings. Some failures may occur as these ideas are brought to the marketplace; but progressive companies are prepared to cope with a reasonable proportion of failures. They recognize that an internal review process designed to extract all possible failures before market testing will probably root out many innovative, potentially profitable inspirations at the same time.[3]

Ideas in government are tested in interdepartmental committees. Failure, which might embarrass ministers, must be avoided. The situation in the United States has been described as follows:

In the private sector . . . taking chances is part of the game. It is hardly a feather in an executive's hat to be the patron of a corporate flop, but neither is it invariably fatal. In the public sector, though, errors [of modest proportions] . . . can lead to exposes, Congressional investigations, and ruined careers. Open admission of error is thus to be avoided at all costs. . . .[4]

In parliamentary democracies, public servants have, by and large, been spared the pain of the public exposure and embarrassment that can accompany a Congressional investigation in the U.S. Nonetheless, it is generally recognized that public service environments are inimical to innovative, risk-taking behaviour. This is not just a matter of some managers' personal style. It is engrained in the system, deriving from the conventions of ministerial responsibility and Cabinet solidarity. Because ministers are expected to assume collective responsibility for the policies of the Cabinet, it is considered important that all policies should be reviewed at the official level through interdepartmental consultation to ensure that each minister's interests are taken into account. An observer of the British scene has noted:

> [Work in the civil service] is, supremely, the kind of work that stresses the need to avoid mistakes, rather than the impulse to suggest bold new initiatives. . . . [A] minister's signature over an Assistant Secretary's error can cause acute embarrassment. So ministers rely on Assistant Secretaries to check the information — and to get it right.[5]

Mistakes are to be avoided wherever possible because the principle of ministerial responsibility tends to lay the responsibility for mistakes at the minister's feet; hence risk-taking and dramatic innovation are implicitly discouraged.

The Primacy of Policy

Another traditional feature of the civil service environment has been the belief that policy is what matters, and that policy is something different from administration or management. Until the period of management change, which in Ottawa began in the early 1960s and in Whitehall somewhat later, it was more or less an article of faith in the public service that an individual expecting to advance had to be skilled in policy development, and that competence in any other area was secondary.

The argument in favour of policy priority ran — and to some extent, still runs — like this. The essence of the role of the senior public servant is to advise the minister on policy. The public servant must assist the minister by becoming cognizant of the many different interests which may bear on a policy issue, must avoid becoming the captive of any particular interest group, and must try to balance competing concerns. The job of the top public servant is to serve the minister by identifying issues that require attention or by developing and testing ideas about policy advanced by the minister, while keeping him or her out of political difficulties that could arise from a failure to anticipate adequately the implications of a proposed initiative. A corollary often associated with this belief is the view that administration – the implementation of policy – is both less difficult and less demanding than policy, and that it can be safely delegated to subordinates.

The person good at policy tended to have strong conceptual skills and was reflective and thoughtful in temperament. The truly effective public servant would be a "generalist", someone uncommitted to any partisan viewpoint, with a sound understanding of the conventions of public administration and a broad grasp of issues. These ideas had important implications for recruitment and advancement. For new recruits with potential for the top jobs, the "classic" (pre-1960s) public service looked for articulate, broad-thinking, literate young people who could see more than one point of view on any given issue. This orientation led fairly directly to individuals with university degrees in the liberal arts, rather than professional or technical specializations. The successful candidate had to have poise, an ability to debate effectively and write convincingly; administrative competence was low on the list of requirements.

Advancement was usually facilitated by an individual's experience in one of the central agencies, where a deft hand at drafting policy was especially important, and where younger public servants could be exposed to the breadth of public service activity and the collective interests of the government. Experience in the office of a deputy minister, or possibly a minister, was also considered to be an asset, as this too provided a better appreciation of the interests of the collectivity. Policy-intensive departments often acted as a kind of spawning ground for candidates for the senior posts in the rest of the public service, providing officials with the exposure and contacts required for a successful career.

These traditions surrounding the recruitment and training of policy officials helped to establish the good reputations enjoyed by both British and Canadian civil service organizations during the first half of the 20th century. However, as the range of public service responsibilities grew and the resources under government administration expanded, the shortcomings of the generalist tradition began to become apparent. Government was, increasingly, in the business of running things. Departments were bigger; programs were larger; government involvement in the affairs of the country was more pervasive; and government activities were growing more complex and technical in nature.

The idea of the public servant as generalist was founded on the assumption that a policy generalist, unimpressed by dogma and able to examine each new proposal on its merits, could function equally well as a general manager, able to direct any function: in other words, a good general education which taught someone how to think clearly, was thought to equip a civil servant for almost *any* kind of senior responsibility – designing or supervising major programs, directing financial administration, administering regulations, personnel management or public relations.

This exaggerated notion of generalist abilities was dealt a resounding blow in Britain with the publication of the Fulton Report in 1968, which suggested that the civil service was making a virtue out of its weaknesses, that the generalist tradition had turned into a sort of cult of amateurism, and that professional or other specialist training might actually be a disadvantage to officials hoping to advance in the British civil service.[6] Not surprisingly, the Fulton Report was afforded a very chilly reception in Whitehall. Civil servants took exception to being called amateurs, and many apparently shared the view of the senior official who claimed that the chapter in the Report dealing with generalists was "piffle".[7] (See appendix 2.)

Loyalty to "The Public Interest"

Closely allied to the belief in the priority of policy is another feature of the public service, namely, a loyalty to something elusive known as "the public interest". The public interest is usually thought to represent some kind of amalgam of partisan interests, a whole which transcends its parts. Many more senior public servants feel (although they would be unlikely to admit it publicly) that their education, training and exposure to a wide range of policy fields in the course of a career in government have given them special skills and aptitudes to ascertain where the public interest lies. It is a little like belonging to a special club: years of experience in the traditions and patterns of thinking of the public service provide the member with the confidence to walk with greater assurance through the fields of public policy.

Even for the most self-confident public servant, discerning where the public interest lies on any particular issue can be a problematic exercise. Public servants naturally bring their own values to their job, which may or may not be representative of the values of the voting public. They tend to develop a vested interest in the status quo and in existing institutional structures, even though they may not believe this to be true. Determining what is the "right" point of view on a policy matter raises a lot of questions: is "right" to be decided on ethical grounds; if so, whose view of ethics should prevail? Is the policy which is "in the public interest" a sort of homogenization of all the competing viewpoints on the issue: a course of action that satisfies no one, but offends the fewest number of parties? Or is the public interest represented by the view of the majority (however defined) which may override and even offend the interests of minority groups? Another consideration is the time consequences of the policy: is the public interest best served by the policy that caters to the short term or to the long term? There are no easy answers to such questions; but wrestling with them is what makes some civil servants believe that their jobs are more interesting and challenging than those of many managers in business.

Paradoxically, loyalty to this ill-defined public interest is often a source of tension between public servants and ministers. Ministers, duly elected by the public, understandably feel that they know where the public interest lies, and that they are best qualified to assess the claims of competing interests and to make the trade-offs required between short- and longer-term considerations. While recognizing the special insights and experience which a minister brings to decision-making, public servants worry that ministers (particularly those who are new to government) may lack exposure to the interplay of interests in government. Ministers may know their own constituency, but are they sufficiently informed about others? Are they used to thinking through the consequences of policy proposals before acting? Since their term in office is only four or five years, will they give sufficient priority to the longer-term? Although some ministers (particularly those in newly elected Governments) feel that public servants can—and should—contribute little or nothing to identifying where the public interest lies on matters of policy, many experienced ministers appear to respect the special perspective which the public servant contributes to policy formulation, and they seem to believe that successful policy emerges from a blending of the experience of politicians and public servants.

Equity and Consistency

Another feature of the government is the strong value attached to a second ill-defined concept, that of fairness or equity. Politicians have found that political longevity is enhanced if the public believes people are being treated evenhandedly. Constituents are angered if they feel that some interest group is receiving more than its due, or if they perceive that some region comparable to theirs is getting a bigger slice of the pie.

As a result, there is considerable stress in government upon managing both administrative activity and public perceptions to ensure that justice is both done and seen to be done. Government strives to ensure that people in different parts of the country are, as far as possible, treated the same. Business does not bear this responsibility unless it chooses to. The administrative consequence of this policy is to increase substantially the burden of bureaucracy in government, because achieving consistency of administrative behaviour requires regulations and procedures. To ensure that services in one part of the country are delivered in the same way as in another, administrative manuals are needed. (Sometimes, this search for consistency can lead to extremes—for instance, the personnel policy manuals of the Canadian government, at time of writing, fill more than 30 volumes, a vast body of material with which no single official could be expected to be familiar.) The "bureaucracy" of which government is so often accused is in many instances a direct consequence of the political priority attached to equity and fair play.[8]

The Public Servant as Custodian

Up to the 1960s, and to some extent beyond, the prevailing view both in the U.K. and in Canada seems to have been that, since policy was much more difficult and demanding than management, presumably anyone who could handle policy could handle management. The task of management could in any event be delegated to some other official with an administrative bent. This belief reflected another pre-1960s concept, that of the public servant as custodian, and the allied notion that "administration" in this custodial sense was the same as management. Custodians are trustees: they do not take initiatives. They do what they are told; they follow the rules and expect to be provided with procedures.

This custodial view of the public servant's role was reinforced by the detailed regulations and procedures which for years characterized many of the laws passed by Parliament. Through such legislation, Parliament instructed public servants not only upon goals to be achieved but also upon how work was to be done. Little discretion was permitted to deal with special cases or circumstances, little room for managerial judgement. Often such legislation was drafted by lawyers who, while well versed in the law, probably did not understand the managerial consequences of such detailed legislation. Seeking to ensure consistency and fairness in the application of laws, members of Parliament often created legislation that was ponderous, complicated and difficult to administer and took an army of clerks, armed with volumes of procedures to execute; it did not require people with flair or imagination. This approach to legislation perpetrated the distinction between policy (where the interesting action was), and administration (where the drones worked).

Since the 1960s, much has changed in both the Canadian and the British civil services. The view that policy is the essence of the public servant's job appears to be gradually giving way to a different view which allows more room for management. Nonetheless, traditions die hard, and misconceptions of management are, in my experience, still widespread. Furthermore, the culture of the civil service remains strongly oriented toward policy. Because ministers are, in general, uninterested in management issues, and because the direction of any major or politically sensitive government program inevitably raises policy questions (which are often intrinsically more important than questions of departmental administration), the need for senior officials skilled in policy development will remain a permanent feature of the public service environment.

For example, few deputy ministers, given the choice between trying to determine on the one hand how to create the right national regime for the promotion of oil exploration or, on the other, how to manage the finances of a department, would choose to spend their time on the latter. Energy policy is clearly more important, and to most people, more interesting. Moreover, the boss (in this case, the minister) will typically have a very keen interest in oil exploration and little interest in financial administration. Given the same option, the informed business executive would make the same choice. In business, it is a good idea to pattern your priorities on those of the boss, and government in this respect is no different.

Clearly, policy work is not going to disappear, nor should it. Any attempts to improve management in the public service must take account of the legitimacy and importance of the policy function in government; otherwise, such attempts will fail.

Anonymity, Neutrality and the Merit Principle

A basic feature of the culture of the public service in parliamentary democracies, and one that many business executives must find hard to understand (especially in an era when chief executives from the private sector are taking to advertising their own products on television) is the belief that public servants must adopt a low public profile. It is recognized that they must advise ministers; but in doing so they must not be publicly associated with a particular policy stance. Perhaps even more important, they must not steal the ministers' thunder by pre-empting opportunities for ministers to make a public impact.

Anonymity and the concept of a neutral, apolitical public service are still powerful traditions in Ottawa and London although at time of writing, concerns about "politicization" of the public service are being expressed in both cities.* Most government officials have been trained to understand that these traditions define what it means to be a public servant in a parliamentary democracy.

---

* Other Western democracies, such as France and Germany, do not share this tradition, and in fact, seats in the legislature may be (and are) held by civil servants.

In some jurisdictions (not Britain), the concept of an independent professional civil service is enshrined in legislation which is supposed to place the power of appointment outside the direct reach of ministers. In Canada there exist two acts, the Public Service Employment Act (PSEA) and the Public Service Staff Relations Act (PSSRA), which define a community known as the "public service of Canada" and which set forth the legislative protections for public servants.[9] This community comprises, basically, all departments and agencies lying between the political institutions of government (Parliament, Cabinet) and the outer circle of Crown corporations. The PSEA also confers on the Public Service Commission the exclusive right to make appointments to positions within that community.

Originally, the merit principle was thought to be a rampart against politicians who ignored the concept of a neutral public service by trying to place their own favourites in key positions, or trying to dismiss public servants because of suspected partisan sympathies (or sometimes for lack of same!). The principle was protected by a variety of procedures designed to ensure selection in accordance with objective criteria, and a fair and open process of competition for vacant posts. (More recently, in Canada, efforts have been made to broaden the concept of the merit principle to ensure that the selection of the best-qualified person for a position is based not only upon professional qualifications, but also upon the personal attributes of candidates taking account of both the organizational unit in which the position to be staffed is situated and the clientele served by that unit.)[10] Although the civil service in the United Kingdom is not defined in a statute comparable to the PSEA, the merit principle is vigorously defended in Whitehall as an integral part of British constitutional tradition, and the British Civil Service Commission plays a role somewhat analogous to Canada's PSC in ensuring that candidates for entry to the civil service are appointed on merit.

The argument in favour of a neutral public service has been well stated by Mitchell Sharp who, as a former deputy minister and later a minister in the Canadian government, brings a special perspective to bear on this issue. Sharp points out that while ministers may be professionals in the field of politics, they are mostly amateurs when it comes to governing. They need people more experienced in government to implement their ideas, not a lot of equally inexperienced advisors who might be long on ideas but short on the ability to translate those ideas into action in a large, complex bureaucracy. Furthermore, Sharp asserts that competent people will see little attraction in entering the public service if they know that the top jobs are being held for political appointees. He also suggests that if ministers spent less time in Cabinet and in committees of Cabinet reading and discussing each other's proposals, and if they delegated more to the public service, they would have a "better perspective on events and more time for politics. . . . [A] first class non-partisan public service . . . is one of the bulwarks of parliamentary government."[11]

The argument in favour of a non-partisan, anonymous public service has been further bolstered by a former Canadian secretary to the Cabinet, Gordon Robertson. Robertson warns against a tendency to see anonymity as "simply another fringe benefit: irresponsibility and un-accountability in disguise". Often it is perceived by the media as "secrecy". Public servants have to accept the implications of anonymity:

> [I]t involves a substantial act of self-denial. It means an unwillingness to hint at influential associations with policies or decisions; refusal to give the private briefing of a journalist that can lead to a benevolent or admiring story; avoidance of photographs with the great; and, within reasonable limits, eschewing the physical trappings of status that are demonstrations . . . of power and importance.[12]

The concept of neutrality is subtle. It does not mean that the public servant is devoid of ideas or input on matters of policy. As noted earlier, participation in policy is viewed as a key part of many senior officials' jobs. Neutrality envisages active involvement in policy (to the degree desired and welcomed by ministers), but strictly within the anonymous privacy of the public service. Officials must not engage in the promotion or defence of policy publicly. And, within the public service, they must be prepared to carry out the minister's wishes once a decision has been made, whether or not that decision is in accord with the advice proffered by officials. They must also be able to contend with the changes in policy that may accompany a change of elected Government.

Coping with Changes of Government

The concept of a neutral public service often bothers newly elected politicians (and their staff advisors). How, they ask, can one reasonably expect officials who have been assiduously serving a previous administration to be able to change gears intellectually, to develop policies for a new administration with a different direction and perhaps different ideologies? Politicians used to committing themselves publicly to an election platform and to making partisan attacks on the previous Government may have trouble understanding a bureaucracy where officials shift from one policy thrust to another. Such behaviour must seem bizarre and perhaps faintly unprincipled. Not uncommonly, a new Government will come to office deeply suspicious of the public service, an attitude that leads to a desire to draw all decision-making up to the political level. In addition, public servants are sometimes treated with a thinly disguised mixture of hostility and distaste, as if they were leftovers from the previous administration (as occurred, for example, in 1957 when the new Conservative Government of John Diefenbaker took over in Ottawa after 22 years of Liberal rule, and similarly when Prime Minister Brian Mulroney assumed power in 1984).

Such developments can gradually poison relationships between the new Government and the public service. The resulting resentment within the service can lead to reduction of performance which, in turn, confirms the suspicions of the new Government. As the climate of suspicion deepens, more authority is centralized at the political level. It then becomes evident that this is not a workable formula — the responsibilities of government are too great, and the public service too large in most modern provincial or national governments for massive centralization of decision-making at the political level. The decision-making process clogs up; public criticism rises; and the Government is faced with the unpleasant choice of having to delegate more to the public service or having to replace senior officials with new appointees with whom they feel more comfortable — a course of action that may lead to charges of patronage and of tampering with the tradition of public service impartiality.

The handling of relations between the political and administrative levels is a critical challenge for a new Government. Unfortunately, such Governments are generally unskilled at the job (especially if they have been out of power for some time), and as a result relations go from bad to worse. In the longer term, relations may improve as confidence grows on both sides, but for the first year or two the new Government often needlessly loses momentum. This occurs because new ministers and their advisors do not understand the basic concept of public service neutrality, and they find it difficult to accept that public servants might be ready and willing to provide effective support to an elected Government with a different platform from the previous one.

An argument sometimes advanced against the concept of non-partisan public service is that such a tradition would crumble in the event of the election of a party with a fundamentally different political philosophy from previous Governments. The concept was severely tested in the Province of Quebec with the election in 1976 of the Parti Québécois, dedicated to the separation of the province from Canada. The experience has been described by a Deputy Minister of Finance from Quebec who served through the years in question:

> The accession to power of [Premier René] Lévésque created a...delicate problem in 1976. Here was a government sustained by a political party with strong ideological tenets and which was assuming power not only to assure the betterment of the population following the maxims of good administration but also to realize a political option which was clearly set apart from that of the traditional parties.... Yet even in that case, the principle of the permanent public service prevailed. It must be said...that the officials adequately backed the government, in recognition of its legitimacy and of the choice that the population had made, whatever their personal sentiments on the question [of sovereignty] may have been.[13]

While the Quebec experience does not establish that every public service could accommodate itself to a Government of every hue, it does provide evidence of the resiliency of the concept of a non-partisan service. It also emphasizes that, although there is no guarantee of unanimity of view on any policy issue within a public service, this does not prevent it from executing a clearly defined policy articulated by ministers who know what they want.

THE ENVIRONMENT AND CULTURE OF GOVERNMENT

Ministers seem to have trouble understanding that not only is the public service itself not a homogenous entity, but it actively works at not becoming too committed to any particular policy. The culture of the public service promotes a certain detachment. Edward Bridges, former head of the Treasury in the U.K., has written of how a civil servant has to be able to adopt "a somewhat coldly judicial attitude" in his work. "Detached, at times almost aloof, he must be if he is to maintain a proper impartiality between the many claims and interests that will be urged upon him."14 A former Canadian deputy minister has stated,

> [T]he department head must try to develop a feeling of participation in policy formulation, without invoking a sense of paternity for ideas. After all he is seeking to develop a range of possibilities for his minister to consider.... The deputy minister finds himself in the curious position of being exposed to the political process, without... being a part of it. He must not permit himself the luxury of becoming too attached to ideas or positions. Somehow he must find a way of maintaining a cordial relationship with those who assist and advise him without ever losing sight of the fact that his first loyalty is to his minister.15

Writing of the British scene, journalist Peter Kellner tells the story of how a top official once commented on a member of his staff, saying, "He gets emotionally involved." This was not a compliment, as it might have been in industry, but a criticism. One of the great motivational difficulties in the public service is to determine how to foster commitment and detachment simultaneously.16

In Canada, a rather subtle process of adjustment at the top levels of the bureaucracy often begins soon after a new Government has been elected. Wholesale resignations and replacements of the type practised in Washington (where the top civil servants are politically appointed) are not acceptable. However, if the new Government brings with it a policy orientation in certain areas that is radically different from that of the previous administration, and if (as is usually the case) the public service was actively involved in developing the prevailing policy in concert with the previous Government, there will be some discomfort on both sides. Usually within a few months of taking over, the new prime minister will move some deputy ministers, perhaps retiring some, perhaps bringing in some new blood from the private sector or other levels of government.

Some months later, a few other adjustments may occur. At the same time, quietly, some people at the assistant deputy minister, or deputy secretary, level, and perhaps some officials one level below that, will also be shifted. A limited reordering of people and positions allows those officials with whom the new administration is more comfortable to move gradually into certain positions of influence. (A much less salutary practice is the periodic general shuffling of deputy ministers every year or so – see chapter 5.)

All this happens rather quietly and diplomatically, making it difficult to assess how widespread the practice is. It appears to be more common at the federal level in Canada than in Britain where changes of Government are not usually accompanied by changes of permanent heads. This situation has led recently to a call for a more realistic policy by the head of the Royal Institute of Public Administration. In a lecture to the Royal Society of Arts in 1985, William Plowden predicted a long-term trend toward a loose form of increased political control of the civil service – a trend he described as both "necessary and desirable" (and which would appear to be more in line with Canadian practice):

> ...I do not believe that thoughtful individuals...
> can...support with equal enthusiasm governments with
> totally dissimilar ideologies; or that they can prevent the
> relative intensity of their enthusiasms from influencing
> their behaviour. Alternatively, an intolerable strain can be
> placed on conscientious officials compelled to implement
> policies with which they personally disagree.... The rela-
> tionship between politicians and bureaucrats...in
> Whitehall...has for long been unsatisfactory, and...is
> deteriorating. I suspect that some Ministers' aggressive
> attitude towards officials derives from their feeling of
> insecurity when faced with these serried ranks who may
> not be on their side. They believe that only the brutal
> approach will carry them through; or more moderately, that
> it is prudent not to consult the mandarins for fear of
> becoming engulfed in a treacly consensus.

Plowden continues,

> Politicians in power should be able to carry out the policies to which they are pledged, and then judged by their electorate . . . . They should not be obstructed by unaccountable permanent officials guided by some inexplicit private conception of the national interest.
>
> I suggest that we should now reject, reluctantly maybe, the myth of the wholly dispassionate, totally effective administrator . . . . Instead of instinctively resisting any increase in political control of the civil service, we ought now to start thinking about how to bring this about in a controlled and constructive way.17

Plowden's proposals may help to facilitate the tasks of both ministers and officials in certain instances, but, as he points out himself, he proposes no wholesale attack on the basic principle of a neutral civil service.

Frugality

Although the public and the media may have trouble believing it, because of widely publicized instances of government over-spending or political boondoggles, another value to which public servants are – at least were – expected to subscribe is that of frugality. There is some evidence that this value is waning; however, certainly frugality was classically considered a standard of conduct in many civil services. The taxpayer's money had to be spent with constant regard for economy. Frugality was reflected in policies related to matters such as salaries, (which were kept below comparable jobs in business), travel (use cheaper modes of transport, stay at less expensive hotels) and accommodation (building and furnishings were generally functional, not luxurious). Departments provided – and in many cases, continue to provide – no budget for hospitality or entertainment for staff; senior officials who wished to reward their colleagues for good work by taking them to dinner or hosting a reception may find it necessary to pay the costs out of their personal income.

More recently, affluence is increasing in public services, and standards in relation to such areas as travel and accommodation are less rigidly utilitarian than they used to be. Some old hands of the Ottawa civil service feel that the virtues of frugality are being forgotten, and that an important government ethic is being abandoned. While frugality may be less prevalent than it used to be, public servants are still typically subject to numerous restrictions designed to prevent profligacy. They have little or no flexibility to extend small generosities to their staff unless they finance them personally, and they are constantly reminded by central agencies of the need to observe efficiency, economy and value for money in their day-to-day work.[18]

Two-Ended Program Delivery

A basic difference between public-sector and private-sector organizations relates to where and how services are delivered. In business, the delivery of services or products is the clear responsibility of the lower levels of the organization. In government, it is not. Because of ministerial responsibility, and ministerial inexperience in management, many ministers wish to be kept informed of quite detailed matters of administration. Moreover, ministers find it politically advantageous to be seen to be personally associated with individual cases. As a result, it is an accepted feature of the public service environment that many government programs are delivered on a "two-ended" basis. A good deal of the work of program administration goes on directly between lower level officials and the public. At the same time, a significant proportion of the corres- pondence and communication associated with the delivery of programs may have to flow up through the bureaucracy to the minister's office.

When a request for information or financial assistance, or a complaint reaches a minister, the minister or his or her office has to decide who should respond. In many cases, it will be determined that the minister, or personal staff member from the office, should reply directly. Constituents like to get letters on impressive ministerial letterhead. Ministers like to be seen to be in touch with the public. As a result, the correspondence is routed into the department so that a reply may be prepared, and then sent back up to the minister's office for approval and signature. Large quantities of paper are constantly flowing down into the organization and back up again, with considerable time of quite senior officials taken to review such correspondence. In some departments, a sort of parallel organization of executive assistants and staff units develops alongside the main line of command, the principal purpose of which is to remove the less critical paper from the desks of top officials and to keep the flow of letters and related documents (e.g., replies to questions in the House of Commons) moving alongside the more important material.

The minister's desire to be visibly involved applies not only to correspondence but to events such as the opening of a new regional office or the inauguration of a new service. In business, most senior managers would appreciate the importance of helping subordinates get on with the job. Delays involve costs and foregone income. Therefore, if they wish to be involved in such an event for ceremonial reasons, there is some incentive to make the arrangements expeditiously and to accommodate the priorities of the people on the spot. However, the situation in government is different. Ministers have many other priorities. Often officials have to arrange administrative events to suit the minister's calendar, holding up needed decisions until the minister is available, and holding press conferences or other events in locations or at times that are politically attractive, perhaps providing a good "photo opportunity", but administratively inconvenient.

Ministers' reasons for wishing to be associated with the delivery of programs and services are entirely understandable. However, what makes good political sense may make less sense from the viewpoint of efficient management. Nonetheless, two-ended program delivery is an established feature of the public service.

Summary

This chapter has considered some of the established traditions of the public service. The concept of a professional public service, free from patronage, has long been considered one of the cornerstones of parliamentary democracy. This concept rests on the traditions of anonymity, impartiality and neutrality which are accompanied by other key features of responsible government such as the concept of ministerial responsibility, discussed in more detail in chapter 4.

The traditions of Cabinet solidarity and the public accountability of the public service — "managing in a fishbowl", — creates a special need for consultation which complicates the formulation of policy and slows its implementation. In addition, they create a bias against risk-taking and innovation, lest a minister be inadvertently embarrassed. Another reality with which public servants must cope is two-ended program delivery. All this occurs in an environment where civil servants have to cope with many regulations designed to prevent abuse or impropriety and to promote frugality, and where consistency and the need for fairness tend to create a need for bureaucracy and procedures.

Some government traditions are coming under scrutiny, if not attack. William Plowden has suggested that neutrality should allow for some flexibility. Others have wondered to what extent public servants can or should retain their anonymity in a situation where ministerial responsibility has been diluted. The growth of government and the expansion of its responsibilities have led to a situation where some of these traditions may be hard to sustain without modification. Adaptation may be necessary, but it must not lead to thoughtless unravelling of key parts of the fabric of parliamentary government.

Clearly, working in the public service is different from working in business. This is not because public servants are different from "normal" people, nor is it because politicians are ill-intentioned. Government is simply not business. There are legitimate and important reasons behind many of the values, conventions and norms of the public service, and these establish a particular kind of organizational culture. In such a culture, the task of management poses different challenges from those in another organizational culture such as that of business.

Footnotes:

1. Committee on Government Productivity, *Report No. Nine,* (Toronto: Government of Ontario, 1973), p. 9.

2. Peter Drucker, *Managing for Results,* (London: Pan Books, 1967), pp. 211ff.

3. "A special attribute of the success-oriented, positive, and innovating environment is a substantial tolerance for failure." Thomas J. Peters and Robert H. Waterman, *In Search of Excellence,* (New York: Harper and Row, 1982), p. 23.

4. Irving S. Shapiro, *America's Third Revolution: Public Interest and the Private Role,* (New York: Harper and Row, 1984), pp. 79-81.

5. Peter Kellner and Lord Crowther-Hunt, *The Civil Servants,* (London: Macdonald General Books, 1980), p. 63.

6. *Report of the Committee on the Civil Service,* Cmnd. 3638, (London: Her Majesty's Stationery Office, June 1968).

7. Author's interview, June 1986.

8. See Lawrence E. Lynn, Jr., *Managing the Public's Business: The Job of the Government Executive,* (New York: Basic Books Inc., 1981), pp. 6-37.

9. The Public Service Employment Act (PSEA), R.S.C. 1970, c. P-32, s.2(1), and the Public Service Staff Relations Act (PSSRA), R.S.C. 1970, c. P-35, s.2.

10. Interview with Edgar Gallant, former Chairman, Public Service Commission of Canada, May, 1986.

11. Mitchell Sharp, "The Role of the Mandarins," *Policy Options,* vol. 2 no. 1, (May/June 1981), pp. 3-44. See also Thomas D'Aquino, "The public service of Canada: the case for political neutrality," *Canadian Public Administration,* vol. 27 no. 1, (Spring 1984), pp. 4-23.

12. Gordon Robertson, "The Deputies' Anonymous Duty," *Policy Options,* vol. 4 no. 4, (July/Aug. 1983), pp. 1-13. For a perspective on the disadvantages of a partisan civil service of the type in

Washington D.C., see James P. Pfiffner, "Political Appointees and Career Executives: the Democracy-Bureaucracy Nexus in the Third Century," *Public Administration Review*, 47, (January-February 1987), pp. 57-65. (This reference thanks to an anonymous reviewer of this book.) See also the article by Chester A. Newland in the same volume of PAR, pp. 45-56.

13. Robert Normand, "Les relations entre les hauts fonctionnaires et le ministre," *Canadian Public Administration*, vol. 27 no. 4, (Winter 1984), p. 36. Author's translation.

14. Sir Edward Bridges, *Portrait of a Profession*, (Cambridge: Cambridge University Press, 1950), p. 8.

15. A.W. Johnson, "The role of the deputy minister," *Canadian Public Administration*, vol. 4 no. 4, (Dec. 1961), p. 71.

16. Peter Kellner and Lord Crowther-Hunt, *The Civil Servants*, (London: Macdonald General Books, 1980), pp. 161-162.

17. Lecture published as William Plowden, "What prospects for the civil service?" *Public Administration*, vol. 63 no. 4, (Winter 1985).

18. The Zussman/Jabes survey cited later in this book documents differences in values between private and public sectors in that regard.

Part Two:

Management at the Centre of Government

Introduction to Part Two

The Scope of Part Two

Management is the art of making institutions work effectively. It starts with mandates, leadership, vision, objectives . . . all those concepts which have to do with defining goals and getting other people to want to realize them. In most business organizations, leadership and direction come from the top of the structure. Usually, it is not too difficult to find the top. For government departments, the "top" or centre is more elusive, more difficult to define.

Government departments are led by ministers. They are legally in charge and accountable for the broad lines of departmental policy to the prime minister and to Parliament. However, they have a very complex job, and running the department is only one facet of this job. They are often quite inexperienced at running anything. The prime minister may rotate them so frequently that they do not have time to learn the substance of their responsibilities before they are whisked off to their next portfolio. They may not understand the concept of public service neutrality and, if they are newly elected, they may be suspicious of the motivations and commitment of the officials who are there to support them. By experience or temperament, they may be inclined to the view that it is preferable to be ambiguous and tentative about their objectives and intentions. Some may have only vague ideas about what they wish to achieve in their present post. They will likely find that their job leaves them little time for sober reflection or longer term planning.

Officials seeking clear direction and vision from ministers are often frustrated, and the relationship between ministers and their departmental staff is as variable as the personalities of the major players. Understanding ministers' jobs, making relationships with them work, and providing effective support to the political level of government is one of the central challenges facing officials. "Supporting" and "advising" a minister in a big department — or in a smaller one with important policy responsibilities — is in certain respects quite a different task from that of managing a large business corporation.

The first chapter in this part of the book discusses the role of the minister and the impact of the political level of government upon the public service. The next chapter, 5, considers the job of the department head, known as the deputy minister in Canada and the permanent undersecretary, or more colloquially, the permanent secretary in the U.K. It discusses the "classic" view of the department head as top advisor on policy to ministers, and examines other dimensions of the head's job. It points out that the top official of a government department faces a complicated web of relationships. Unlike business chief executives, who usually are clearly accountable in the first instance to their boards of directors, department heads are concurrently accountable to several different individuals and institutions, not all of whom will necessarily agree on objectives or priorities. It's not a job for persons who are uncomfortable with ambiguity. Chapter 6 deals specifically with the question of the accountability of department heads and concludes that, in a parliamentary democracy, there is no neat formula for simplifying the framework within which they must work.

Next to the relationship with the minister, one of the key relationships which department heads must maintain is with central departments or agencies. These organizations exercise great influence over how departments operate and over the resources available to them. However, their relationship to departments is, once again, more complicated and ambiguous than the relationship between a corporation's head office and its divisions or subsidiaries. Chapter 7 discusses the nature of this relationship and suggests that it is changing in response to the pressures of size and complexity in government. It also suggests that some central departments may have to rethink their mandate and their relationship to departments, and perhaps to restructure themselves to some degree, in order to manage the relationship with departments more effectively.

Policy and Management

It is impossible to discuss role and relationships at the centre of government, the subject of this section of the book, without encountering the concept of policy. One of the big differences between the private sector and government is that, in the former, one hears the word "policy" relatively seldom, whereas in the latter one can hardly escape it. To understand management in government, it is necessary to understand the relationship between policy and management (or administration).

Just what is policy? One wit has suggested — with considerable insight — "Policy is anything you want to decide yourself. Routine details are anything you don't want to be bothered with."[1] As we shall see, this definition may be one of the best available.

Although traditionally viewed as the most interesting and important domain of public administration and political science, policy seems imbued with a slightly mystical and paradoxical quality: it defies description, but you can always tell when you encounter it. One author of a book on management in government decided that the only way to deal with this subject was not to mention it at all![2] However, the relationship between policy and management cannot be ignored since perceptions of that relationship have an impact on key aspects of government. For example:

(1)   What is the relationship between the public service and the political level of government with respect to policy? Who formulates it; who is accountable for it? Does the public service have any role in policy or is this the exclusive preserve of ministers?

(2)   What are the appropriate staffing, promotional and human resource development practices in government, particularly at the senior levels of departments? What kinds of aptitudes are required at different levels of the bureaucracy?

Policy: Creating the Socio-Economic Context

To answer these and related questions, the point of departure must be a definition of policy. The word is used to mean different things in business and in government. In business, a policy is usually an internal operating rule or procedure. The word "strategy " is a closer private sector analogue to "policy" in government.

In government, people use "policy" in several ways. People at senior levels of government or in policy departments sometimes employ it to describe new initiatives to be recommended to ministers (e.g., a new agricultural policy) in order to create a certain type of social or economic situation in the country. People at middle management or supervisory levels tend to think of policy as the approved method of running a program. Experienced government hands learn to be sensitive to the different shadings of meaning, realizing that what the word is intended to convey often derives from the context in which it is used. Learning the meanings of policy is part of the process of acclimatization through which every new public servant must pass.

At the most basic level, policy has to do with creating the kind of society – economically, socially, morally, legally – within which we want to live. A policy may be something the government wishes to do – "It is our government's policy to privatize the air transport industry." Policy may refer to intentions at quite grand levels (economic policy) or at more mundane levels (policy regarding parking on the street). A policy may refer to a particular goal that the government wishes to achieve – "Our policy is to achieve a free-trade agreement with the United States." Or it may refer to a condition or a relationship which the government wishes to sustain, or a course to which it wishes to hold – "We have a policy of non-alignment." In all these conceptions of policy, the notion of *intent*, or *purpose*, is never far below the surface.

Policies emerge from organizations in several ways. Some are the result of the rational, orderly process of planning which first year students of administration are often taught, whereby goals are formulated, information is collected and analyzed, alternatives are identified, options are costed and the optimal course of action is selected. However, others emerge in a much less predictable and obvious way. They are not the result of some well-engineered process. They emerge, for example, from a tortuous process of inter-departmental negotiation where the result is not what anyone expected when the process began, or they arise from action deep within the organization where a committed individual pushes an initiative along without formal sanction from above.

Professor Henry Mintzberg has suggested that many policies appear like weeds in a garden, unexpectedly; they "take root in all kinds of strange places", and may spread until they cover much of the terrain.[3] Mintzberg notes that many weeds are not noxious. Part of the art of managing strategy or policy development is judging when these unexpected or unplanned policies should be nipped in the bud or should be allowed to develop and even be encouraged, in the interests of exploring new ways of doing things.

In summary, one useful definition of policy ties it to what the government intends to do or achieve in future. In this definition:

> A policy consists of intentions or objectives, to be given effect through law, regulation, expenditures, or in other ways, that define the government's view of how some aspect of society should evolve or of conditions that should prevail. A policy may prescribe how certain institutions or individuals are expected to behave, or it may define certain benefits members of the public will receive (or penalties they will suffer) under specified conditions.

Policy: Pattern in Action

The second definition of policy is more retrospective in its focus. It emphasizes what actually exists as opposed to what is, or was, intended. Thus, a policy may be a framework or context that has already been established through past decisions – "Our policy is to help industries locate in areas of high unemployment," or "We have a policy of non-discrimination in immigration."

There is often a gap between what some organizations intend to do and what occurs in practice. Sometimes organizations may be pursuing a policy in a general sort of way without really being strongly aware of it. A policy in this sense may be implicit, undetected, and even unintended. For example, an elected Government may discover that some of its decisions are leading to unexpected consequences — or opposition parties may bring the fact to its attention. ("Your Government's policy is to use the welfare system to destroy the will to work in this country!")

Organizations' (or people's) policies may be inferred even when they do not have an explicit document or plan recording their intentions, or a clearly articulated view of where they are going. Mintzberg suggests that policy in this sense can be defined as "pattern in action". A policy which the government wishes to implement is *intended*; one which emerges from an organization organically or unexpectedly rather than as a result of conscious, planned intentions is *emergent*. A policy which gets implemented, whatever its origins, is a *realized* policy; if it is realized as intended, Mintzberg calls it *deliberate*. Not all realized policies arise from intended policies — some develop from emergent roots. Exhibit II-1, adapted slightly from Mintzberg, illustrates these relationships.[4]

A definition of policy to accommodate this retrospective aspect of the word is as follows:

> A policy is an underlying pattern or logic discerned in past government actions (legislation, programs, regulations, institutions or other instruments of government), likely to lead to the realization of certain social or economic consequences.

Modern governments operate in the context of a host of existing policies — a sort of legislative and administrative coral reef that has gradually grown up over the years. The scope of government activity has become so broad that no newly elected party, unless it is committed to radical changes affecting the basic premises of government, can hope to alter more than a small percentage of existing policies.

EXHIBIT II - 1

From Conception to Implementation

Different types of policy (1)

CONCEPT

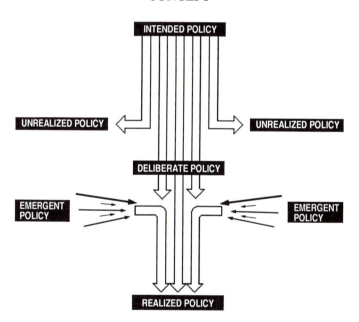

IMPLEMENTATION

BEYOND THE BOTTOM LINE (1988)
(1) Diagram adapted from Henry Mintzberg.

Much of what government does, as Edward Bridges has pointed out, consists in updating policies already in effect.

> [T]he work of Government at any given moment of time is being carried on in accordance with policy decisions, or directions given by Ministers, at some date in the past. The time comes when these former policy decisions need renewal, nearly always in a rather different form. This may be the result of changes in social habits or economic conditions. Or it may come from the sudden pressure of events, which makes it obvious that some existing line of policy can no longer be made to work or has ceased to be acceptable to public opinion.... [T]he work of Ministers and their senior staffs is concerned with the continuous task of keeping the policies of departments in line with the needs of the day ....
>
> In this kind of work the traffic in Government affairs moves both up and down .... Policy and management ... are inseparable.[5]

Policy and Administration: A False Dichotomy

In the late 1960s, the Fulton Report criticized the British government for maintaining a civil service divided into horizontal as well as vertical classes. This restricted mobility and tended to reserve the upper ranks of the service to "generalists" with rather vaguely-defined policy skills. The prevalent view in the U.K. for many years was that policy was the job of the top officials, and execution, administration or management, was the job of the lower levels. A CEO (chief executive officer) was a recognized rank in the British civil service at the time ... but it fell about half a dozen levels below that of the permanent secretary, because the "executive class" was thought to be concerned with "execution", not with policy.[6]

The problem with the notion that policy sits above administration, like a sort of cream on the milk, is that there is just enough truth in it to make it difficult to refute. As exhibit II-1 illustrates, policy *does* precede implementation, and much of management theory is about implementation. There is thus a certain plausibility to the notion that senior officials need to be knowledgeable about policy, while subordinate ones should be skilled in management.

INTRODUCTION TO PART TWO

Nonetheless, there are several difficulties with this idea. For example, there is no way of defining what "policy" is in the abstract. After reviewing 50 years of management literature,[7] Herbert Simon, one of the deans of writers on management, concluded, "No clear-cut criteria or marks of identification have been suggested that would enable one to recognize a 'policy question' on sight, or to distinguish it from an 'administration question'."*

The most common way of trying to distinguish policy from administration is to assert that policy has to do with ends, while administration is confined to means (or implementation of ends). The attempt to differentiate between means and ends has been a puzzle for many philosophers, so it is not surprising to find that in a management context, it still engenders confusion. The problem with the ends-means approach is that one person's (or one department's) means are another's ends.

Most government officials work within the confines of a particular "policy field" or framework. A policy field is an arbitrarily defined sphere of public concern, such as defence or transportation or industrial promotion. Ministers and officials who work in a given field tend, over time, to draw an intellectual map for themselves where destinations are defined in terms of certain policy objectives. However, what is "policy" in the Department of Transport (an end or objective) may be "administration" in, say, the Department of the Environment, and vice versa. A Minister of Transport might, for example, consider whether to build a road to connect two locations a policy issue. How it is built would be a matter of implementation or administration. However, for members of Parliament through whose constituencies the proposed road would pass, such questions as the size of the motorway, where it would be sited, what arrangements would be made for diminution of noise and other forms of pollution, would clearly be questions of policy.

---

* Simon considered confining policy issues to those decisions involving values (administration would thus be restricted to decisions on matters of a factual nature). However, the difficulty with this is that different persons have different values. Thus Simon concluded, "In practice the separation between the ethical and the factual element in judgment can usually be carried only a short distance . . . ."

Another practical difficulty with the ends-means argument is that of knowing where to draw the line between ends and means. This is a classic conceptual problem: how does one differentiate between planning and implementation? Anyone involved in the process of moving an initiative from conception to execution is engaged in both the formulation of objectives and in actions directed toward the attainment of those objectives. However, there is no way to draw a clear dividing line between the "policy" aspects of a new initiative and the "administrative" or "managerial" aspects. One shades gradually into the other.

Moreover, the definitions of these terms, "policy" and "administration", are fluid. To return to the example of the road cited above, when the possibility of building the road is in its early stages, senior officials will tend to define the "policy aspects" of the question as those related to whether it should be constructed; "administration", not an imminent possibility, will be those considerations related to when and how it is built. Thus "administration" hangs on policy, because nothing will happen until the basic issue (should the road be built?) has been decided.

The way bureaucracies work, however, once this decision has been taken, senior officials may not deem that the "policy aspects" have been dealt with ... what used to be "administration" gets reclassified as "policy". Now, the policy question is where to build the road; the administrative issue is, who builds it and when? Further along toward the completion of the project, the policy question may be, who builds the road? and the administration issues will relate to the materials to be used. In the real world of bureaucracy, policy is a word often used by senior officials to hold on to an issue until they feel that they are ready to delegate it. Thus it often transpires that policy is, indeed, "anything you want to decide yourself," and administration is "anything you don't want to be bothered with."

A related objection to the policy/administration dichotomy is that most policy problems are infused with administrative implications. People at upper levels of departments must clearly possess conceptual abilities. However, they are not responsible simply for building abstract castles in the sky. Someone has to live in these castles. The plumbing has to work. To be responsible for "policy" does not constitute a leave of absence from the realm of administration.

Good policy is policy in which the general administrative consequences have been anticipated and thought through. A senior government official who is good at "policy" but who has no administrative sense (the breed is not unknown!) will create endless problems for those who have to make the policies work. There is not much "pure" policy in government, in the sense of decisions with no administrative consequences. In fact, now that government plays a proactive role in society and in the economy, most of its policy decisions involve quite extensive administrative arrangements (offices, staff, procedures, criteria, job descriptions, computers, etc.).

Whether or not new policy proposals entrain administrative consequences, senior officials working in a department of any size — even one whose primary role is the development of policy proposals for ministers, rather than the deployment and direction of a large administrative apparatus — still possess managerial responsibilities. Policy departments may employ hundreds, perhaps thousands, of staff members. Such large organizations would be considered a substantial company in the private sector. No one would think of suggesting that its senior staff did not require managerial ability in order to direct and motivate staff. Policy development is itself a generic function in government, just like marketing or production in the private sector; yet little has been written about the management of this function. As a group of senior British civil servants observed in a submission to the Fulton Committee, "So far, the methods of management consultancy have been applied surprisingly little to the policy-making function of government."[8]

Summary

Policy has many meanings. The word is frequently used to allude to a Government's legislative objectives or platform, particularly its major plans and intentions — "It is our policy to privatize the air industry." Policy is also often used to describe agreed methods governing the operation of existing programs — "Our policy is to provide assistance only to people over 60." Policy has likewise been defined in a retrospective sense as pattern, or intentions, discerned in decisions already in place — "The policy of the Government was clearly to discourage immigration, even though this was not explicit."

Policies do not emerge solely from rational, carefully engineered planning processes. Many policies are "emergent", developing from unexpected origins and in somewhat unpredictable ways. Some policies which are "realized" or implemented derive from clear intentions ("deliberate policy"), while others derive from emergent roots.

Governments just elected to office fall heir to a "coral reef" of previously adopted policies. Governments which are not intent upon radical change to the existing social order will usually alter only a small percentage of these policies during their term of office.

It is very difficult to separate policy from administration for the following reasons:

- one department's policy is another's administration;

- policy shades into administration. Even when an initiative appears to have moved beyond policy into execution or administration, people often redefine "policy" progressively, to allow them to retain control of a situation or an issue;

- most policies in today's government involve substantial administrative implications, which must be thought through if the policy is to be effective in practice.

Business administration is sometimes thought to comprise a number of basic functions: production, finance, marketing and perhaps human resource management might be viewed as the key ones; others might include strategic planning and corporate relations or corporate affairs. The notion that there constitutes a set of basic functions in the public sector is less well established. However, if one were to develop a list of this type for a government organization, policy development might be first on it. Developing policy is seen as a key role in many if not most government agencies. This function must be managed, just like the finance function or the marketing function in business. Later in this book, a full chapter (chapter 10) is devoted to the management of policy development. The fact that policy development must itself be managed is another reason why the concepts of policy and management cannot be viewed as falling into two different spheres or worlds. They are inextricably linked.

Footnotes:

1. Cited in T.L. Martin, *Malice In Blunderland*, (New York: McGraw-Hill Book Company, 1973), p. 106.

2. Desmond Keeling, *Management in Government*, (London: George Allen and Unwin Ltd., 1972), p. 36.

3. Henry Mintzberg, and Jan Jorgensen, "Emergent strategy for public policy," J.J. Carson Lecture, presented at Ottawa University, 26 September 1985.

4. See Mintzberg, *op. cit.*, also Mintzberg and James A. Waters, "Of Strategies, Deliberate and Emergent," *Strategic Management Journal*, vol. 6, (1985), pp. 257-272. It should be noted that Mintzberg uses the word "strategy" rather than the word "policy," but he points out that the words are virtually synonymous in the public sector.

5. Lord Bridges, "The relationship between ministers and the permanent departmental head," *Canadian Public Administration*, vol. 7 no. 3, (September 1964), pp. 271-272.

6. *Report of the Committee on The Civil Service, 1966-68*, (Fulton Report) vol. 1, Cmnd. 3638 (London: Her Majesty's Stationery Office, June 1968), p. 11, p. 17.

7. Herbert Simon, *Administrative Behaviour*, 3rd ed., (New York: Collier Macmillan, 1976), pp. 52ff. See also Charles Lindblom, *The Policy-Making Process*, 2nd ed., (Englewood Cliffs: Prentice Hall, 1980), p. 116.

8. *Submission of the Association of First Division Civil Servants to the Fulton Committee*, "The Civil Service and Government Policy," (London: April 1967), p. 17.

Chapter Four:
Politics, Ministers and
Management

Because convention has it that ministers are responsible for policy, and officials for administration, ministers are often ignored in a discussion of management in government. However, as we have seen, there is no clear dividing line between policy and administration. As every fan of the popular BBC television series "Yes, Minister" knows, officials are intimately involved in most policy matters. What emerges rather less clearly is that ministers strongly influence the culture and working practices of the public service. Ministers do not preside magisterially from a distance, like some detached chairman of the board in the private sector, but frequently intervene in detailed aspects of departmental administration. Thus, any realistic discussion of the problems of management in government must start with ministers and their relationship to the public service. In jurisdictions such as Canada, the role of ministerial staffs, which have been growing in size and influence in recent years, must also be taken into account.

This chapter reviews the objectives of ministers, comparing their goals with those of a top business executive. It discusses Cabinet as the top decision-making body in the executive arm of government, describes the role and relationships of the minister, and concludes with a discussion of how Cabinet, ministers and their staffs affect the practice of management in the public service.

Ministerial Objectives

Cynics like to argue that politics attracts people who are devious, ambitious and untrustworthy. Media reporting which focuses on politicians' errors and gaffes rather than their achievements enhances this impression. However, there is little hard evidence to suggest that, as a breed, politicians are any worse or any better than the rest of us. Reminiscing about his political life, Henry Hicks, a former provincial premier and later president of Dalhousie University said,

> [I]n my experience in the Legislature of Nova Scotia, the quality of the average [Member]... compares favourably with that of any profession or group of citizens within the province. I have often felt that my fellow Members were less well informed than I wished they were or that their judgment was not as good as it ought to have been. But I have seldom had occasion to impute to any of them wrong motives or attitudes less worthy than one would expect to find in a representative group of doctors, lawyers, businessmen or labour leaders or even civil servants themselves. On the whole, my observation would be that the public... has chosen representatives of itself who are fully as worthy and as good as any other group that can be singled out in the community.[1]

However, politicians do tend to compromise, a quality that often draws criticism upon them.

> I have met many well meaning citizens who seemed genuinely concerned with this aspect of public life.... I believe the concern arises from a misunderstanding of the nature of compromise itself. The government of men cannot be accomplished if each is to have his way in every particular.... The stable government of mankind certainly requires a compromise between the interests and views of conflicting parties.... Generally speaking, the politician tries to secure the best decision which he believes will be supported by the majority....

[The acts of politicians] must be judged with constant and due reference to the limitations under which the government of men is of necessity carried on. Too often the politician is tested by ideal and quite impractical standards of accomplishment.[2]

Most politicians seem to find that politics is, indeed, the art of the possible. Many prefer not to be too specific about their intentions, as this allows them room for manoeuvre and compromise if they encounter opposing views. Asked to specify where they stand, they manage to occupy the entire terrain, as the former president of Mexico once indicated in a classic political response: "We're not left wing. But then we aren't right wing either. We're quite the contrary."[3]

Even once established on a course of action, they are often prepared to double back, reconsider, and adjust if the situation demands it. Studies of American politics have shown that Congress sometimes passes legislation whose goals are not only unclear, but even contradictory; Congress leaves it to the hapless public service to try to sort out its intentions and mount a sensible program. Other politicians often behave the same way.[4] Thus, trying to implement — indeed, trying to identify! — a politician's objectives is no easy task. Public servants, attempting to follow their leaders, sometimes have great difficulty knowing where they are going. Often ministers are themselves not too sure where they want to wind up, and they advance carefully, sniffing the political wind as they go.

This is one of the central differences between government and business. It is all very well for the purveyors of techniques such as management by objectives (MBO) to tell public servants that the way to manage is to start with clearly articulated strategic objectives at the top of the organization. There is some doubt as to whether business itself really functions in this simplistic manner; and certainly in government, the public servant waiting for an unambiguous public statement of departmental goals may retire before the goals are revealed. Such simple, structured recipes for management are useless to most public servants, because they relate to the environment as "management experts" would like it to be, not to the swirling realities of government.

Government leaders pursue many goals in addition to that of efficiency. Business people who understand the political environment know that,

> important as it is to have the facts, arguments based solely on economic efficiency, technological imperatives, and statistical probabilities . . . have limited power to predict outcomes . . . . Politicians are less likely to ask, "Is it true?" than "Will it sell back home?" and "Does it sound fair?" . . . On one issue, cold facts do carry the day and the government process seems to make eminently good sense. The next time round, an equally convincing set of facts seems to get lost . . . . [5]

Politicians are not by nature corrupt or illogical. They respond to different imperatives than do business people. There is a tendency in a capitalist society to assume that behaviour conventionally associated with business success (e.g., economy, competitive drive, entrepreneurial aggression) should serve as a sort of template to judge behaviour in other contexts. "Why don't politicians behave in a more business-like manner?" To understand political behaviour, one must understand power. In politics, power is the sine qua non of all other ends — without it other objectives cannot be achieved.

Politicians' behaviour is constantly directed toward the attainment, preservation and consolidation of political power. This is a basic objective. Over the years, ministers' abilities to realize economies or to show evidence of tight administrative systems have not been known to enhance their performance at the polls. What does contribute to electoral success, and hence to the retention of power, is an ability to balance competing interests, to be perceived as just, or at least to offend as few people as possible. " 'Fairness' is a universal touchstone in politics, one of the few."[6]

A Canadian DM made the following observation about the relationship between ministers and officials and the goals which they pursue.

> Ministers [who often have little preparation for their departmental responsibilities] form a perception of what they want to do, but they are influenced by a desire to get personal kudos and support for the Government. These

considerations may obscure, to a greater or lesser degree, their interest in the longer-term context. The best policies . . . come from an exchange of ideas between the DM and the professional bureaucrats and the professional politicians. The best of all possible worlds would arise from a professional relationship between the two, each searching for the best solution that would accommodate the various [short-term and longer-term] interests.[7]

Ministers are not functioning in a commercial environment and should not be expected to behave as if they were. Ministerial behaviour and motivations have a fundamental impact on the managerial environment in government departments. It renders some of the more simplistic formulae for improving management unhelpful in a public-sector context. Any realistic approach to management in government must take uncertainty and ill-defined objectives as a given. The problem is not how to "fix" this situation, but how to operate effectively within it.

Cabinet

As the senior decision-making body next to Parliament, Cabinet exercises an extraordinary influence on all the workings of government. It is a powerful vortex drawing towards it the policy proposals of the public service.[8] As an executive body its "outstanding duty . . . is to provide the country and Parliament with a national policy and to devise means for coping with present emergencies and future needs", constantly gauging, as it does so, where it stands in relation to public opinion. As a legislative entity, it generally controls the House of Commons; it dominates legislation in Parliament; and it enacts "subordinate legislation" in the form of orders-in-council or minutes dealing with a huge range of matters, not least of which are the numerous appointments to top positions of departments, agencies, government corporations and boards of directors.[9]

In Britain, a distinction is drawn between the "ministry" and the Cabinet. There may be several dozen ministers at any time, but not all are in the Cabinet, which is restricted to about 20 of the most senior ministers. In Canada, however, all ministers are, by convention, in the Cabinet, the result of which is an unwieldy, inefficient body for decision-making. The issue of the size of Cabinet has been an ongoing object of debate. When Canada's first Cabinet was formed in 1867, the Opposition argued that 13 ministers were too many and suggested that seven or eight would suffice. However, when the Government changed, the former Opposition found it necessary to create a Cabinet of 14 members. Ever since, efforts to diminish the size of Cabinet have foundered on the need for representation of a broad cross-section of interest groups, of French and English interests, and of the many geographic regions of a sprawling country.[10]

Since the selection of Cabinet members is based as much upon representational considerations as upon experience or ability, a Canadian Cabinet usually comprises a mixed bag. Particularly in a newly elected Government, Cabinet members may have had only superficial exposure to the many complex issues of public policy before assuming their posts. In administration, many Cabinet members (and members of Parliament as well) often have very limited background. In the 40-member Cabinet of Prime Minister Brian Mulroney in 1987, for example, more than half the members come from backgrounds in the professions or small business; only half a dozen or so have had senior managerial experience (such as holding the position of a president or vice-president of a large institution).* A Canadian deputy minister who had worked with ten different ministers over the years observed, "Most ministers are not as bright as the officials they are leading. This may be different in the U.K.; however, in my experience, a minister in Canada is typically a former small businessman or a walk-up lawyer or a farmer; he or she has little or no executive experience and little by way of shared values with a department."[11]

---

* A rough analysis of the occupation backgrounds of Cabinet members, based on summary information prepared by the Library of Parliament, suggested that 12 members were "professionals," (and ten of these were lawyers); nine others might have been called "small businessmen" (chicken processor, importers, sales manager, farmer, farm equipment dealer, etc.) Another seven were engaged previously in teaching or academic administrative posts. The remainder came from a variety of occupational backgrounds: mayors, professional politicians, voluntary organizations, etc.

Because Cabinet is so large, much of its work is transacted in committees. In the last two decades or so, Canada has had between nine and 12 Cabinet committees, dealing with such issues as priorities and planning (the most influential committee, sometimes referred to as the "inner Cabinet"), government expenditure and management (Treasury Board), legislation and the planning of House of Commons business, foreign policy and defence, communications, security and intelligence, economic policy and social policy. (The British tradition is that the composition of Cabinet committees should be secret.)

Most of the work of Cabinet and its committees involves proposals contained in memoranda to Cabinet, or Cabinet documents, formally sponsored and signed by ministers, but nearly all prepared by public servants. Once a document has been considered by committee, and subsequently approved by Cabinet, a record of decision conveying ministerial intent is prepared by central agency officials and forwarded to the responsible department(s). Knowledge of these procedures constitutes the stock-in-trade of any moderately senior government official.[12]

As governments grow, so do the number of Cabinet documents and the complexity of the issues they address. In the decade from 1957 to 1967, the number of Cabinet documents considered in Canada rose from around 400 to 800 a year.[13] More recent statistics indicate that by the early 1980s, about 900 documents a year were being processed, resulting in about 750 records of decision.[14] One source suggests that in Britain, Cabinet was coping with about 1,800 documents a year as of 1977.[15]

In any large government, the volume and length of Cabinet documents present a dilemma. Almost two decades ago, a former Secretary to the federal Cabinet in Canada was lamenting "the relentless daily servitude our ministers now face when Parliament is in session", pointing out the "enormous difficulties" associated with the volume of legislation and Cabinet material.[16] Departmental officials, in attempting to do justice to complicated policy questions, produce long and detailed memoranda. Seeking to reduce ministers' workload to human proportions, central agencies call for shorter documents and executive summaries. Departmental officials protest that such summaries are superficial and inadequate as a basis for decision-making. It is a problem with no obvious solution. A modern

Cabinet is severely stretched, if not seriously overloaded. Cabinet members just do not have the time to do justice to the host of complex issues brought before them.

Most ministers read the documents on a highly selective basis, depending on their officials to notify them of difficult or topical issues. Increasingly, for less contentious issues, the Cabinet document system is primarily an instrument to ensure effective interdepartmental consultation before the confirmation of a decision by Cabinet. Ministers, of course, retain the power to intervene, and they do on important issues; but on less significant questions, the Cabinet document serves as a record of agreements struck and compromises evolved through channels subordinate to the Cabinet itself. Cabinet simply provides the final seal of approval — often with a rubber stamp.

It seems unlikely that ministers have ever been able to afford much time for abstract strategic policy issues or for conceiving grand schemes. Running one portfolio is more than sufficient challenge for most. Efforts to engage the Canadian Cabinet in a form of corporate planning during the 1970s, under Prime Minister Pierre Trudeau, were judged by many observers to have been unsuccessful.[17] Similar attempts in the same period by Prime Minister Heath, and later Prime Minister Wilson, with the help of Whitehall's Central Policy Review Staff (since disbanded), got very mixed reviews. A former Permanent Secretary of the British Treasury, Douglas Wass, has indicated that even though Cabinet members possess a collective responsibility for government policy, this does not necessarily mean that Cabinet has a collective view as to the strategic directions that policy should take. On the contrary:

> Ministers in Cabinet rarely look at the totality of their responsibilities, at the balance of policy, at the progress of the government towards its objectives as a whole .... The form and structure of a modern Cabinet and the diet it consumes almost oblige it to function like a group of individuals .... No minister I know of has won political distinction by his performance in Cabinet or by his contribution to collective decision-taking. [As a result] ... the ordering of priorities is discussed in only the most general terms .... Fifty years ago Leo Amery, himself an experienced minister, was writing that "a Cabinet consisting of a score of overworked departmental Ministers

is quite incapable of either thinking out a definite policy or of securing its effective and consistent execution."[18]

Cabinet is ill-constituted to provide an overall strategic plan for governmental activity or even a framework of assumptions that could be used by departments as a basis for their own planning. There are important areas of public policy where Cabinet cannot easily afford to communicate its assumptions, even within the bureaucracy. For example, planning in some areas of the public service is significantly affected by future movements of the exchange rate, by the pay which government is prepared to offer its employees, by interest rates and by the rate of inflation. It could be useful to some departments if Cabinet were to tell them its assumptions on such topics. However, there is too great a risk that the market could learn Cabinet's expectations, and take action that might undermine government efforts to attain critical policy objectives.

In any event, Cabinets tend to operate on an issue-by-issue basis in planning and formulating policy. In many areas of policy, departments have to make their own assumptions, groping as best they can for indications of intent in the Government's actions and announcements, hoping that their own plans and policies will result in some sort of co-ordinated thrust and some consistency of direction.

Participation in Cabinet and its committees is hard work for ministers. Issues brought before Cabinet are often complicated, involving difficult technical points derived from scientific disciplines; complex financial or economic assessments related to major government investments, monetary policy or international negotiations; subtle legal points embodied in agreements with other levels of government or foreign powers; or critical political calculations that could affect the balance of power in the next election. Many documents are the result of years of preparation and countless hours of staff work within the public service. Yet Cabinet must dispose of them within the course of one or two meetings.

Ministers' Relationships

Cabinet is only one dimension of a minister's job. As well, ministers maintain a bewildering array of relationships outside Cabinet: with the prime minister and his or her office, with colleagues, with constituents, with party officials, with regional interest groups, with other interest groups of particular relevance to their portfolio, with the media, with other members of Parliament including opposition parties, with their departments, and with Crown corporations and other advisory bodies for which they may be responsible (including the members of the boards of those bodies).

Maintaining these relationships and acting as a spokesman for the Government demand a great many public appearances at which the minister must be able to articulate and defend not only the policies for which he or she is directly responsible, but also the general thrust of the Government's stand on other issues. The principle of Cabinet solidarity requires a minister to stand fast with the key directions of government policy, even on issues of a moral or ethical nature with which they might not personally agree. From time to time, Cabinet ministers are publicly reminded of their responsibilities in this regard, as happened in March 1985 when the Premier of Nova Scotia instructed his Cabinet on its response to the abortion issue:

> HALIFAX (CP) — Premier John Buchanan has defended his threat to expel any Cabinet minister who publicly disagrees with the government's stand against Dr. Henry Morgenthaler's plan to open a Halifax abortion clinic. The Progressive Conservative premier made the threat in the legislature Wednesday . . . . Questioned by reporters, Buchanan denied he is tampering with his ministers' freedom of speech.
>
> "They have a right to free speech but not in a matter which is a government decision," Buchanan said . . . . "That is Cabinet solidarity . . . ."[19]

Constant pressure from the media can make a ministerial job extremely stressful. One minister from the Cabinet of former Prime Minister Pearson, Maurice Lamontagne, stated that

> the mass media have . . . a great deal of influence on the politician . . . . If a minister enjoys a good press, he will be envied and respected or feared by his colleagues. If he has no press, he has no future. And, if he has a bad press, he is in serious trouble, because he will be viewed even by his

own associates as a political liability, in spite of the qualities he may have.[20]

Lamontagne suggested that the increasing complexity of Cabinet business, the growing role of the state, and the unending demands for personal appearances are gradually rendering ministers ineffectual, turning them into figureheads for the Government. He argued that ministers succumb to maintaining a positive image, responding to the media's superficial stress on sensation and on "surface" rather than on "performance". Competent ministers are sometimes destroyed simply because they show themselves to be human; conversely, ineffectual ministers may continue to have good ratings.

With respect to their constituents, ministers must exercise caution. With the exception of the rare minister appointed to Cabinet from the upper house, ministers can never forget that they are members of Parliament first, and members of Cabinet second. Although travel to and from a riding can be time-consuming and physically exhausting, ministers must appear in their constituencies frequently. Those who do not, often fail to secure re-election.

It is a rash minister who will tell electors that constituency concerns take second place to regional or national issues. Some relatively inconsequential local issue may be the determining factor on how an important group of voters will mark their ballots at the next election. Henry Hicks tells of his experience with voter priorities. A constituent explained to Hicks that although he had been a Liberal Party member for years, as had his father and grandfather before him, he did not vote for Hicks in the previous election. On investigation, it transpired that,

> the week before the election a road-grading machine had passed by [the constituent's] house and knocked over his mailbox — which was located on the highway right-of-way in any event. He had written to the county highway office but had received no reply nor had his mailbox been restored by election day. He thereupon concluded that if, after years of support, the Liberal Party could not look after him better than this, he would no longer vote for its candidate.

The moral of this story, for Hicks, was that,

> in a democracy the politician must deal with people as they
> are and not as he would wish them to be. Furthermore, the
> party which hopes to receive support from all sections of the
> public, must be able to show that the government it forms
> can attend to the wants of the citizen who sees no further
> than the road in front of his house . . . as well as . . . address
> itself to the great problems of state.[21]

Ministers must also maintain good relationships with members
of their own party, especially if they have long-term political
ambitions (such as party leadership) which will make it necessary to
seek the support of party members at some future date. The bigger
the Government majority in the House of Commons, the more party
members there are to consider.

Ministers who pay attention to their relationship with the House
of Commons as a whole, and who maintain good relations with the
opposition parties, can find their role greatly simplified; an arrogant
or uncaring minister may often encounter heavy weather. "[F]rom
the viewpoint of almost all parliamentarians, question time in the
Commons is central to the principle of parliamentary government . . . ."[22] This is when the opposition tries to score debating points
against the Government, and perhaps tries to force it to reveal
damaging information, or to embarrass a minister who is ill-prepared.
Question period is the focal point of House of Commons activity, and
in general tends to attract much more attention than other debates.
Ministers go to considerable lengths to avoid embarrassment by
preparing to cope with even the most trivial question (and many of
them *are* trivial) related to their portfolios.

The need for ministers to be able to deal personally with queries
raised by voters, either from their own constituencies or from
elsewhere, through questions raised in question period or perhaps in
caucus, has very important implications for the operation of the public
service. In business, chief executives can afford to delegate less
important matters to subordinates; such matters, once delegated, are
usually off their desks for good. Not so a minister of the Crown. As
noted in chapter 3, much of the trivia comes back to the minister's
office.

By comparison with the private sector, the problem of "two-ended program delivery" creates a much greater need for staff support positions, such as assistants-to, at top levels of departments. It clogs up the priorities of organizational units, such as planning offices or policy shops, with relatively unimportant paper. It consumes more of the time of ministers and senior officials than they would like. It gets in the way of line managers trying to run their programs on a systematic basis. It is a classic example of the urgent driving out the important. But it is a fact of life in government.

In summary, above and beyond their Cabinet responsibilities, ministers maintain an extraordinary range of relationships. The 1977 schedule of a particularly active British minister, Anthony Wedgwood-Benn, included roughly 70 engagements in his constituency, 150 meetings with people from the Labour Party, providing replies to over 200 questions in the House, attending over 150 meetings with non-governmental groups, plus another 150 meetings of Cabinet and Cabinet committees, reviewing 1,750 Cabinet documents and presenting some 45 of his own to Cabinet committees, 19 visits abroad, presiding over sessions of the Energy Council of the European Community, giving 80 speeches around the country, 83 radio interviews, 57 television appearances, 34 press conferences and 30 interviews with individual journalists, dealing with 1,000 letters outside his constituency mail and ministerial work, plus various other responsibilities too numerous to mention.[23]

As this example indicates, ministers' time is constantly under siege. At such a killing pace of work, a minister typically has only "a few hours a week to spend on his department,"[24] according to a Canadian study.

Ministers and their Departments

New ministers — who have often never run anything larger than a law office, a political campaign or a small business — suddenly find themselves at the head of an organization which may have many decades of history, engrained traditions, several thousand employees, and operations that extend across the country. Many ministers are quite unprepared for their departmental responsibilities. They have no experience in directing a big institution, and have difficulty understanding that ocean liners do not change course as easily as dinghies.

Sometimes ministers are appointed to portfolios for which they are well prepared, as when, for example, an MP who was the party's critic of industrial policy while in opposition is named to an economic development post. However, often ministers are selected to lead a department without much warning. Since the prime minister must consider many factors besides the personal interest or suitability of the potential incumbent, often an MP is assigned to a portfolio in which he or she has little background or even interest. With little time to prepare, new ministers may arrive at their post with scant knowledge of departmental policy concerns and with no clear agenda of what they wish to accomplish. One former deputy minister of finance commented on his minister's views on policy: "My experience as often as not was that the minister had no view . . . and I don't say that critically."[25]

As a result, new ministers, especially those of a newly elected Government can be somewhat unpredictable, and may treat their departments with a mixture of intense suspicion and distrust. One Canadian deputy minister characterized this aspect of government as a sort of "institutionalized unfriendly takeover" in the private sector.[26] If ministers do not grow to trust their departments, relations with the public service can be tense, tiring and frustrating for both sides throughout the tenure of the minister. Fortunately, in most cases, departments and their ministers reach an accommodation that is mutually acceptable if not entirely satisfactory; and sometimes, a highly successful partnership emerges.

Some ministers make the mistake of thinking that it is their job to run their department—to direct the day-to-day work, hire staff, structure the organization. Such ministers have to be gently educated by their officials and by central agencies in such mysteries as the merit principle, the responsibilities of the collectivity and the role of central agencies. Most ministers are not managers in any event, either by temperament or experience. While managerial questions occupy rather more ministerial time than they used to (at least according to one former British minister),[27] most ministers would probably agree with former Saskatchewan Premier Allan Blakeney:

"If there is one thing a minister should not be, it is the administrative head of his department."[28]

Blakeney has proposed two roles for a minister in relation to a department: to explain departmental policies to the public, and to interpret to officials public reaction to the department's policies. In his view, the first role is well understood by officials whereas the second is less so. Blakeney believes that the essence of the minister's job is to ensure that policies in place are those which "are in the range of public acceptability," not necessarily those which are technically ideal.

The key aspect of the minister's relationship to his or her department has to do with the development of policy. If ministers and departments share common views about this aspect of their work, the relationship is generally happy. If they do not, it is more difficult. Sometimes there is some doubt as to who is running things. A former British and a former Canadian prime minister, Edward Heath and Joe Clark, have expressed rather different views on this issue.

Heath:

"I would say quite clearly and definitely that civil servants were under ministerial control. I have absolutely no doubt about it. In my ministerial life this has always been the case."[29]

Clark:

"Without anyone willing it to happen, our system has changed to the point where most policy decisions are taken by the public service, even if they are approved by the politicians. The appointed government decides more than the elected government does. That runs exactly contrary to the theory on which our system is based."[30]

Ministers are clearly in charge of the development of new policy: they are obviously in a position to enforce their will over the public service but within certain constraints. Most important, they must be able to carry their Cabinet colleagues with them.

Except for those exceptionally gifted, it is difficult for ministers to provide leadership in policy fields with which they are unfamiliar. Public servants with years of experience in a particular area of policy usually have quite strong ideas about what works and what does not.

Ministers who come to that field with no background and few preconceptions of their own, inevitably have a lot of catching up to do. Catching up is almost impossible, as former British minister Anthony Wedgwood-Benn has pointed out.

> Cabinet members are soon overwhelmed by the insistent demands of running their departments. On the whole, a period in high office consumes intellectual capital; it does not create it . . . . [The less ministers] know at the outset, the more dependent they are on the only source of available knowledge; the permanent officials.[31]

According to Benn, ministers inevitably come to depend on "civil service policy". He defines this as follows:

> Civil service policy . . . is an amalgam of views that have been developed over a long period of time. It draws some of its force from a deep commitment to the benefits of continuity, and a fear that adversary politics may lead to sharp reversals by incoming governments of policies devised by their predecessors, which the civil service played a great part in developing.[32]

Ministers clearly can prevail when they want to; but wise ministers pick their issues. Those who seize a few strategic objectives, and who are not overwhelmed by day-to-day pressures, can undoubtedly have a major impact on policy.[33]

From time to time, politics attracts individuals who make a mark because of their vision and their strength of character. Leaders tend to be characterized by focus and by persistence. Ministers who come to office equipped principally with the generalities of their party's election platform and some rather vague ideas of their own will have to take cues from officials, perhaps more often than they would like. But that, after all, is hardly a reasonable basis upon which to criticize public servants, nor does it suggest that there is (as is sometimes suggested) a public service "plot" to stifle the elected Government. The fact is, some ministers are more able than others. The able ministers lead; the less able ones are carried with the tide. This does not necessarily result in poor government, but it obviously places a very important responsibility on the public service to ensure that the policy proposals they advance are soundly analyzed and sensitive to public opinion.

Gordon Robertson, a former Canadian deputy minister and Cabinet Secretary, has articulated this view of the civil servant's policy role.

> Any civil servant much above clerical or stenographic grades who has spent any substantial time in a job without contributing to some degree to the policy he administers in a job should be fired .... Since we, as administrators, must execute the policies ultimately decided upon by our political masters, we have an enormous interest in the quality of those policies and in the efficiency of the decision-making process by which they are arrived at.[34]

Even in areas of policy where they do not have background or strong personal views, ministers may often make important contributions such as the ability to exploit connections with a lot of "leading public figures", to sense the currents of public opinion, to assess the likely response of Parliament to proposed legislative change, and to present a new proposal to Parliament if warranted.[35]

Former Premier Blakeney argues that the minister's function is to be attuned to public views; he must circulate, consult and listen. In addition, Blakeney recommends that "the minister must hold himself aloof from the decision-making process until that process is in its final stages." Not all ministers would agree with this; some believe it is critical to affect the shape of policy at an early stage, before it goes through the interdepartmental mill. However, Blakeney's belief is that if ministers get involved too early they do not have time to perform what he calls their political function – that is, they lose the capacity to criticize proposals from a public perspective. "This has the effect in many cases of making the minister a captive of his department," (and therefore less effective in his other roles as a member of Cabinet, as a department leader or as a representative of his constituents).[36]

It must be said that elected Governments do not make it easy for ministers to be effective departmental leaders. The great impediment is the Cabinet shuffle – the practice of shifting ministers from one portfolio to another every year or two. Shuffling ministers is a technique used by prime ministers to "launder" a Cabinet sullied by

133

crises and misjudgment. It helps to create a fresh face with which the Government can confront the public. It may also be thought to give the public an illusion of action and to keep the Government's name in the headlines. In addition, shuffles may be initiated because prime ministers want to prevent ministers from becoming too committed to the interest groups associated with their existing portfolio. Ministers too long in one portfolio may be thought to be in danger of becoming the "prisoners" of their department.

Cabinet shuffles occur several times during the normal four- or five-year term of many Governments. Most people need a year or so in a new job before they can start to be fully effective. Thus, ministers are often just starting to hit their stride – and officials are just getting used to working with them – when they are hustled off to a new portfolio. This diminishes ministerial effectiveness while leaving public servants in a state of recurring uncertainty as to what the appropriate policy emphasis should be for their department. Ministers are seldom in place long enough to complete the initiatives they start.[37] Even though, following a shuffle, a new minister will come from the same party as the previous one, he or she is likely to have different views about priorities and about how the department should operate. The prevailing practice of "musical chairs" may entail short-run political gains for a Government, but it impedes ministers' ability to achieve anything of substance in their portfolios, and it is extraordinarily disruptive for public servants trying to administer programs consistently and efficiently.[38]

To summarize, ministers are, in principle, able to prevail powerfully over their departments. However, their ability to provide substantive, rather than cosmetic, leadership on major issues is often constrained by too many other responsibilities and by Cabinet shuffles. They are forced to rely heavily upon the public service in the development of new policies. There are times when ministers must feel like the pilot of a large aircraft, ultimately in charge, but inadequately prepared for the job and overburdened with other tasks, therefore having to accept advice and guidance from the ground simply in order to stay in the air.

Ministerial Responsibility

Ministers' functions relate not only to new policy but also to policy already in place. It is here that the doctrine of ministerial responsibility particularly applies. Like the doctrine of Cabinet solidarity, that of ministerial responsibility originated when government was smaller and simpler. In those days, legislation was often written in great detail, specifying not only the broad objectives of government policy but the detailed procedures for its implementation. Ministers were deemed to be personally responsible for everything that went on in their departments. An administrative error of any consequence could be cause for resignation. More recently, the growth of government and the pace of socio-economic change have made it impractical for Parliament to specify the administrative arrangements appropriate to every policy. The delegation of more administrative discretion to the public service has diluted the doctrine of ministerial responsibility.

In business, it is recognized that the chief executive has to be accountable for the overall conduct of the business, and above all, for its bottom-line performance. However, no one would think of suggesting that, in the normal course of business, a CEO should be personally accountable for, say, poor service delivery by a remote sales office. Indeed, if a board of directors found that a CEO was spending time dealing with matters on this level of detail, there would be concern about his or her sense of priorities and suitability for the top job.

Governments are gradually recognizing the logic of this view. According to a recent examination of ministerial responsibility, except for situations involving personal culpability or direct ministerial involvement, "it is now almost universally accepted that it is unreasonable to hold a minister personally responsible in the form of resignation for the administrative failings of his subordinates."[39] Ministers retain, of course, a responsibility in respect of major lines of policy. Where they sponsor an important policy which turns out to be unsuccessful, they are expected to shoulder the blame in the same manner as a CEO who institutes an ineffective business strategy. Resignation may be necessary if the failure is sufficiently serious.

However, ministerial responsibility is not dead. What has passed away is the rather dated and foolish notion that a minister should automatically resign for relatively inconsequential administrative errors. Ministers are still expected to answer for their departments publicly. They are still expected to maintain the traditions of civil service anonymity and neutrality, and not drag civil servants personally into public debate on matters related to their departments' internal operations. However, in controversial situations, it has become a matter of judgment and politics as to when the circumstances are so grave as to warrant the minister's own resignation.

Ministers' continuing responsibility to answer for their departments' activities in Parliament, combined with the opposition's tendency to inquire into many detailed aspects of departmental administration, results in patterns of behaviour in the public service that are inimical to a carefully planned, well-organized approach to administration. Contrary to popular belief, bureaucrats are not all circumspect and cautious by temperament, nor are they bad planners. However, officials do respond rationally to their environment. There is little incentive to plan activities when the minister's office keeps intruding upon day-to-day work with requests for information on minor matters, (or for assistance in arranging some apparently politically-motivated initiative). Further, no official wishes to be responsible for an action that could embarrass his or her minister. New public servants, particularly those in subordinate administrative positions, tend to learn that, when in doubt, follow the book, and avoid initiatives that could lead to trouble.

Dilution of the doctrine of ministerial responsibility has raised new questions about the accountability of public servants themselves. If it is accepted that the minister can disclaim knowledge of, and personal responsibility for, administrative errors in a department, then presumably the responsibility for some mistakes and misjudgments should fall on the public service. How should public servants be held to account?

There are two lines of thinking on this subject. One stresses the development of better methods for holding public servants to account within the bureaucracy—clearer lines of authority, performance measures, improved management information systems, new budgeting systems tied to responsibility centres, internal audits, program evaluation—in short, many of the instruments discussed in this book. The other approach stresses the external relationships of the public service. The main vehicles for achieving this in a systematic way have been the enlargement of mandates of national auditors (a movement by no means confined to Canada)[40] and the attempt to establish a direct accountability for permanent secretaries or deputy ministers to committees of the House of Commons (particularly the Public Accounts Committee) on matters of administration. The prospect of greater external accountability of public servants, however, conflicts with another cherished doctrine of parliamentary democracy, namely, that of the anonymity of the civil service. (Accountability to parliamentary committees is discussed in more depth in chapter 6.)

The Minister's Office

In Britain, ministers receive relatively little staff support. In Canada, however, the "exempt staff" (so called because they are not part of the neutral public service, and not governed by the merit principle) has been a growth industry in the last two decades. By the late 1970s, most federal ministers had, in addition to a "departmental assistant" seconded to their office from the public service, one executive assistant, at least a couple of special assistants (sometimes more) plus, in some cases, other staff at the constituency level.

The election of the Progressive Conservative Government of Brian Mulroney in 1984 led to the invention of the chief-of-staff concept and a further enlargement in the size of the ministers' offices. The chief-of-staff concept provided for a substantial increase in pay for the most senior ministerial assistant (formerly the executive assistant), to a level roughly equal to that of an assistant deputy minister (ADM). For a while, people in Ottawa began to talk about the chief-of-staff as a kind of political ADM Policy.

How much assistance should be afforded to ministers, and of what kind, has been a subject of continuing discussion in the literature of public administration. The argument in favour of enlarged staffs points out how ministers are often ill-prepared for their jobs; they tend to become "captives" of their departments; they need advice on the political dimensions of new policy proposals that the civil service is unable to provide; they have large quantities of correspondence and many representations to handle, well beyond the capacity of one or two support staff; they require individuals to help with constituency-related duties and obligations; they need support to handle aspects of their ministerial role not directly related to the mandate of their department; their job is so big no one could do it without strong staff assistance.

The counter-arguments are that ministers persistently tend to hire staff without sufficient regard for their qualifications; many staff members do not in fact have the background to give the minister the kind of mature political advice that is required; the nature of the job (short term, ill-defined, resented by the public service) is such that it is unlikely to attract the type of people wanted in such a position; ministerial aides tend to be ambitious individuals who, lacking supervision, develop private agendas unrelated to the minister's interests, thereby causing the minister more harm than good; assistants interfere in the work of the department in ways that serve partisan political purposes, unrelated to the general public interest.

In principle, it seems difficult to resist the conclusion that ministers need more help. Two authors who reviewed the Canadian scene in the 1970s and early 1980s concluded that more staff was desirable.[41] The premise underlying most studies that call for more staff is that the minister needs help in the area of policy development. The problem, as stated by one Canadian minister, is, "By the time something is brought to my level, the die is cast. Essentially I have two choices: I can go along with what the department is proposing or I can refuse to sign. That is the only real power I have to check the department. It is a negative power and consequently I very rarely employ it."[42]

While the minister's observations are valid, they raise a more basic question as to whether the role of the minister should be to check the department or to lead it. It is unlikely, even with a dozen assistants, that a minister would be able to "check" a big government department effectively. Simply enlarging the minister's staff for this purpose would have little impact on the minister's ability to provide direction on the key issues of departmental policy, especially if the minister (and his or her staff) are shuffled to a new department every year or so.

It is difficult to generalize about the role of ministers' staffs. How ministers hire and use their assistants tends to be a highly personal decision. Some use them wisely and effectively. Some staff members make a very useful contribution, but on the other hand, some ministers employ staff members with no aptitude for the key elements of the job simply to satisfy patronage obligations. Some even hire individuals of questionable integrity. (It was revealed in 1987 that a Canadian Minister of Public Works had employed two staff members with criminal records.)

One of the persistent problems with many ministerial assistants is that they are unable to resist dabbling in departmental affairs without adequate justification. Staff members whose supposed role is to help the minister with his or her private office and with constituency matters interfere in departmental administration in ways that are clearly designed to further the minister's (or their own) personal careers, rather than the general public interest. Public servants in many departments in Canada can tell numerous tales of ministerial assistants who abused their positions. Such examples include contracts directed to bidders who were not competitive; the ministerial assistant who held up a departmental publication for months simply so that a letter with the minister's picture could be included (the idea was ultimately abandoned and the document released, late, with no change); a costly film that had to be re-shot at a cost of $10,000 lest a trifling incident on camera embarrass the minister; the chief of staff who demanded that a minor cosmetic change be made to the cover of a completed departmental booklet, resulting in a supplementary cost of $15,000.

Such occurrences will be inevitable unless and until political parties institute procedures that introduce an element of merit into the selection process for ministerial staffs. As one of the studies cited above pointed out, most of the Canadian assistants in ministers' offices in the early 1980s had sparse intellectual qualifications. Most would not have been able to secure a relatively junior post in the full-time civil service. Many seemed to have come to the job as a first step in their career, bringing little knowledge of government or public policy issues to their positions.[43]

Regrettably, ill-qualified or over-ambitious ministerial staff members can do a lot of damage to the permanent public service, for they speak with the minister's voice and are often in a position to override the judgment of individuals of greater experience selected according to more rigorous criteria. This undermines the sense of professionalism of the full-time public service and promotes cynicism about the motives of the elected Government. In extreme cases, the public servant who feels unable to fight back inside the bureaucracy against blatant abuse may fight back outside the service through leaks to the media or "whistle-blowing". This can ultimately prove damaging to all concerned: to the minister, to the assistant, to the Government, and to the reputation for neutrality of the civil service itself.

Politics and Management

Ministers function within a political environment, an environment from which the public service is intentionally insulated, particularly as regards the selection and appointment of staff. However, the principles of anonymity and neutrality do not isolate the civil service from the broader influences of politics. Public servants operate in an environment which is constantly awash in the realities of political life. The closer a government is to the municipal level, the more political considerations tend to intrude on management action. A provincial civil servant responsible for running a research institute told me,

> I had a disastrous period of working for a minister who felt that he had to direct and approve everything personally, including "routine" departmental management items .... The predictable result was a high degree of paralysis, along with a number of strategies employed by the public servants to bypass the lengthy ministerial approval processes, and thus get on with the job.[44]

While such circumstances may be somewhat extreme, most public servants have experienced them at one time or another in their careers. Politics is always intruding to one degree or another in "administration"; ministers (and, in particular, their political staff members) do not hesitate to exercise their influence over many administrative matters. In short, the idea that there is a dividing line between policy and administration, and that ministers stay on their side of that line, is a fiction. The reality of management in government is as follows.

- Ministers who form part of a new Government will often be inexperienced, inexpert at wielding power, suspicious of the civil service and unwilling to accept advice. It may take 6 to 18 months to establish a relationship of trust with a minister, by which time the minister may be changed. Moreover, as the term of elected Governments advance, ministers become increasingly preoccupied with the issue of re-election (thus, frequently less interested in departmental priorities). Some ministers never trust the public service.

- Frequent changes in ministers must be expected, but will have a generally unsettling impact on departmental operations. Changes in ministers tend to paralyze many aspects of departmental operations – only routine activities are carried out, needed changes are not made and no initiatives are set in motion for fear of misunderstanding ministerial desires or alienating the new boss. Even an experienced minister may need a year or so to get to know a new department well enough to be able to provide effective direction.

- Different ministers will bring to the position different priorities and styles. Some may be interested in the long-term public interest, others concerned only with the short-term personal advantages to be derived from the portfolio. Some may be attracted to the substance of the department's responsibilities, while others may view their present department merely as a way-station en route to a more senior appointment.

- Since ministers have many non-departmental responsibilities, their time for dealing with departmental priorities or learning about the intricacies of programs and policies is at a premium.

- For some ministers, the appearance of what is done may be as important as the substance (or even more important). Some officials, less sensitive to appearances and public impressions and more concerned with "facts", resent what appears to them as political meddling and interference in "rational" solutions to policy problems.

- Departments cannot anticipate clear leadership from most ministers. Since the elected Government may wish to appear all things to all people, politicians often avoid commitment to explicit goals. One of the key challenges of management in government is how to function in this context.

- Ministers pressed by the opposition may have to devote a fair amount of the limited time available for departmental issues to briefings on relatively trivial matters of administration rather than on more substantial policy questions.

- Departments have to live with the realities of two-ended program delivery and the need to process the quantities of relatively unimportant information that constantly flow down from, and back up to, a minister's office.

- Departments have to reach an accommodation with ministerial staff assistants. Although some of these can be very helpful to officials, others with explicitly political goals may well conflict with, and impede the attainment of, the objectives of the neutral public service.

Footnotes

1. Henry Hicks, "Civil servants and politicians—a defence of politicians," *Canadian Public Administration*, vol. 6, no. 3, (September 1963), pp. 267-269.

2. *Ibid.*

3. Quotation attributed to Luis Echeverria by Ronald Buchanan in "The Rising Cost of Austerity," *Maclean's* magazine, 11 March 1985.

4. Lawrence E. Lynn, Jr., *Managing the Public's Business: The Job of the Government Executive*, (New York: Basic Books Inc., 1981), pp. 29-30. See also Irving Shapiro, *America's Third Revolution: Public Interest and the Private Role*, (New York: Harper & Row, 1984), pp. 113-115. On the subject of the Clean Air Act and of industrial safety legislation, Shapiro describes how Congress framed vague, inherently contentious regulations to satisfy the competing interests concerned with the bills. Also see Graham White, "Bill Davis—Intensely Political Style of Governing," *Financial Post*, (20 October 1984), p. 9. An assessment of the career of Ontario's Premier William Davis attributed his success to his "intensely political outlook." What were Davis' objectives? "[O]ne lacks any sense of the Davis government's vision of what Ontario society should look like at the turn of the century .... it is all but impossible to divine a consistent Progressive Conservative ideology .... In consequence, it has not always been easy for labour, business, or any other group to know just where it stands ...."

5. Shapiro, *op. cit.*, p. 33.

6. *Ibid.*, p. 82.

7. Author's interview, March 1987.

8. For a thorough discussion of the role of Cabinet, see any of the many standard references, such as W. Ivor Jenning's classic, *Cabinet Government*, (Cambridge: Cambridge University Press, 1965), or R. MacGregor Dawson, *The Government of Canada*, (Toronto: University of Toronto Press, 1957).

9. MacGregor Dawson, *op. cit.*, ch. 10.

10. Unpublished lecture notes by Dr. Eugene Forsey, "Le Cabinet fédéral," p. 116. See also the *Royal Commission on Government Organization*, vol. 5, (Ottawa: Queen's Printer, 1963), p. 34.

11. Author's interview, November 1985.

12. For a description of the main features of the Canadian Cabinet document process circa 1980, see Audrey D. Doerr, *The Machinery of Government in Canada*, (Toronto: Methuen Publications, 1981), pp. 88-97. For a more recent discussion, see Ian Clark, "Recent Changes in the Cabinet Decision-making System," paper by the Deputy Secretary to the Cabinet (Plans), (Ottawa: Privy Council Office, 6 December 1986).

13. R.G. Robertson, "The Canadian parliament and cabinet in the face of modern demands," *Canadian Public Administration*, vol. 11 no. 3, (Fall, 1968), pp. 272-279.

14. Ian Clark, "A New Look Into the Privy Council Office," notes for a presentation by the Deputy Secretary to the Cabinet (Plans) to the Third Annual Canadian Chamber of Commerce Seminar on Business-Government Relations, (Ottawa: Privy Council Office, 20 December 1983).

15. See Peter Kellner and Lord Crowther-Hunt, *The Civil Servants*, (London: Macdonald General Books, 1980), pp. 211ff.

16. Robertson, *loc. cit.*

17. For an assessment of Canadian central planning, see M.J.L. Kirby and H.V. Kroeker, "The Politics of Crisis Management in Government: Does Planning Make Any Difference?" in C.F. Smart and W.T. Stanbury, eds., *Studies in Crisis Management*, (Montreal: Institute for Research on Public Policy, 1978), pp. 179-195; Richard D. French, *How Ottawa Decides: Planning and Industrial Policy-making 1968-80*, (Toronto: James Lorimer and Company, 1980), p. 157; Christina McCall-Newman, in "Michael Pitfield and the Politics of Mismanagement," *Saturday Night*, (October 1982). On the CPRS see William Plowden, "The British Central Policy Review Staff," in Peter R. Baehr, and Bjorn Wittrock, eds., *Policy Analysis and Policy Innovation*, (London and Beverly Hills: Sage Publications, 1981), pp. 61-89; Douglas Wass, *Government and the Governed*, BBC Reith Lectures 1983, (London: Routledge and Kegan Paul, 1984); Peter Hennessy, Susan Morrison and Richard Townsend,

"Routine punctuated by orgies: the Central Policy Review Staff, 1970-83," Strathclyde Papers on Government and Politics, no. 31, Jeremy Moon, ed., (Glasgow: University of Strathclyde), p. 10, also Appendix A.

18. Douglas Wass, "Cabinet: Directorate or Directory?" in *Government and the Governed*, BBC Reith Lectures 1983, (London: Routledge and Kegan Paul, 1984).

19. *Ottawa Citizen*, 29 March 1985.

20. Maurice Lamontagne, "The influence of the politician," *Canadian Public Administration*, vol. 11 no. 3, (Fall 1968), p. 263.

21. Henry Hicks, *loc. cit.*

22. Kellner and Crowther-Hunt, *op. cit.*, pp. 165-166.

23. *Ibid.*, pp. 211-217.

24. Donald J. Savoie, "The minister's staff: the need for reform," *Canadian Public Administration*, vol. 26 no. 4, (Winter 1983), pp. 509-524.

25. Discussion with author, September 1986.

26. Author's interview, July 1985.

27. See quotation from Lord Soames, Minister for the Civil Service, in Hugo Young, and Anne Sloman, *No, Minister*, (London: British Broadcasting Corporation, 1982), p. 41. "There's more emphasis on tight-ship management . . . . Certainly management plays a far greater part today in the thinking of ministers and occupies ministers much more than it did in my first incarnation as a minister in the fifties and sixties."

28. Allan Blakeney, "The relationship between provincial ministers and their deputy ministers," *Canadian Public Administration*, vol. 15, no. 1, (Spring 1972), pp. 42-45.

29. Former British Prime Minister Edward Heath, in 1977. Quoted in Kellner and Crowther-Hunt, *op. cit.*, p. 204.

30. Speech by former Canadian Prime Minister Joe Clark to the Victoria Chamber of Commerce, 28 February 1983. Quoted in Thomas D'Aquino, G. Bruce Doern and Cassandra Blair, *Parliamentary Democracy in Canada — Issues for Reform*, (Toronto: Methuen, 1983), pp. 43-44.

31. Quoted by Flora MacDonald in "The Minister and the Mandarins," *Policy Options*, (September/October 1980), pp. 29-30. See also Henry Kissinger, *White House Years*, (Boston: Little, Brown and Company, 1979), chapter III: "Any statesman is in part the prisoner of necessity. He is confronted with an environment he did not create, and is shaped by a personal history he can no longer change . . . . [T]he convictions that leaders have formed before reaching high office are the intellectual capital they will consume as long as they continue in office . . . . The public life of every political figure is a continual struggle to rescue an element of choice from the pressure of circumstance."

32. *Ibid.*

33. Similarly with prime ministers. See Jeffrey Simpson, "The PM's Strategy," *Globe and Mail*, Tuesday, 26 January 1988, p. A6.

34. R.G. Robertson, *loc. cit.*, p. 272.

35. Lord Bridges, "The relationship between ministers and the permanent departmental head," *Canadian Public Administration*, vol. 7 no. 3, (September 1964), p. 276.

36. Blakeney, *loc. cit.*

37. Lord Bridges, *op. cit.*, p. 279.

38. See D'Aquino *et al.*, *op. cit.*, p. 43, also Kellner and Crowther-Hunt, *op. cit.*, pp. 211ff.

39. Kenneth Kernaghan, "Power, Parliament and Public Servants in Canada: Ministerial Responsibility Reexamined," *Canadian Public Policy*, vol. 3, (Summer 1979), pp. 383-396.

40. For a summary of auditing functions and practices in 10 western countries, see the *Report of the Independent Review Committee on*

the Office of the Auditor General, (Ottawa: Information Canada, 1975), Appendix II, pp. 129ff.

41. Cited in Donald J. Savoie, *loc. cit.*, pp. 509-524; see also Thomas D'Aquino, "The Prime Minister's Office: catalyst or cabal?" *Canadian Public Administration*, vol. 17 no. 1, (Spring, 1974), pp. 55-79.

42. Cited in Savoie, *loc. cit.*, pp. 519-520.

43. *Ibid.*, pp. 514-516.

44. Letter to the author, February 1987.

Chapter Five:
The Role of the Department Head

The Context for the Job

Recent decades have been unsettling ones for department heads.* A 1985 study of accountability in Ontario noted a prevailing climate of uncertainty about "what the scope and emphasis of responsibility in each portfolio should be and what counts for a job well done."[1] To understand the job of the department head, it is necessary to understand its environment. The head is, of course, subject to the usual traditions of the public service such as anonymity, neutrality and ministerial responsibility. However, in addition, there are special pressures on the top public service post. First, the deputy minister has to accept the difficulties involved in functioning between political and bureaucratic cultures. Next there are the uncertainties associated with the multiple accountabilities of the position. Third, there are the

---

* As there are several different ways of describing the position of the head of a government department, the terms "deputy minister", "DM" or "department head" in this chapter will be used interchangeably to designate the position; they are equivalents of permanent secretary, permanent undersecretary, or undersecretary of state.

difficulties arising from the policy of rotating deputy ministers which has afflicted some jurisdictions.

Between the Politicians and the Bureaucrats

Many deputy ministers emphasize the difficulties of working between two environments with different values and methods of operation. Above, there is the political culture, where optics and impressions are often more important than "objective" reality. Below there is the bureaucratic environment, composed of large administrative operations that rely on stability, constancy of purpose and professional, "rational" analysis of public issues. Ministers have cause to worry about perceptions; but perceptions will not make highways accident-free, get pension cheques out on time or cure disease.

The deputy minister functions "like a hinge between the political world and the administrative world."[2] The job involves a host of ambiguities. Perhaps most severe are those associated with a change in the party in power, when a Government appears uncertain of its direction or when ministers are being changed from portfolio to portfolio. One deputy, who when interviewed was in this situation, spoke with some passion of the difficulties of the job:

> [U]nlike the private sector, you wind up at the top levels being subordinate to someone who may have no business knowledge, no experience in management, who has never run a big bureaucracy, and who may have very different values from you. The deputy minister is at a point of extraordinary tension between the two universes .... The provision for changes of minister in government is almost like institutionalized unfriendly takeovers in business. The new minister may not know you, may come from a different background, and may have different objectives ....

> A deputy minister is extremely vulnerable — for example, you may get an incompetent minister to serve, or you may invest a lot of time and commitment in a major program thrust and then face a new Government or minister who wants to go in a totally different direction. Or you may suddenly find yourself reassigned to a portfolio that is not of great interest to you .... If, as a senior official, you do a hell

of a good job, this may or may not be to your advantage tomorrow.[3]

Relationships with the minister are greatly dependent on the personalities of the two incumbents, and upon the circumstances at the time. One deputy noted that when he took over his department, the minister had already been in place for several years and knew the department and its programs intimately. The deputy had never worked in the department before. "My first priority was to gain the confidence of the minister. My second had to be to get to know the department."[4] Jack Pickersgill, who served as a top public servant in Ottawa before turning to politics, has cautioned against any attempt to codify the ministerial-deputy relationship: "As a minister, I had four deputies and my relationship with each depended far more on his temperament and method of work than on any set of rules."[5]

Inevitably, given the differences in the backgrounds of many ministers and department heads, there can be sensitivities and frustrations in their relationships. Asked about his relationship with a certain minister, Paul Claudel, former Secretary General at the Quai D'Orsay in Paris once lamented:[6] "Mon ami, quand je lui parle, il ne m'entend pas. Et quand il m'entend, il ne me comprend pas. Mais quand il me comprend, il oublie."*

Accountabilities

Some authors cite the multiple accountabilities of the deputy minister's job as its most challenging aspect. Exhibit 5-1 illustrates the reporting relationships of a department head.[7] A deputy minister is usually appointed by the prime minister, (in the U.K., the minister appoints the permanent secretary on instructions from the prime minister), but his or her principal role is to serve a minister. This creates a "ménage à trois" — a three-cornered relationship among the prime minister, the minister and the deputy minister.[8] In addition, the deputy minister is, in reality if not in principle, accountable to the

---

* "My friend, when I speak to him, he doesn't hear me. And when he hears me, he doesn't understand. But when he understands, he forgets."

EXHIBIT 5 - 1

ACCOUNTABILITY RELATIONSHIPS

*Formal and informal accountability relationships
of a Canadian Deputy Minister*

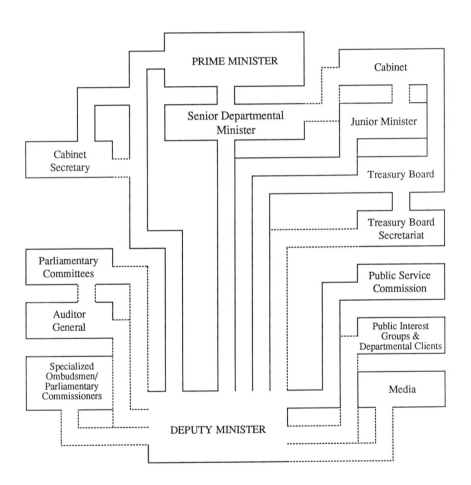

BEYOND THE BOTTOM LINE (1988)

Solid lines denote formal relationships, usually embodied in legislation.
Dotted lines denote informal relationships. Depending upon the issue and the
circumstances, some informal relationships may be more important than some formal ones.

Secretary to the Cabinet (or the Deputy Minister to the Premier in a provincial context). The nature of this accountability depends to a considerable extent on the seniority of both parties: new Cabinet secretaries may be cautious in dealing with old hands with solid reputations. Nonetheless, as the secretary exercises considerable influence over appointments and advancement, every deputy is careful with this relationship.*

In addition, the DM is formally or informally accountable to the Treasury Board and to the Public Service Commission (or their equivalents). In Canada, certain aspects of both these accountabilities are framed in legislation and flow directly to the DM, not through the minister. The DM is also answerable, if not formally accountable, to numerous other constituencies, including the Public Accounts Committee, other parliamentary committees, the auditor general, special commissioners or ombudsmen, and interest groups concerned with his or her department. The DM must likewise contend, from time to time, with the intrusive interest in his or her department's affairs that may be manifested by the Prime Minister's Office (PMO), or in some jurisdictions, with occasional attempts by the minister's personal staff to interfere in departmental administration.[9]

The Lambert Commission reported that because there are so many of these accountabilities, "[s]ome deputies maintain that they are, in effect, accountable only to themselves, and claim to measure their performance against their own standards of excellence."[10] In Britain, William Plowden, Director General of the Royal Institute of Public Administration, has alluded to the problem of "unaccountable permanent officials guided by some inexplicit private conception of the national interest."[11]

The ambiguities associated with the deputy's job mean that it is not an occupation for someone who wants a clear mandate. Typical

---

* This illustration depicts the accountability relationships of a Canadian DM. In Britain, because of the formal accountability of the permanent secretary to the Public Accounts Committee of Parliament, a solid line would have to be drawn to this Committee. Conversely, in the U.K., the solid line from the department head to central agencies might have to be replaced by a dotted line, because the relationship between the department head and central departments is not legislated in Britain as it is in Canada. (See chapter 6.)

was the deputy who observed, "No one ever told me what I was supposed to do." (Recently appointed DMs in Ontario, however, did note that when the new Liberal administration took power under Premier David Peterson, the Premier took the unusual – and appreciated – step of discussing mandate personally with the DMs he appointed.)[12] Effective deputies seem comfortable with ambiguity. They figure out what needs to be done – for the PM, the minister, central agencies, the department, and others (and also for their own self-preservation). Then they get on with doing it.

Rotation of Postings

An increasing concern in some jurisdictions during the 1970s was that of tenure of deputy ministers (not a problem in Britain since there, permanent secretaries usually serve from five to ten years in one post, usually at the end of their careers in government). In both Ottawa and Toronto, however, there has been a tendency to move top officials within two or three years of their appointments and sometimes even more often.* (A former Canadian deputy minister of Finance noted in an interview with the author that in the century from 1867 to the early 1970s, there had been seven deputies at Finance; and that in the subsequent decade or so, there had been seven more.)[13]

Perhaps changing DMs is thought by the prime minister to help put a new face on the government, rather like shuffling ministers. Some politicians may have a somewhat perverse fear that if DMs are too knowledgeable about their departments, their expertise could overpower that of their ministers. Some turnover of deputy ministers

---

* A 1985 study at the provincial level observed, "In general, deputies no longer spend their careers in the ministries they head. [Of 28 deputies in Ontario as of April 1984,] ... only eight have had previous experience in their present ministries...." At the federal level in Canada, the Lambert Commission found that, "[n]early 80% of present [1979] deputies received their initial appointment since 1971, and about half have neither worked at lower levels in the department they administer, nor have had the benefit of significant similar experience in related fields before joining the federal government." Subsequent research indicated that as of 1986, the average time spent by DMs in their jobs in Ottawa was 1.4 years.

is doubtless needed to prevent some departments' policies from becoming too set in a particular course.

The policy of rotation may also have been legitimized by a belief about general management that gained a certain currency in the 1960s and 1970s. According to this thinking, management ability consists of certain aptitudes which are universally adaptable to any kind of job. Good general managers can be groomed and then moved about anywhere without damage to the organizations they lead. This concept has since been largely discredited, and there is increasing recognition of the need for managers to know the substance of their organizations' work if they expect to be effective at their jobs, even at senior levels of the organization.[14]

The policy of rotating DMs is not entirely perverse. According to some DMs, in at least one province, deputies are sometimes rotated in order to ensure that a policy decision is seen through to implementation. Where a new policy cuts across departments, its implementation will necessitate initiatives in several organizations. If old methods of thinking are deeply entrenched, an elected Government may find that simply instructing existing deputies in these departments to change their priorities or behaviour yields an inadequate response. To counter this problem, the Government may assign a trusted DM to, in effect, "chase" a policy issue from department to department until all the required changes have been instituted — a process which will be facilitated by the periodic rotation of DMs. "In some jurisdictions, if you watch the pattern carefully, you may find that only certain DMs are rotated, while others may stay in their jobs for years."[15]

No doubt there are some circumstances that necessitate changing DMs from time to time. However, routine, wholesale rotation of deputy ministers is highly disruptive. The problem is compounded by Cabinet shuffles. The resulting turbulence in departments can lead ultimately to cynicism and a "who cares?" attitude to work. A middle-level official who joined the government of Ontario for a few years on secondment from academia described the view from below.

> [What] I found most difficult to fathom was the change in leadership . . . . Four months after I joined the ministry, the deputy minister left. We had to adjust to the style and

philosophy of the new deputy. Approximately a year went by, the minister left and a new minister came. Another year went by, the second deputy left and a new one came. I ended my secondment with government in June 1983. Had I stayed a week longer, I would have been on to my third minister; and six months later, my fourth deputy!

Since each change represents a shift in course, you wonder about such things as commitments, goals, mandates, policies, morale – and the effective serving of the citizens . . . .[16]

The Lambert Commission argued that switching deputies every two years or so "is a partial but vital explanation of low morale in the public service, drifting departments, and the lack of a sense of direction in management. Unless deputy mobility is reduced, the prospects for sound management are slim."[17]

The Policy Role

Much has been written about the job of the deputy minister.[18] The classical view, predominating up to the 1980s, characterized the role almost entirely in terms of the responsibility to serve the minister in the field of policy formulation.

Department heads often use "policy formulation" as a shorthand meaning "the provision of advice to the minister". Deputy ministers and permanent secretaries interviewed for this chapter consistently placed "liaison with the minister" or "serving the minister's needs" among their top priorities – advising a minister how to cope with emerging issues or explaining the likely consequences of courses of action the minister may be contemplating. Some of these initiatives may involve matters of great consequence, such as a redesign of the country's social benefits program, a new tax system, or a major international commitment in the field of defence. Other questions upon which the minister may want advice will be more mundane, but will nonetheless be sensitive as they could lead to political embarrassment, and perhaps a question in the House. For example: who should be appointed to a particular position? Where should a certain speech be delivered? Who should be invited to a conference? What stance should be taken in negotiations with an interest group?

Many of these questions will concern political relationships between the minister and the several constituencies to which he or she is accountable.

Nominally, the advice of the deputy minister is restricted to matters outside the realm of politics, but inevitably, to some degree, "objective" advice on questions of public policy and counsel on matters of a political nature become intertwined. Deputy ministers have to learn how far to go in approaching the political aspect of the minister's work. However, the political dimension of policy is inescapable: "To be 'above politics' in public management is a contradiction in terms."[19]

While deputies and permanent secretaries are careful to point out that they do not make decisions, it is taken for granted that they are actively involved in policy development, and some will even admit that they are involved in assisting ministers on political questions (recognizing that any policy matter will obviously involve political implications). According to the theory of public administration, what deputy ministers do not provide is partisan advice — that is, advice on matters that directly affect the question of re-election of the party in power. (In practice, deputies will from time to time offer advice to ministers on the partisan dimensions of policy options. As one minister said in an interview with the author, "The most useful advice I got was when the deputy would say to me, 'Minister, you can do that if you want, but it will cost you ten seats at the next election!'" However, this type of advice would only be offered when a relationship of mutual trust had been established, and it would almost certainly never be committed to paper.)

In general, being a deputy minister requires a capacity to understand the subtle shadings of meaning surrounding the concepts of "policy advice" (a legitimate and critical part of the job), "political advice" (goes with the territory, but a mine field), and "partisan advice" (formally, off limits). These are shadings ministers, particularly new ones, may have trouble grasping and, at least until they become more conversant with the notion of a neutral public service, they doubtless wonder why deputy ministers sometimes back out of important discussions, or refuse to commit themselves to a point of view in public.

The DM who is effective in this policy role will be expert at building and maintaining personal networks. It is the external intelligence gathered through such relationships, rather than the internal data provided through computerized management information systems, that will constitute the key source of information for much of the DM's policy work. Former Saskatchewan Premier Allan Blakeney cites the story of two deputies who worked for him. One placed little emphasis on monitoring public reactions to the department's programs, while the other "had an intelligence system that was marvelous to behold." In the first case, there were always delegations on the minister's doorstep raising problems; in the other,

> [I]t was a rare day when a delegation met me as minister where the deputy had been unable to brief me in advance on what position the delegation was likely to take, and not infrequently what position individual members of the delegation would assume.... There is not much doubt in my mind which of these departments was best organized to serve the minister and to serve the public.[20]

The DM's principal policy responsibilities relate to his or her department's programs. However, the operation of many of these programs involves interaction with other institutions and other jurisdictions. To be knowledgeable about the positions and plans of other organizations, a deputy minister must maintain appropriate relationships with Crown corporations and other agencies at varying degrees of "arm's length" from the government that may report to the minister directly. Ensuring, on the one hand, that the independent character of these agencies is respected and, on the other, that their activities are at least broadly consistent with government priorities can be a challenging task. It calls for a finely tuned ability to read ministerial intentions (and sometimes, to help guide them), tact, sensitivity to jurisdictional concerns, and a capacity to rein in departmental officials over-eager to provide "policy guidance" to other organizations. Similar capacities and sensitivities are required in the maintaining of relations with other jurisdictions.

Traditionally there has been a strong personal dimension to the job of the deputy minister — the professional's emphasis on the quality of his or her personal advice to the minister. A former secretary to the

THE ROLE OF THE DEPARTMENT HEAD

Cabinet has stated that the role of the deputy includes a responsibility "to point out the traps . . . [and] to include elements of personal judgment about the feasibility of policy or public reaction to it that are similar, in substance, to the kinds of judgment politicians must make."21

As in other professions, what the public service has traditionally valued above all else is that elusive quality called judgment – the skill to see to the heart of an issue, to know when to jump or hang back, to balance conflicting priorities, to notice a parallel, or analogy, where none is apparent, to spot unexpected implications, to summon wisdom rather than formulae to the process of making decisions, to know when experience is a reliable guide to the future and when it is not. Judgment and policy competence have always been inextricably linked, and deputy ministers are expected to possess both.

Some deputy ministers in big departments claim that the traffic of proposals to the minister is too heavy now for the head to be able to place a personal stamp on each one. There are too many issues (and increasingly, too many ministers relating to one department). DMs have to pick the issues in which to get directly involved; the rest of the policy traffic has to run past their office to that of the minister(s) through deputy secretaries or assistant deputy ministers, with the deputy minister kept informed through copies of correspondence and periodic briefings.

This problem is likely to become more common in future. Deputy ministers will have to serve as policy *managers* in addition to being policy *advisers*. They will have to ensure that their senior colleagues are better than ever briefed on the priorities of the Government and the views of other ministers; that the decision-making processes in the department provide for an adequate review of proposals as they move up the chain of command; that the appropriate parties are involved; that sound training, hiring and promotional practices are observed to ensure that competent policy officers develop in the department; and that appropriate consultative relationships are maintained with clients of the department and with other departments. In addition, the DM must make sure that the department has adequate methods of monitoring issues, and a way of setting a policy agenda so that organizational attention is directed to the areas of higher priority. In complex departments a process for planning policy engagement and intervention which is separate from, but linked to, the process of expenditure planning and control, will be increasingly important.

Expenditure Planning and Control

The idea of the deputy minister as a manager has often been equated with his or her responsibilities for the planning and control of expenditures, broadly interpreted to include both money and person-years (a role also called "resource allocation"). The need for the DM to be effective in this sphere has been highlighted, first by a period of dramatic growth in government spending during the late 1960s and the 1970s; and second, more recently, by the need to "downsize" and to supervise the process of "cutback management" that began a little before 1980 in many jurisdictions.

New procedural tools in departments were needed for better expenditure planning and control, especially improved methods of budgeting. Previous budgeting techniques had been designed around line objects of expenditure or inputs. New budgeting techniques — initially program budgeting and later zero-base budgeting — stressed the need for budgets to pertain to the results to be achieved by government programs. Many deputy ministers had to preside over major revisions to the traditional budgeting systems (see chapter 9). The planning process in many departments became more formal and bureaucratic. There was experimentation in several jurisdictions with various forms of centralized planning and with greater use of tools of quantitative analysis.

Throughout the last two decades, control has been a continuing theme. Central agencies urged upon departments the triple virtues of economy, efficiency and effectiveness. Better control was to be attained through the adoption of new forms of performance measurement, through more precision in program goals, through the transition to program budgeting referred to above, through new forms of audit, through new techniques for monitoring policy such as program evaluation, through improved reporting methods to Parliament via the annual Estimates, and through the institution of computerized management information systems. Deputy ministers who were more comfortable with Byron than bytes had to ensure that these new systems were installed professionally and economically.

The principal emphasis in most of the reforms instituted in this period was on the control of resources as objective, or impersonal, "things". Expenditure control is an important component of management, but it is not management. Because so much stress was placed on resource control, many public servants came to interpret management in an impersonal and mechanical way, the economist's or accountant's way.

The difficulties with this conception of management are several and serious: it treats people like factors of production; it obscures the co-ordinating and motivational responsibilities of senior managers; it invites delegation of management to subordinate officials who can install the procedures and make the systems work, thereby suggesting that the deputy minister can somehow get rid of management responsibilities and take refuge in the classic policy role.

Stress upon better administration of resources formed an overlay to the classical policy role of the deputy minister; it did not supersede this role (though some deputy ministers must have thought the demands of "management" were such that the policy role was being eviscerated). The period of change from about 1960 to 1980 transformed the deputy minister into a policy advisor *and* a controller of expenditures and operations. However, the scope of the job clearly extends beyond this. The DM is also the leader of an organization and of the people who work within it, with important responsibilities for morale, motivation and organizational performance.

The DM as Organizational Leader

The literature of management tells us that making an organization function productively involves a variety of mechanical or procedural arrangements — a sound structure, appropriate technology, systems to plan and control expenditures, internal rules and operating policies. However, people have to want to make these things operate, and therefore staff must be motivated, a process requiring skill, patience and persistence that is not susceptible to mechanization.

Because systems and procedures are always imperfect, people inside organizations invariably create their own networks, an informal organization which may complement and even overtake the formal organization. Thus, to build a high performance organization,

161

the right systems must be in place but leaders must also understand what affects attitudes to work. They are called upon to convey a sense of purpose beyond operational goals. They must know how to exploit the subtle dynamics of the informal organization as well as how to operate the formal levers of control. The leader must adapt people to positions, positions to people, and elicit the will to work from colleagues and subordinates, tying their discrete activities into an effectively-functioning whole, a function described in this chapter as "organizational leadership". This type of leadership requires a subtle understanding of how organizations work.

Elliott Jaques has written compellingly about the economic and social responsibilities inherent in organizational leadership. Using the term bureaucracy in its non-pejorative sense, Jaques argues,

> The general evidence and the most widely held opinion are of course in favour of the view that bureaucracy, in spite of its practical value, tends to become socially and psychologically stultifying.... But this pathology is not necessarily inherent in bureaucracy *per se*. Bureaucracy is not only a rational and efficient type of human organization,... but it has the potential to provide the setting both for constructive human relationships and for individual creative expression and satisfaction. To gain this creative setting, however, requires that we learn enough about the properties of bureaucratic organization to use and control these institutions and to avoid being controlled by them....[22]

Anyone who has worked in an institution can hardly fail to be struck by the key role of the top executives. And among those executives, the most important is clearly the chief executive. An effective CEO in the private sector can powerfully affect the organizational culture, pick the key people, determine the strategic goals, decide what businesses the company will be in, and manage the sensitive relationships of the enterprise. Such a CEO balances the interests of board directors, top managers, shareholders, and employees, as well as key external relations with customers, governments, unions and competitors. Although there are some important institutional differences between the deputy minister and the CEO, in this regard the requirements of the positions are similar.

THE ROLE OF THE DEPARTMENT HEAD

A recent study has examined the qualities of successful leaders in a variety of settings. The sample of 90 included business chief executives, university presidents, the head of a government agency, athletic coaches, symphony orchestra conductors, the heads of public interest groups and a non-profit society, and an astronaut. The study was searching for "kernels of truth about leadership — the marrow, if you will, of leadership behaviour."[23] Four themes emerged.

One was a leader's ability to secure attention through vision. "All of the leaders to whom we spoke seemed to have been masters at selecting, synthesizing, and articulating an appropriate vision of the future."[24] A related capacity was the ability to communicate that vision effectively, a process involving not just the transfer of information but the richer function of organizing and focusing meaning within the organization, often through the use of images and metaphors. The establishment of a climate of trust was a key leadership function. "Trust is the lubrication that makes it possible for organizations to work." Allied to this was the need for the leader to "position" the organization appropriately — "to design, establish and sustain a viable niche in its external environments."[25] Finally, there was a need for the leader to design and direct the organization in such a way that it was capable of learning and innovating.[26]

This study stresses the importance of the leader's ability to mould the organization and to "empower" other people by pulling rather than pushing them. "It motivates by identification, rather than through rewards and punishments." The study portrays the leader as a "social architect who understands the organization and shapes the way it works."[27] This includes influencing the organizational values and the way people relate in the workplace.

Peters and Waterman describe the leader as a shaper of values, with two functions: that of pathfinder and that of implementer.

> [E]xcellent companies are driven by coherent value systems.... The value-shaping leader is concerned, on the one hand, with soaring, lofty visions that will generate excitement and enthusiasm.... On the other hand,... leaders implement their visions and behave persistently simply by being highly visible. Most of the leaders of the excellent companies have come from operational backgrounds.... [T]hey are comfortable in the field....

They travel more, and they spend more time, especially
with juniors, down the line."28

Although there has been little explicit recognition or analysis of
organizational leadership in the literature on public administration,
the resolution of organizational problems is often a major
preoccupation of deputy ministers, an exercise, of course, complicated
by the DM's relationship with the minister. The minister is, by
tradition and law, the person in overall charge of the department. Yet
public servants know that ministers come and go. When a strong,
effective minister is appointed to a department, he or she may well
assume some of the organizational leadership role. However,
ministers with powerful preconceptions about major policy matters do
not appear to be very common. Many ministers appear to be well
intentioned and reasonably receptive to advice, but relatively
uninformed about the department, with few concrete ideas about
policy. (One deputy minister whose portfolio was apparently seen as a
stepping stone for advancing ministers, said, "I trained a new minister
every year, and I ran the department.")29 In these circumstances, the
organizational leadership role, if it is to be exercised at all, must fall to
the DM whose responsibility it is to ensure a good relationship
between the minister and the department, and to provide intellectual
leadership on policy issues. (Being just a good administrator, without
policy strengths is not enough to be a credible leader.)

Many of the problems of organizational leadership involve people
and how they can be adapted to organizational functions – or vice
versa. The challenge of achieving the right fit between people and
senior organizational responsibilities is often intimately connected to
issues related to the mandate and strategic priorities of the
department. Two illustrations may help to illustrate this point.* In
reviewing her departmental mandate, a deputy minister embarked on
a new course involving a move away from "giveaways" of government
money towards an increased emphasis on the provision of certain

---

* In both examples which follow, minor adjustments have been made to protect the
confidentiality of the organizations and individuals involved. However, both are
based on actual events and the minor changes do not alter the nature of the situations
in any material way.

services to the public. This required changes in some functions and certain aspects of organizational behaviour and a transfer of responsibilities from headquarters to the field offices. One of the deputy minister's senior associates was temperamentally unsuited to the emerging context and was disrupting the operation of the top management group. Additionally, a survey had revealed that many of the employees believed the department could be achieving a good deal more within the existing resources.

The problems of organizational leadership facing the deputy minister were: (1) how to adapt the structure and decision-making processes of the organization to the new mandate, (2) how to transfer power from headquarters to the field in the face of entrenched resistance and the additional hurdle of the resulting reduced pay and status for some officials' (some of whom would have to help carry out the transfer), (3) how to tap the productive potential that employees believed to be latent in the department, (4) how to achieve the right combination of people on the top management team, (5) how to co-ordinate the working of the department by promoting greater sharing of information among different organizational units (which had started hoarding information) and (6) how to make this all happen at a time when there was likely to be a change of the minister.

In another case, a department had commissioned a pilot project to investigate new computer technology that would support all key organizational functions in future. The project had been quite successful, although marred by somewhat erratic leadership, and strained relations had developed between the project team and the rest of the organization. It was clear, however, that the way ahead for the department lay in adopting a new system, a development that would have a major impact on the way the organization worked and on the jobs of its employees. The deputy minister was faced with the problem of integrating the members of the project team into the fabric of the department. He knew that the organization had had a history of indifferent management of change, and there was considerable cynicism about senior management's commitment to address the people-related problems associated with the realignment of jobs. In addition, the proposed integration was vigorously resisted by the project leader, who forecast the collapse of the project and dire consequences for morale if it were put into effect.

In this instance, the deputy minister faced several problems of organizational leadership. His most immediate challenge was how to redistribute responsibilities among the management team members, some of whom were adversely affected by the change. He had to overcome the legacy of cynicism to effect change in a positive manner; he had to resolve technical problems arising from the integration of functions; he had to establish a more positive climate of staff-management relations. It was apparent that the design of the new organization had to include new members in top management if the general fabric of the institution was to be strengthened to cope with certain emerging long-term problems.

Effective organizational leadership requires an understanding of both the subtle ecology of organizations—how they *really* work as opposed to how the organization charts and the flow diagrams say they do—and of the demands inherent in leadership. It is unlikely that many individuals attain the rank of deputy minister without being, or becoming, highly astute about the functioning of organizations and the dynamics of power. It is less clear, however, that all DMs are knowledgeable about, or interested in, how to be effective in their capacity as organizational leaders. Some DMs take this aspect of their responsibilities very seriously, others, either because of other responsibilities or, perhaps, because of personal disinterest, devote little attention to being an effective leader.

Subordinate officials take their cues from the deputy minister on many matters affecting organizational culture and climate. Senior appointments send important messages to staff on all sorts of issues—policy priorities, the degree to which hard work of existing staff is likely to be rewarded, to what extent the DM values open communication among staff, and so forth. Skilled deputies can have a significant impact on their organizations' productivity through their strategies for selecting top officials, the way in which they handle unsatisfactory performers, the degree of attention they give to communication among branches, the time they devote to operational problems (especially those in regional offices), the ways they choose to divide up responsibilities at top levels, the encouragement that they give to new ideas, the priority they accord to issues such as career development which are typically important to staff, or the ways in which they recognize outstanding achievement. Conversely, DMs who are unaware of or uninterested in this aspect of their role may have little impact — indeed, through oversight, their impact on the organization may even be damaging.

In short, organizational leadership is not just policy formulation, nor is it just expenditure control as conventionally understood in government (although it certainly affects productivity). Whether they are aware of it or not, all deputy ministers exercise organizational leadership. It cannot be delegated, though it may be abdicated. Some DMs exercise it consciously and constructively. Some do not.

Responsibilities on Behalf of the Collectivity

Although the main functions of most deputy ministers relate to their department, they are also members of the larger "collectivity" of government. Appointed by the prime minister and subject to central agency policies, they are expected to play a corporate role on behalf of the government as a whole. Such a role may include serving on a special task force investigating some new policy question or perhaps a matter of government organization.

A Canadian DM has observed,

> The PCO [Privy Council Office] is concerned with the performance of the governmental machinery as a collective organism. It expects deputies to look beyond the relatively narrow horizon of their own departmental mandate and interests, even though that area may require the bulk of their time and effort; and to contribute, to the extent they are qualified and free to do so, on matters of an interdepartmental or government-wide nature. Indeed there are some deputy ministers, just as there are some ministers, whose strictly departmental responsibilities are relatively light. Their value to the government rests mainly on the contribution they make outside the area of their specific appointment.[30]

Deputy ministers must always be conscious of their responsibilities to the broader interests of government. Occasionally, it appears that their sojourn with a department may have relatively little to do with the mandate of the organization in question. Some central agency officials clearly think of deputy ministers as being engaged in special projects on behalf of the prime minister or central agencies – the accomplishment of some specific policy goal within the department's mandate, or applying across several departments. A DM working under direction of this sort would obviously bring a rather different orientation to his or her position than the one who arrived with no instructions, or perhaps simply a general encomium to "get on with the job".

Fitting the Deputy to the Department

The kind of individual needed to fill the deputy minister's job will be – or should be – heavily influenced by the degree to which a department's role is advisory or administrative. The mix of policy and administrative responsibilities varies considerably from department to department. When governments played a less proactive role in the economy, and departments were less complex, perhaps the distinction between policy departments and administrative departments was clearer than it is currently. In many departments today, the line between policy and administration has become less clear; most so-called policy issues are larded with managerial considerations. The "pure" policy department is becoming more and more rare; those that do exist principally to advise ministers are getting bigger and harder to manage; and in the great majority of departments, policy and administration are entangled.

Policy competence and managerial skill do not always go hand in hand. Clearly there are a few key positions in government at the deputy minister level where the ability to develop policy must take precedence over the traditional managerial capabilities associated with running a large organization. However, for most departments today this ability alone is not enough. That many central agency officials now recognize this is an important step forward, since a deputy minister's position cannot be divorced from its managerial and leadership responsibilities. Contemporary DMs have to be selected, not only for their incisive skills of analysis, but also for their ability to provide vision and direction for staff and to operate organizations that may be highly complex and far-flung.

The Deputy as CEO

Outside the public service, most individuals are more conversant with the role of the private-sector chief executive officer (CEO) than with that of the deputy minister. Even within the public service, many public servants are sufficiently removed from the deputy minister's office that they are more familiar with business models than those of government. Thus a comparison of the CEO's job with that of the DM may shed further light on the nature of the DM's role.

Studies portray the successful CEO of a large enterprise as an individual with a strong self-image who typically exhibits excellent abilities to take charge, who interacts with constituencies supportively, provides permission to take risks to those inside the corporation, and is a thinker as well as a doer.[31] Effective CEOs are able to set directions in circumstances of great uncertainty and can impart a vision to their subordinates that transcends simple ambition and material advantage. They are concerned with the organizational climate and culture; they are dedicated to their particular enterprise; and they work constantly at promoting, disseminating and reinforcing key beliefs and values that both define what the corporation is and how people are expected to work within it.

CEOs are effective at balancing the long- and short-run interests of their corporations. They maintain networks both inside and outside the company; they elicit co-operation from people over whom they do not exercise any direct authority; they husband their time but are not afraid to become immersed in detail when it matters. Particularly in the larger corporations, there is evidence of a growing involvement of CEOs in important issues of public policy that have a bearing on their companies. One survey of 40 CEOs by the American academic, George Steiner, argues that the public dimension of the CEO's responsibilities will occupy more and more time in years to come, and Shapiro, the former Chairman of Dupont, strongly advocates such involvement. Such conclusions suggest that there may be a gradual convergence between some of the characteristics of top jobs in industry and in government.

A review of the literature on CEOs, suggests that there are many similarities between the role of the CEO and that of the deputy minister; there are also several important differences:

DMs, in public, are more self-effacing. Many deputy ministers would be uncomfortable describing themselves as the chief executive officers of their departments. They would point out that the minister is in charge, setting policy and assuming responsibility publicly for all the key decisions. However, the business CEO position is full-time: a minister has many preoccupations other than departmental affairs. Rather, the minister's position is more comparable to that of a chairman of a board of directors who provides overall direction to the organization but has other interests outside it. But a CEO, the minister is not.

Nonetheless, deputy ministers are constrained by tradition and training to give the limelight to the minister. The conventions of public service neutrality and anonymity dictate that no matter how strong the DM's influence may be, the minister should be front and centre when the interests of the department have to be defended or represented in a public forum or the media. Thus DMs do not "personify" their departments publicly in the same way that an effective CEO might represent his or her corporation.

DMs must spend more time on vertical relationships. An important difference between the job of the deputy minister and that of the CEO lies in the nature of their upward relationships. In business, a company president can usually expect to report to a board of directors whose objectives for the company are broadly similar to his or her own. Further, members of the board are usually content to let the president run the company within the broad parameters set by the board. Other than in exceptional circumstances such as, say, a takeover bid, managing the relationship with the board of directors occupies a relatively small percentage of most presidents' time.[32] While Steiner's study of American CEOs indicates that boards of directors are becoming more probing in their relationship with top corporate management,[33] business boards are miles away from demanding the kind of care and feeding that ministers require from their departmental staffs — and, in particular, from the deputy minister.

The minister may have different objectives from the department. Unlike the CEO, the deputy minister has to face the fact that his or her superior may not fully share the objectives of the department. The department and its officials usually expect to be around for many years. Longer-term plans can be seen through to fruition, and satisfaction derived from their achievement. Ministers can expect to be around until the next election, or for an even shorter time, until the next Cabinet shuffle (in Canada, these have been occurring recently more than once a year). Departments have a vested interest in the status quo; ministers may not. Ministers may bring little personal interest to their current portfolio, seeing it as a stepping stone to some preferred position; officials have often spent much of their careers in their department, and may have a powerful personal commitment to its objectives. Ministers worry about re-election; officials do not. Thus, the community of interest and relative stability that typically prevail between most boards of directors and company presidents may not exist, or not to the same extent, in the relationship between a minister and his or her department; the deputy minister has to act as a moderator or interpreter in this relationship to a much greater degree than does the CEO.

Deputy ministers function in a much more ambiguous context. In addition to the relationship with the minister, the deputy minister has key relationships that must be maintained with the prime minister, the PMO, PCO, the minister's staff, other central agencies, the Public Accounts Committee and other powerful groups. Many DM positions are highly political, using "political" not, of course, in the sense of party politics, but in the sense that the DM must be adept at defining and balancing priorities among several interests, and at maintaining relationships with many more constituencies than those with which most CEOs must cope.

CEOs have more opportunities to define organizational beliefs and values and instill a corporate vision. As noted previously, recent literature on the private sector has made much of the importance of values and vision in contributing to the performance of successful businesses. Irving Shapiro asserts that the management process "hinges on vision and on the ability of the people at the top to capture support and build institutional loyalty."[34] Another study of CEOs asserts, "the leader ... comfortably holds himself or herself out as a model. By doing so, he or she offers clarity of direction for himself or herself and for his or her followers ...." "All [CEOs] assumed that they were responsible for making their organizations the best .... They tied people together by repeatedly urging their tradition and their own values and by policing their enforcement." The concept of vision is linked to this; vision is more than objectives or specific goals: "Meaning is derived from purpose beyond goals."[35]

The effective CEOs appear to see themselves as institution-builders, not just profit-makers. They have a deep affection for their particular organizations. Building enduring corporations is seen as

> ... a continuous socialization process: the training and indoctrination of those new to the organization, the continuous articulation and reinforcement of what customs, values and beliefs the organization held and what models it honoured...[36]

In addition, although they may well find the decision difficult, an effective CEO is prepared to sideline members of the top management team who do not support his or her vision.

In government, all deputy ministers must function within the broader framework of public service values — neutrality, objectivity, anonymity. To some extent, these traditions constrain the scope for organizational leadership. A senior official who anticipates a possible change of government has to be careful, even within the department, not to become too powerfully identified with a particular policy position or point of view. A former DM has written of how the deputy must "try to develop a feeling of participation in policy formulation, without invoking a sense of paternity for ideas. After all he is seeking to develop a range of possibilities for his minister to consider...."[37]

Some practical constraints also arise from the relationship with the minister. The demands imposed on ministers by Parliament make it difficult, while the House is in session, for the minister or for some deputy ministers to be absent from the capital for more than a few days. The greater number of interests and constituencies with which the DM must interact, relative to the CEO, also reduces the time available for management by wandering around. (Peters and Waterman relate with approval the case of one chief executive who, with his top management team, was on the road for 65 per cent of his time during the first 18 months of his tenure. This option would not be feasible for the head of a government department with sensitive policy responsibilities.) Deputy ministers are also constrained from perceiving themselves as institution-builders, perhaps, by the practice of rotating DMs; (they may tend to be more committed to the public service as an institution rather than their current department).

Despite all these impediments, DMs can play a value-shaping and institution-building role at the level of the individual department. Subtly, and sometimes not so subtly, the deputy minister can shape his or her organization. Being in the public service does not make the task impossible, but it certainly makes it harder and less predictable.

CEOs have more power to allocate resources. A key role of the CEO is the allocation of organizational resources. Here a distinction needs to be drawn between the deputy minister's personal prerogatives and his or her sphere of influence, and between committed "organizational" resources and public resources generally. The deputy minister's personal authority relative to organizational resources probably comes out well behind that of most CEOs. The DM's main responsibility is to ensure control of resources previously allocated by the minister or Parliament. Even minor reallocation can be a policy matter outside the deputy's own authority. Central agencies will seek to channel 'free' resources into deficit reduction or some pressing priority in a department unrelated to the one with the 'surplus' funds. The DM is also constrained in the allocation of people. The public service is typically fraught with regulations and rules related to classifications, reorganizations, staffing and dismissals. In short, as a manager of committed resources, the deputy minister's role is highly — some think too highly — circumscribed.

On the other hand, some (not all) deputy ministers' influence, (as opposed to direct authority), over resource allocation will far exceed that of most CEOs. Some exercise huge influence over key aspects of macro-economic policy, and over decisions in social policy, transportation policy or resource development that involve massive investments by both public and private sectors. Paradoxically, it is sometimes the smaller departments that have the largest role in resource allocation in this sense.

DMs' influence on public policy may compensate for their lack of control over organizational resources. It might seem that, given organizations of roughly equal size, a deputy minister has less power than a CEO. This would be an accurate conclusion were it not for the central importance of the policy function and the influence which it accords deputy ministers, a function that finds no parallel in business. What encourages many deputy ministers to continue to work in an environment so replete with ambiguities and frustrations is the potential to exercise, as part of the democratic process, a significant impact on important public policy. (One former minister, who later became a top business executive, believed that over the long term, the job of the deputy minister was both more satisfying and more influential than that of most ministers.)[38]

In addition, most deputy ministers are motivated by the intrinsic interest of the work and by the rather old-fashioned belief that they are engaged in something worthwhile, something of public benefit. Interest in public policy is like an obscure tropical disease which, once acquired, can never be entirely shaken. Opportunities for public service are, of course, not restricted to "the public service". Nonetheless, for deputy ministers, and indeed for many public servants, interest and a sense of service are two of the main reasons that keep them coming back to work through the travails of ministerial incompetence or self interest, central agency nit-picking, budget cuts and public vilification of their profession.

Conclusion

In principle, the department head's position comprises four elements: policy advice, expenditure planning and control, organizational leadership and special assignments on behalf of the collectivity of government. The balance among these elements will depend upon the mandate of the department and the type of legislative framework within which it operates, as well as the temperament and experience of both the current minister and the deputy and the direction received from the PM and central agencies. There is, in fact, no such thing as *the* job of the DM, but several rather different sorts of jobs at the head of department level, all of which exist within a common framework of traditions and constraints.

Because of changes over the course of the last generation or so, many DMs have had to become policy managers to some extent, rather than personal advisors to their ministers on all policy questions. While expenditure planning and control are key aspects of management, they represent only a portion of the DM's managerial responsibilities. Whether a department is small or large, the DM has important organizational leadership responsibilities. Greater priority must be devoted to the organizational leadership dimensions of the DM's role. (The literature of public administration emphasizes the classic policy role and, more recently, the procedural, expenditure management-related elements of the job, but it devotes little attention to the leadership aspects.)

Morale in many government organizations has suffered from the turbulence of the last two decades: the tide of rising public expectations and the politicians' inability to stem it, the heaping of new responsibilities upon the public service in the 1960s and 1970s, the difficulties experienced by senior officials in digesting unfamiliar managerial responsibilities and in making the transition to an era of big government, the enlarged mandates being accorded to auditors general leading to fresh public criticism of public servants; and more recently, governments' attempts to cut back on expenditures and person years while assuring the public that programs will not be eliminated and that levels of service will not be impaired.

Governments need leaders who are able and willing to guide their organizations through these difficulties, who have the commitment and interest to see to the human dimensions of management, who are prepared to work at sustaining morale and providing a sense of "purpose beyond goals" for their staff. It is up to the department head, with the help of his or her key associates, to assume this challenge.

Footnotes:

1. Price Waterhouse Associates/The Canada Consulting Group, "A Study of Management and Accountability in the Government of Ontario," (Toronto: January 1985), p. 55.

2. Robert Normand, "Les relations entre les hauts fonctionnaires et le ministre," *Canadian Public Administration*, vol. 27 no. 4, (Winter 1984), p. 528. Author's translation.

3. Author's interview, July 1985.

4. Author's interview, February 1987.

5. J.W. Pickersgill, "Bureaucrats and politicians," *Canadian Public Administration*, vol. 15 no. 3, (Fall 1972), p. 420.

6. Quoted in David Kirkwood, "Accountability and the deputy minister," *Optimum*, vol. 13 no. 2 (1982), pp. 17-29.

7. Normand, *loc. cit.*

8. Cabinet secretaries also recommend dismissals, as revealed by the leaked letter from Paul Tellier to Prime Minister Brian Mulroney recommending the firing of a DM who was thought to be "insensitive to the minister's role" and to have "lost control of the department ...." *Globe and Mail*, "Letter urging high-level firing leaves top mandarin red-faced," 28 February 1987.

9. Hubert Laframboise, "A note on accountability," *Optimum*, vol. 13 no. 4, (1982), pp. 82-84.

10. Royal Commission on Financial Management and Accountability, (Lambert Commission), *Final Report*, (Ottawa: Supply and Services Canada, 1979), 188ff. See also Ted Hodgetts, "The Deputies' Dilemma," *Policy Options*, vol. 3 no. 4, (May-June 1983), pp. 14-17.

11. William Plowden, "What prospects for the civil service?", *Public Administration*, vol. 63 no. 4, (Winter 1985), pp. 393-414.

12. Author's interviews, September 1986 and March 1987.

13. For statistics on DM tenure, see Price Waterhouse/Canada Consulting Group, *op. cit.*, p. 54; Lambert Commission, *op. cit.*,

p. 194; and Gordon Osbaldeston, "The myth of the mandarin: the role of a deputy minister in the parliamentary-cabinet system of government," (undated: 1987?), available from the National Centre for Management Research and Development, University of Western Ontario, London, Ontario.

14. See in this connection, John P. Kotter, *The General Managers*, (New York: The Free Press, 1982). Also Robert L. Katz, "Skills of an effective administrator," in *Paths Toward Personal Progress*, reprints from *Harvard Business Review*, (1983), pp. 23-33, esp. the "Retrospective Commentary," pp. 34-35. Kotter's study debunks the notion of the generalist business manager who can step into any organization and run it.

15. This interesting insight into the workings of government arose at a seminar held to discuss a draft of this chapter at the annual meeting of the Institute of Public Administration of Canada in Vancouver, September 1986.

16. George Bancroft, "Government Hitch," in the University of Toronto *Graduate*, vol. 12 no. 2., (November-December, 1984).

17. Lambert Commission, *op. cit.*, p. 194.

18. In addition to references cited elsewhere in this chapter, see V.S. Wilson, "Mandarins and kibitzers," *Canadian Public Administration*, vol. 26 no. 3, (Fall 1983); Hugo Young, and Anne Sloman, *No, Minister*, (London: British Broadcasting Corporation, 1982); Honourable W. Darcy McKeough, "The relations of ministers and civil servants," *Canadian Public Administration*, vol. 12 no. 1, (Spring 1969); Privy Council Office, "The Office of Deputy Minister," (Ottawa: June 1984), unpublished paper describing statutes and conventions that define the role of the deputy minister in Canada; Herbert Balls, "Decision-making: the role of the deputy," *Canadian Public Administration*, vol. 19 no. 3 (Fall 1976); Mitchell Sharp, "The Role of the Mandarins," *Policy Options*, vol. 2 no. 2, (May/June 1981); Robert D. Carman," Accountability of senior public servants to Parliament and its committees," *Canadian Public Administration*, vol. 27 no. 4, (Winter 1984).

19. Gordon Chase, and Elizabeth C. Reveal, *How to Manage in the Public Sector*, (Don Mills: Addison-Wesley, 1983), p. 93.

20. Allan Blakeney, "The relationship between provincial ministers and their deputy ministers," *Canadian Public Administration*, vol. 15 no. 1, (Spring 1972), pp. 42-45.

21. Gordon Robertson, "The Deputies' Anonymous Duty," *Policy Options*, vol. 4 no. 4, (July/Aug. 1983), pp. 11-13.

22. Elliott Jaques, *A General Theory of Bureaucracy*, (London: Heinemann, 1976), pp. 1-21.

23. Warren Bennis and Bert Nanus, *Leaders: The Strategies for Taking Charge*, (New York: Harper & Row, 1985), p. 26.

24. *Ibid.*, p. 101.

25. *Ibid.*, p. 43; also ch. III, esp. pp. 153-156.

26. *Ibid.*, p. 158; pp. 158-203.

27. *Ibid.*, p. 80; p. 110.

28. Thomas J. Peters and Robert H. Waterman, *In Search of Excellence*, (New York: Harper & Row, 1982), pp. 287-288.

29. Author's interview, February 1987.

30. David Kirkwood, *loc. cit.*, pp. 17-26.

31. The view of the CEO employed here is informed by several sources. These include the Bennis and Nanus study, *op. cit.*, a variety of journal articles, mostly from the *Harvard Business Review*, as well as the following books: Henry Mintzberg's *The Nature of Managerial Work*, (New York: Harper & Row, 1973), which examines five top managers' jobs (including two public sector posts, but no government departments); Peters and Waterman's *In Search of Excellence, op. cit.*, a study of top-performing U.S. corporations; George Steiner's *The New CEO*, (New York: Macmillan, 1983), which looks at the future of CEOs in big companies; Irving Shapiro's *America's Third Revolution*, (New York: Harper & Row, 1984), reflections on CEOs' public responsibilities; John Kotter's *The General Managers, op. cit.*, which analyzes the jobs of 15 managers with multifunctional responsibilities in nine U.S. corporations, and Levinson and Rosenthal's *CEO — Corporate Leadership in Action*, (New York:

Basic Books, 1984), a study of six leaders of major American companies.

32. Mintzberg, *op. cit.*, p. 45 indicated that seven per cent of his CEOs' time was spent with company directors; only one per cent of mail came down from "above" in the organization and only two per cent of what the CEO originated was directed to superiors.

33. Steiner, *op. cit.*, p. 69: "Not many years ago the typical board meeting dealt with operational and financial matters. Today, the territory covered is far wider and the probing is more penetrating."

34. Shapiro, *op. cit.*, p. 251.

35. Levinson and Rosenthal, *op. cit.*, pp. 263-286.

36. *Ibid.*

37. A.W. Johnson, "The role of the deputy minister," *Canadian Public Administration*, vol. 4 no. 4, (December 1961), pp. 363-373.

38. Discussion with author, 1970.

Chapter Six:
The Accountability of
Department Heads

In the attempts to improve management in various jurisdictions, one of the recurring preoccupations has been accountability, especially in Canada, where some authors have suggested that it is the most important issue in public administration at present.[1] In Britain, the Fulton Commission devoted several pages of its report to the need to establish "accountable units" in the civil service "where individuals can be held personally responsible for their performance."[2]   More recently, two controversies, one associated with "whistle-blowing" by an official, Clive Ponting, during Britain's Falklands war, and the second with the Government's refusal to allow civil servants to appear before Parliamentary committees in the context of the "Westland Affair", have drawn the issue of accountability of both ministers and civil servants into sharp focus.[3]

There are three levels of accountability in government. The first concerns the relationship between the public and the elected Government. The processes, systems and conventions for ensuring accountability here are the province of political science as well as public administration. They include the written constitution and amending formulae, electoral procedures, parliamentary procedures and rules of order, constitutional conventions, the role of the opposition parties and parliamentary committees, ministerial responsibility and freedom of information legislation. Accountability at this level takes effect through the basic processes of democracy itself; the concept of responsible government is the public sector analogue to that of shareholder supremacy in the private sector.

The second level has to do with the accountability of the individual department of government and, in particular, of its head. For many years, there was not much concern about accountability arrangements at this level. However, the dilution of ministerial responsibility (see chapter 4) has led to greater concern with accountability at the level of the head of the department. How can top officials be held to account for their performance? And to whom should they be accountable? Concern over departmental accountability has been heightened by the growth in the size and complexity of government. In earlier days, informal, back-of-the-envelope approaches to accountability were perhaps adequate; today, something more formal is required. At the root of the problem are the ambiguous, multiple reporting relationships of department heads: how can anyone be held to account if he or she serves so many masters?

The third level has to do with accountability within individual departments. Just as there is a need for appropriate mechanisms and relationships at the level of the deputy minister or permanent secretary, there is a parallel requirement to ensure that officials below this level are held to account for their performance. How can this be done in the fluid environment of the public service?

Defining Accountability

Like the concept of management, that of accountability is often misunderstood. In normal English usage, accountability is a synonym for responsibility. It is a type of relationship that comes into existence when an obligation is taken on by an individual (or corporate entity), such as the responsibility to assume a role or discharge a task. Accountability is obviously facilitated to the degree that the task is clearly defined; the more vague and ambiguous the responsibilities, the more problematic it becomes to try to hold individuals to account for performance.

THE ACCOUNTABILITY OF DEPARTMENT HEADS

A key aspect of accountability is the notion that the individual assuming the responsibility is bound to give account. The obligation assumed in an accountability relationship thus contains two elements: the substantive task or responsibility, and the obligation to report back on how it is discharged. In such a relationship, arrangements may legitimately be made by the person conferring the responsibility to monitor what is going on, and to step in if required. Accountability may also extend to the idea that a sanction, (such as a loss of certain privileges or other disciplinary action) may be exercised if the responsibilities are not properly discharged.*

In summary, accountability involves the following elements:

(1) a responsibility conferred

(2) an obligation to report back on the discharge of that responsibility

(3) optional monitoring to ensure accountability

(4) possible sanctions for non-performance.

Strictly speaking, accountability describes a state or absolute condition that either does or does not exist. It is like pregnancy: you either are, or are not, accountable; you cannot be more or less accountable. However, there are obviously many different ways in which individuals may be monitored or held to account. Thus, colloquially, we speak of individuals being "more or less" accountable in different situations. Accountability in this sense becomes a synonym for control. This narrow usage of the word can lead to problems, as we shall see.

"Accountability" is employed in rather different ways. Accountants and auditors focus on the control aspect: financial auditors are trained to look for documentary evidence of procedural

---

* It is arguable whether sanctions are an intrinsic part of accountability, as there are certainly situations where people feel they are morally or ethically accountable but where they are not subject to conventional sanctions (i.e., those imposed by some outside party.) In bureaucratic contexts, however, accountability involves the exercise of direct or indirect authority, and this usually includes the possibility of sanctions in the form of reprimands or discipline if duties are not properly performed.

rectitude, and deem accountability to exist only if an "audit trail" provides written records of why decisions were taken, who was involved, what judgments were brought to bear on a situation, whether authority was exceeded, and so forth.

There are two problems with this approach. First, it places entirely too much emphasis on documentation. Written reports for purposes of control have their place, but not in all circumstances and in all management functions. A good manager controls operations by considering such factors as the environment of the organization, the kind of people working there, the tasks being performed, and to what degree different sorts of control information are needed for decision-making. That is, the good manager chooses the approach to control most suitable to the circumstances.

The ways of establishing control over an organization are limited only by human imagination. Man has been given five senses for collecting information, and nowhere is it prescribed that the manager is confined to the use of computer printouts, financial reports or other types of documentary evidence to keep in touch with operations. For example, as Peters and Waterman suggested in *In Search of Excellence*, management by wandering around (MBWA) can be a powerful method of asserting control in a non-threatening and personal manner.[4] There may be other methods of control more effective and cheaper than being buried in a mountain of paper.

A second and more serious problem with the narrow view of accountability as control is the danger of responding to "accountability problems" with the wrong policies. Accountability in its broader sense has to do with *delegation* — with conferring responsibility for the execution of a task, with ensuring clarity of role and of reporting relationships, and with devising convenient and effective arrangements for monitoring or reporting back. To the manager, accountability is sound when people know to whom they are accountable and for what, and when the manager is able to follow up on progress. Sound accountability in the sense of effective delegation lies at the core of management.

An Overdose of "Accountability" in Ottawa

If accountability is equated with control, then the solution to an "accountability problem" is clearly to increase controls rather than to deal with the broader aspects of accountability such as clarity of reporting relationships or objectives. The Canadian government fell into this trap in the 1970s.

As mentioned in the Introduction (see also appendix 1), the government responded to its "accountability" difficulties during the late 1960s and 1970s by multiplying the rules to be followed by departments, installing a complex operational performance measurement system, developing audit units within departments, adding special staffing rules and requirements related to bilingualism and affirmative action, enlarging the mandate and staff of the auditor general, introducing program evaluation, and creating a new central agency, the Office of the Comptroller General, to audit the state of management in departments. These were typical government responses, increasing the overhead and the burden of control on departments. As Shapiro has observed, "Government manages, not wisely, but too much."[5]

A top Canadian public servant, Hubert Laframboise, noted in 1982 that "'accountability' has become a faddish word in public service jargon, and accountability is spoken of as if it had never existed."[6] Elsewhere, Laframboise counted nine different accountabilities at the deputy-minister level, making a complex job even more difficult. He became sufficiently exercised by what he perceived as the systematic attempt by Michael Pitfield, the then Secretary to the Cabinet, to obscure the prerogatives and responsibilities of line departments that he took the unusual step of publicly criticizing Pitfield. He suggested that the Secretary was attempting to spin a "web of authorities" around deputies, throwing them off balance, "never sure of the authority they should give precedence to," in order to make them "docile and receptive to ... guidance."[7] Others have criticized the initiatives taken in the name of accountability during the 1970s as excessively theoretical, attempting to make neat and tidy what is inherently disorderly. As another DM commented in regard to the reforms of the Pitfield/Trudeau era, they seemed to have been implemented according to the criterion, "That's all very well in practice, but does it work in theory?"[8]

Undoubtedly, one of the key problems of accountability in the public service is that of devising objective and reliable methods of assessing performance, which would make it easier to "hold people to account". However, in my view, the issue which most profoundly affects performance and productivity in government is not an insufficiency of controls, but rather, the apparent inability of governments to delegate in such a way that officials feel they have the tools they require to perform their jobs effectively and to make adequate use of their own judgment and initiative.

The challenge facing governments is to try to create an environment within which objectives can be less equivocally defined and more consistently adhered to, where responsibility is more clearly focused, and where authority commensurate with responsibility is delegated so that officials can get on with their jobs without constantly looking over their shoulders or checking with central agencies. As Laframboise observed, "In the overall, the pursuit of simplicity and speed, and the reduction of clutter and obfuscation should dominate. Freedom to act, with control measures only to the extent needed to prevent impropriety and gross errors and to ensure general responsiveness to government policies, is the manager's dream."[9]

Had the Canadian government recognized this during the 1970s, it might have paid more attention to the delegation of authority to departments from central agencies, and it might have tried to reduce the confusion of roles and mandates that characterized an increasingly large and complex public service. As it was, however, the government did precisely the opposite. While calling for "improved accountability," it in fact made the situation worse by creating several new "co-ordinating" central agencies which confused and diffused authority in critical policy fields.

If a department has an ambiguous role arising from ambiguous legislation; if its scope for action is encumbered with overlapping mandates from other agencies; if its top officer is accountable in half a dozen different directions; if its objectives adjust with each change of minister; if the DM is reassigned every couple of years; if (as also happened in Ottawa in the 1970s) the role of the deputy minister is clouded by the appointment of "associate deputy ministers" with direct access to the minister, then making the organization subject to various types of investigations and audits may do something by way of control, but it does little to "increase" or "improve" accountability in the basic sense. Indeed, if someone speaks of increasing accountability, it is likely that their objective is to increase control and to centralize power – the converse of delegation.

The "Finan-centric" View of Management

Misunderstandings of accountability have been fostered by the prevalence of what might be called a "finan-centric" view of management, which places accounting and financial administration at its heart, subordinating all other dimensions of management. This misconception is common in government, although it is not confined to the public sector. Shapiro has noted how, for a time, business also went down the "blind alley" of believing that finance was the "hub of the management wheel".[10]

The finan-centric view of management equates accountability with control. An organization afflicted with the finan-centric ideas about management usually displays some or all of the following characteristics:

- authority for the approval of expenditures resides in the financial division of the organization rather than with line managers, thereby emasculating the role of the line manager. The financial people, in effect, run the organization;

- "management information" is thought to mean "financial information," leading to information systems that take insufficient account of managers' needs for non-financial information, and that are thus inadequate as a basis for operating control;

- responsibility for the management of information systems is allotted to the senior financial manager. (Typically, the consequence of this arrangement is that financial systems take precedence over systems needed to support other functions of the organization, including its principal line responsibilities);

-   financial auditors are employed to investigate and recommend solutions to general problems of operational management, on the premise that financial training is the key competence required to analyze management issues;

-   budgets and plans are prepared by officers in the finance division rather than line managers.[11]

The Accounting Officer Concept

It is clear that the accountability of the deputy minister or permanent secretary is fundamental to the question of accountability generally in the public service. If there are problems at this level, they will filter down to lower levels of the organization and create further difficulties there. Several ways have been suggested for coping with what has been called the "lack of accountability" of department heads – or more accurately, the multiplicity of reporting relationships for these officials. All have disadvantages. One proposal is to create a new accountability on administrative matters, directly from the deputy minister to a parliamentary committee. This involves an extension of the accounting officer concept which has been in place in Britain for many years. A second option is to create a stronger formal accountability to central agencies on management matters. A third is to reinforce the prevailing relationship to the minister. Each of these is discussed below.

In Britain an accounting officer is appointed by the Treasury for each parliamentary vote. This officer, usually the permanent secretary of the responsible department, is

> held responsible to Parliament and answerable to the Committee of Public Accounts for the formal regularity and propriety of all the expenditures out of his assigned vote, and for the efficient and economical administration of the organization that he leads. The accounting officer concept helps to establish a distinction between accountability for overall policy . . . and accountability for sound administration.[12]

As accounting officer, the permanent secretary is expected to appear on request before the Public Accounts Committee of the House of Commons to answer questions related to his or her department. The minister is not involved, nor expected to appear at these Committee sessions unless matters of policy are broached. Unlike all other matters of administration or policy, the permanent secretary's relationship to Parliament in the area of financial management does not flow through the minister responsible for the department. The accounting officer concept presumably evolved from the view that financial prudence and propriety are not matters upon which there is, or should be, partisan rivalry. These are questions upon which the House of Commons as a whole shares a united view, and thus on such an "objective" matter there is no violence done to the principle of ministerial responsibility by allowing a permanent secretary to appear before a committee of the House unsupported by his or her minister.

Recently the scope of the accounting officer concept has been informally widened in Britain. The definition of financial management has been expanding, and with it, the purview of the Committee of Public Accounts. When public accounts committees were first created, good financial management meant ensuring that proper accounting procedures were being followed and that due prudence and propriety were being observed in the control of funds voted by Parliament. However, the extension of the mandates of government auditors into value-for-money questions has broadened the field of inquiry of the Public Accounts Committee. Increasingly, the border between financial management and management generally has been obscured. Financial management is now interpreted to mean almost any aspect of administration. In Britain, (and also in Canada), this has made the discussions of the Committee more interesting than in previous years. Opportunities for finding out about departmental activities have improved, as have opportunities for embarrassing the Government. Furthermore, public accounts committees and legislative auditors are pressing for constant enlargement of their mandates; for example, a study commissioned by the Canadian Comprehensive Auditing Foundation has, somewhat predictably, urged that these committees (and the auditors which support them) should have the power to inquire into all aspects of administration and some areas of government policy as well.[13]

To some extent, the accounting officer concept exists already in Ottawa. Although the formal personal accountability of the deputy minister for departmental finances is not enshrined in law, the practical reality is that deputy ministers do appear before the Public Accounts Committee, and they are not always accompanied by their minister. They are expected to answer questions about any matter of departmental administration, but to avoid matters of policy.

It has been suggested that the present informal arrangements should be formalized, both by a former Secretary of the Cabinet and by the Lambert Commission.[14] In principle, it seems difficult to find fault with a proposal that would increase the involvement of members of Parliament in reviewing how tax revenues are spent and in bringing them closer to the delivery of operational programs — which is, after all, the level at which government affects the great majority of the population. However, there are problems with the accounting officer concept.

First, it is not entirely apparent what problem the proposal to formalize the DM's accountability to the Public Accounts Committee is supposed to be solving. It does not clarify the deputy ministers' multiple reporting relationships; it does not suggest that this new approach should supplant existing relationships, but simply adds yet another line of accountability to the many that already afflict DMs. In fact, this proposal promises to make their accountability relationships even more uncertain and potentially contradictory. Committees are usually imperfect and unpredictable organisms to which to be accountable, especially in situations where committee members play politics from time to time, drawing civil servants into controversy simply in order to make headlines.

The proposal, in fact, provides yet another method of monitoring the activities of the public service, and perhaps another increase in control. Serious doubts have been expressed about the idea by top officials from two Canadian provinces. Bob Carman, a former Secretary to the Management Board of Ontario, has asked: Are elected representatives, already overloaded, likely to devote much time to assessing departmental administration? Will the review process be balanced or simply a demoralizing recital of weaknesses? Will it be necessary to hire yet another group of auditors to support the committees' investigations?[15] More fundamental concerns have been raised by a deputy minister of finance from the Province of Quebec, Robert Normand.

> A trend in recent years has been that certain legislation directly attributes powers to deputy ministers or to the presidents of organizations, to the exclusion of the minister. I believe that this new tendency should be checked rapidly, for it leads to the institution of an administrative power parallel to, or even exclusive of, that of politicians, and it requires, as a result, a direct accountability of the deputy minister or the head of agency to elected assemblies. This tendency transforms officials into second-class politicians who become competitors of their immediate superior.16

A proper assessment of the merits of the proposal requires that a distinction be drawn between accountability and answerability. To be accountable implies a formal relationship and, as noted previously, it also implies a prior act of delegation direct from one party to another. This condition does not apply in the relationship between a deputy minister, or permanent secretary, and public accounts committees. A fundamental principle of responsible government is that the line of accountability runs from Parliament to Cabinet to the public service, not directly to the public service from Parliament.

As long as the mandate of public accounts committees was restricted to "financial management," and as long as financial management was interpreted as referring to prudence and propriety, there was not much danger in the notion that DMs should be in some way accountable to public accounts committees. But now, as the mandates of such committees range farther afield, the proposal that there be a direct accountability between a committee of Parliament and a departmental head becomes more problematic. The distinction between policy and financial administration upon which the British accounting officer concept is premised is more difficult to maintain.

Splitting a department head's accountability between Parliament and his or her minister on the basis of the distinction between administration and policy, (or hanging the DM's accountability to a parliamentary committee upon such vague and pliable concepts as "financial administration" or "value-for-money") could have serious consequences for the principle of neutrality and anonymity of the civil service. Developments could ultimately lead to entanglement of deputy ministers in policy debate and an impairment of their relationship to their ministers. (Political entanglement is, indeed, what has been happening to the Canadian auditor general who has, in the opinion of one astute observer, been losing sight of the policy-administration distinction, engaging his office in political issues outside the mandate of his office, and damaging the principle of civil service anonymity).[17]

However, department heads should be *answerable* to the Public Accounts Committee, as indeed they are to other parliamentary committees and to the public generally, for the effective administration of their department.[18] Having a deputy minister appear before the Public Accounts Committee to report on questions of administration does provide one more window on the public service that will help the public know what is going on inside the bureaucracy. If the relationship is not enshrined in law, and if the deputy minister is not made formally accountable to tread the line between a vaguely defined concept of financial administration and matters of policy, the relationship will perhaps be less open to abuse and less likely to lead to constitutional difficulties. Deputy ministers would retain more flexibility to draw their ministers into the committee meetings if they feel that the discussions are ranging beyond appropriate bounds. Moreover, if some precedents or ground rules are established which would discourage MPs from trying to drag public servants into controversy for their own purposes, appearances of department heads before such committees could help to improve the credibility of the public service and increase mutual respect between officials and politicians.

To summarize, I see no problem with DMs appearing before parliamentary committees to answer questions related to departmental administration; but given the various interpretations of the meaning of value-for-money, it seems to me more consistent with constitutional tradition to leave these relationships informal (answerability) rather than formal (accountability). Making the deputy minister accountable to a public accounts committee along the lines adopted by Britain does not solve the basic problem of multiple reporting relationships, in fact it tends to make a confused situation worse. If accountability is to be clarified, the objective should be to channel, not diffuse, the formal relationships of department heads.

Accountability to Treasury

A second "solution" to the problem of department heads' accountability is to create, or reinforce, a direct accountability to central agencies on all management matters. An experienced Canadian official, Michael Hicks, has suggested that there are two lines of accountability that run from Cabinet to the deputy. The line on policy runs directly through the minister to the deputy; a separate line, on management, runs from Cabinet to Treasury Board and thence to the department. Hicks and others have pointed out that, in Canada, there is already legislation related to certain matters of financial administration and personnel where the deputy is directly accountable to the Treasury Board, and not through the minister. "[T]he Board, not his minister, is the effective boss of the deputy head in the vast area of personnel administration"; while in finance, the "function of setting out the rules under which the departments operate is also assigned to the Treasury Board by Cabinet." Hicks concludes: "On balance, it would probably be best to make each deputy minister responsible in law to Treasury Board, not to his minister, for all his management functions, not just those personnel functions now delegated."[19]

The central difficulty with this proposal (which would probably be vigorously resisted by most department heads) is the idea that *all* management accountability should flow to the Treasury Board. Such a split rests on, and indeed would codify, the dubious distinction between policy and management. As long as management is seen as a set of central agency rules and procedures to be followed, then there is a possibility that this suggestion could be implemented. However, its effect might be to perpetuate the "impoverished" understanding of management criticized by observers of the British government.[20]

Consider an example. The government must make a policy decision regarding the incarceration of certain classes of criminal offenders. Suppose the decision was that, subject to good behaviour, more serious offenders were to be moved to less secure types of institution as their prison term progressed; and suppose this decision necessitated the construction of a new medium security prison. The location of that prison would clearly be a matter of administration, not policy, but hardly an issue upon which the deputy could be accountable to a central department or a committee of ministers rather than to his or her own minister. Similarly, it might be argued that the cost of the prison was an administrative matter that could be safely left to the department in consultation with the Treasury Board; however, if there were cost overruns or problems with contracts, it is the responsible minister who would be criticized, not a faceless central agency of government. The basic difficulty, once again, is the impossibility of drawing a clear distinction between policy and administration.

Accountability to the Minister

A third solution to the problem of department heads' accountability would be to make the minister responsible for holding the incumbent to account for management performance. The attraction of this proposition lies in its apparent simplicity and clarity. The DM's relationship to the minister would be reinforced, and it would be the minister's responsibility to make sure that the DM observed sound management practices. Unfortunately, the very simplicity of this proposal is its weakness. The fact is that relying exclusively upon the minister — even with extra staff support — to deal with the complexities of supervising management performance in a big government department would usually not be practical.

Most ministers have a very big job simply learning how their department works. Many have little knowledge of administration. To expect a minister to become conversant with the collective dimensions of government management — such matters as government approaches to financial management, contracting policies, the merit system and other subtleties of personnel management in the public service, performance measurement or program evaluation — would be both unrealistic and unreasonable. Thus, "solving" the problem of a department head's accountability for management by consolidating all aspects of this accountability in his or her ministerial relationship is unlikely to serve much purpose.

Moreover, making the department head accountable to the minister overlooks the fact that the DM is also accountable to the PM. A final objection is that, if pressed to the limit, this proposal would remove the accountability of DMs on matters of appointment to such agencies as Canada's Public Service Commission. The accountability of DMs to central agencies or independent commissions on personnel matters has been created in order to protect the principle of appointment on merit. If all managerial accountability was to be placed in the hands of ministers, the merit principle might soon be prejudiced and with it, the concept of a neutral, professional civil service as well as other collective management policies of the government.

Political Accountability with Central Agency Backup

There appears to be no formula whereby the complex relationships of the department head might somehow be reduced to something clearer without entailing basic changes to parliamentary government. I do not think that the ambiguity of the DM's position has led to problems in public administration so serious as to warrant a major reshaping of existing institutions and conventions.

Unless parliamentary government itself changes, the complexity of the environment within which DMs and permanent secretaries function is not going to change. Within this context, the primary accountability to the minister should be maintained, not just for policy but for many questions of management as well. The DM or permanent secretary must be responsible in the first instance to his or her minister for results within the context of any general direction provided by the prime minister. It is up to the minister, responding through Cabinet to Parliament, to define what those results should be.

Since it seems unlikely that prime ministers will delegate their prerogative to appoint deputy ministers and permanent secretaries, department heads will have to continue to function within the context of the "ménage à trois" described by Robert Normand in chapter 5. Clearly, the job of the DM is made easier if the PM and the responsible minister agree on the tasks to be accomplished. But this depends upon the relationship between the PM and the minister, something that cannot be planned or systematized. In some jurisdictions the prime minister sends a "mandate letter" or some similar document to a newly appointed DM. Premier Peterson's meetings following his election with his new deputies in Ontario (see chapter 5) also helped to clarify expectations. Such documents and meetings should ideally reflect the input and agreement of the minister whom the PM assigns to the department, but obviously there is no way of ensuring that this will be the case.

When expectations are unclear or contradictory, it is difficult to hold a top official to account in a systematic way. However, the whole notion of systematic accountability, applied at the top level of organizations, has a certain mechanical cast to it that does not accord easily with the realities of executive level management. There is not a lot of evidence, even in the private sector, that company presidents or vice presidents are "held to account" according to some list of specific objectives negotiated at the start of each year. The process of accountability in the executive suite, in my experience at any rate, is generally rather subtle, unstructured and inexplicit. In this, as in other spheres of management, it is important not to import private sector myths into public service management.[21]

In the context of the public service, even if the PM, the minister and the DM invest the necessary time to set a suitable mandate for the DM, there is no guarantee that the mandate will continue to be relevant as time passes. A senior deputy minister in Ottawa describes his experience:

> The fact is, senior jobs change all the time. I recall doing a letter setting forth my goals at the beginning of one year. On February 29, the Prime Minister resigned. In June a new Prime Minister took over the Government. My agency was abolished; shortly thereafter there was an election which resulted in a change of Government. This was a bit atypical, but not so far off the mark for senior positions. The idea of objectives set in stone for the senior public service is counterproductive.[22]

Unless the nature of parliamentary democracy changes fairly drastically, DMs are going to have to continue to function in an uncertain, ambiguous context.

Because of the fluidity of the political environment and because of most ministers' disinterest and inexperience in management matters, another line of accountability for DMs is required. A lesser accountability, but an important one nonetheless, should exist from the head and his or her department, to a central agency (or agencies) on issues of management. The central agency should reach agreement with the DM or permanent secretary on management improvements, and perhaps negotiate a contract or mandate letter touching these issues with new DMs. It should ensure that there is internal coherence among the regulations and standards of performance established for finance, personnel management, information management, internal audit, evaluation, and so forth. As discussed in more detail in chapter 7, it should ensure that the nature of the accountability framework established for the department is appropriate to its particular functions.

The relationship that prevails between central agencies — particularly Treasury departments — and line departments is fundamental to the problem of improving management in government. For many years, the principal emphasis in this relationship was upon the restraint of expenditure, and in some jurisdictions this continues to be the main priority. However, changes are occurring. Some Treasury departments are realizing that this emphasis creates a confrontational relationship with departments and necessitates the development and policing of a host of detailed regulations within which departmental managers must function. Some Treasury departments are envisaging their roles in a rather different light, and in several jurisdictions this change of emphasis has been accompanied by a change of title from "Treasury Department" (or something similar) to "Management Board." These developments are discussed in the following chapter.

Summary

This chapter has attempted to clarify the meaning of accountability in government, and to review its application to the job of the deputy minister (and permanent secretary). The concept of accountability is often confused with that of control, when, in fact, it is really concerned with effective delegation. The finan-centric school of management, which perceives financial administration as a sort of template for management in general, places too much emphasis on the control element of accountability. This has led to an unreasonable emphasis on documentation for documentation's sake and upon formal, structured methods of ensuring accountability. If management in government is to improve, it should not be hobbled by restrictive or misinformed ideas about accountability; rather it should move toward greater clarity and simplicity in relationships wherever this is possible.

The "problem" of accountability at the level of the deputy minister and permanent secretary will not be solved by the establishment of a formal accountability from the deputy minister or permanent secretary to a committee of Parliament. Such an arrangement would simply add to the relationships of the DM, perhaps making the job even more ambiguous than it already is. There is little to be gained through formalizing the DM's relationship to public accounts (or other parliamentary) committees: this relationship is best left informal.

The difficulty of holding DMs to account has to do with the ambiguity of their responsibilities and the multiplicity of their reporting relationships. This is unlikely to change; it is inherent in the job.

This chapter concludes that the DM should remain primarily accountable to his or her minister, subject to whatever overall guidance may be provided from the prime minister through mandate letters, occasional meetings and the like. A secondary accountability to a central agency (or agencies) can legitimately and usefully supplement the ministerial relationship. Such an accountability should encompass many, but not *all*, aspects of management. There is no way to establish a clear line of demarcation between policy and management, and it is unrealistic to suggest that ministers have no influence on departmental management. A DM's accountability for managerial matters flows *both* to the minister and to central agencies. This is not very neat, but it is the reality of parliamentary government.

Footnotes:

1. See, for example, Marsha Chandler and William Chandler, "Public administration in the provinces," *Canadian Public Administration*, vol. 25 no. 4, (Winter 1982), pp. 580-602, and P.M. Pitfield, "Bureaucracy and Parliament," speech to the Ottawa Kiwanis Club, 25 February 1983. "Of all the areas that require improvement . . . the one that most officials would regard as fundamental is that of accountability."

2. *Report of the Committee on the Civil Service, 1966-68*, (Fulton Report), vol. 1, Cmnd. 3638, (London: Her Majesty's Stationery Office, 1968), pp. 51-54.

3. See Clive Ponting, *The Right to Know: the Inside Story of the Belgrano Affair*, (London: Sphere Books Ltd., 1985) for Ponting's view, and "Civil Servants and Ministers: Duties and Responsibilities," Cmnd. 9841, (London: Her Majesty's Stationery Office, July 1986) for the Government view re the Ponting Affair; on Westland, see "The Defence Implications of the Future of Westland plc.," Cmnd. 9916, (London: Her Majesty's Stationery Office, October 1986), and "Accountability of Ministers and Civil Servants," Cmnd. 78, (London: Her Majesty's Stationery Office, February 1987). The latter document is a White Paper that seeks to establish firm ground rules for appearances by officials before committees of Parliament.

4. Thomas J. Peters and Robert W. Waterman, *In Search of Excellence*, (New York; Harper & Row, 1982), p. 122.

5. Irving S. Shapiro, *America's Third Revolution: Public Interest and the Private Role*, (New York: Harper & Row, 1984), p. 96.

6. H.L. Laframboise, "The future of public administration in Canada," *Canadian Public Administration*, vol. 25 no. 4, (Winter 1982), pp. 507-519.

7. H.L. Laframboise, "A note on accountability," *Optimum*, vol. 13 no. 4 (1982), pp. 82-84. The nine authorities were the PM, the minister, parliamentary committees, COSO (a committee of senior officials charged with reviewing DM performance and compensation), the Comptroller General, the Treasury Board Secretariat, the merit system of the Public Service Commission, the Auditor General, and assorted other agencies "charged with

ensuring that government operations . . . are meshed together in
a smoothly coordinated manner."

8. Author's interview, November 1985.

9. H.L. Laframboise, "The future of public administration in
Canada," *loc. cit.*, p. 519.

10. Shapiro, *op. cit.*, pp. 250-251.

11. Finan-centric thinking in Treasury reportedly made it necessary
to call the initiative to improve management in Whitehall, the
"financial" management initiative, rather than the
"management improvement initiative." As one senior official
said, "[The FMI] was a program for line managers. We called it
"financial management" tactically in order to engage the direct
interest and support and muscle of the Treasury who have
traditionally not shown particular interest in management, but
who do show interest in financial control . . . . It was a way of
provoking a stronger engagement by the Treasury . . . ." Author's
interview, May 1985.

12. *Report of the Independent Review Committee on the Office of the
Auditor General*, (Ottawa: Information Canada, 1975), p. 76.

13. John J. Kelly and Hugh R. Hanson, *Improving Accountability:
Canadian Public Accounts Committees and Legislative Auditors*,
(Ottawa: Canadian Comprehensive Auditing Foundation, 1981),
p. 13.

14. Pitfield, "Bureaucracy and Parliament," *op. cit.*; Royal Commission on Financial Management and Accountability, *Final
Report*, (Ottawa: Queens' Printer, 1979), p. 189.

15. Robert D. Carman, "Accountability of senior public servants to
Parliament and its committees," *Canadian Public Administration*, vol. 27 no. 4, (Winter 1984), p. 554.

16. Robert Normand, "Les relations entre les hauts fonctionnaires et
le ministre," *Canadian Public Administration*, vol. 27 no. 4,
(Winter 1984), p. 537. (Author's translation.)

17. See Sharon L. Sutherland, "The politics of audit: the federal
Office of the Auditor General in comparative perspective,"

Canadian Public Administration, vol. 29 no. 1, (Spring 1986), pp. 118-148.

18. With respect to permanent secretaries' appearances before other parliamentary committees, the British government has reaffirmed that "they do so on behalf of, and subject to their duty and accountability to, their Ministers . . . . While it may often — indeed generally — be convenient that departmental evidence . . . should be given by civil servants, it is the Minister in charge of the Department concerned who is accountable." See "Accountability of Ministers and Civil Servants," *op. cit.*, pp. 1-2.

19. Michael Hicks, "The Treasury Board of Canada and its clients: five years of change and administrative reform, 1966-71," *Canadian Public Administration*, vol. 16 no. 2, (Summer 1973), p. 196. See also *The Office of Deputy Minister*, (Ottawa: Privy Council Office, June 1984) — a good summary of the legal framework surrounding the position in Canada.

20. Les Metcalfe and Sue Richards, "The Impact of the Efficiency Strategy," *Public Administration*, 62, (Winter 1983), pp. 439-454. "Government is struggling with an impoverished concept of management. We do not suggest that there are no individuals holding sophisticated ideas about management, but those ideas are not yet in good currency; they do not get a ready hearing. Most civil servants define management too restrictively." (p. 441)

21. See in this connection Gordon Osbaldeston, "Job Description for DMs," *Policy Options*, vol. 9 no. 1, (January/February, 1988), p. 36.

22. Author's interview, November 1985.

Chapter Seven:
Central Agencies and Departments
Creating the Environment for Management

Next to the character of the elected Government, the factor most affecting the practice of management in government is the relationship between central departments or agencies and line departments. The traditional posture of most central agencies toward departments seems to be one of control. Every review of management practices in government leads to a fresh examination of this relationship, usually resulting in pleas for greater delegation to departments.

Why Delegate?

Central agencies don't want to see too much authority in the hands of departments because of a number of legitimate concerns: they worry that departments will spend money on programs for which adequate parliamentary authority does not exist, or whose benefits have been overstated, whose long-term implications have not been thought through, or whose costs have been underestimated. Central agency officials have no lack of such examples. Departments do not always properly analyze the need for new programs or initiatives, especially when under the influence of a strong minister determined to respond to constituents' demands; and they sometimes delude themselves when promoting a new initiative which they believe to be in the public interest.

Given their proximity to the political level of government, central agency officials want to protect ministers from embarrassment, which has led to a "better-safe-than-sorry" philosophy. They know that some top departmental officials occupy their positions primarily by virtue of their policy skills, not their managerial competence. Delegating into a void is a risky business. Unless central agency officials believe that a department is effectively administered, they are reluctant to provide greater authority.

Another reason why delegation proceeds slowly is that some central agencies perceive themselves as the custodians of the government's collective or corporate interests. As noted in chapter 4, most elected Governments do not come to power with a grand design or corporate strategy for the country as a whole, nor do they evolve one while in power. In practice, the "collective interests" which central agency officials wish to protect very often mean "expenditure restraint". A government is a little like a large family in which one member worries about income and the remaining members spend. The economizer is constantly having to fend off new spending propositions. Treasury department officials sometimes have a Horatius-at-the-bridge attitude toward their job: all other departments and ministers want to institute costly new programs; only the Treasury stands between them and financial disaster for the government. The "interests of the collectivity" translate into any plausible argument that the Treasury can devise which may make it difficult for spending ministers and departments to get a new program underway.

Another reason for the retention of power at the centre derives from the evanescent nature of much of what government departments produce. The benefits from such activities as research into animal diseases or pesticides, establishing standards for the conduct of economic activity (such as the adoption of the metric system), regulating air traffic or providing services to new immigrants or to veterans of previous wars are not readily quantified. Government agencies have no ready standard by which to gauge the value of their activities or to compare their benefits. Ministers are loath to cut existing programs, and they have an understandable tendency to want to improve and expand them, which leads to constant pressures for more money. The problem, in these circumstances, is how to build checks into the system.

Some central agency officials see themselves acting as a sort of surrogate for market forces. Business products and services have to stand up to competitive pressures; government programs have to stand up to the rigours of Treasury analysis. The action of the market makes business "lean and mean". Treasury officials see it as their role to ensure that government programs are operated on a similar basis: no frills, no surplus staff, just the essentials. Since departmental officials usually believe that they have already done a careful review of program costs and benefits, they often accuse central agencies of simply second-guessing them in order to justify their existence. They point out that central agencies are protected from public scrutiny and the pressure of client groups, and that "when programs fail because they are underfunded, poorly staffed, or inadequately housed, it is the line manager who takes the fall . . . ."[1]

Working in a Treasury department is not a recipe for popularity. An American line manager expresses many officials' opinions of central agencies:

> In theory, these agencies are designed . . . to aid in allocating resources efficiently . . . to ensure a competent, professional, and productive public workforce; and to realize economies while maintaining quality in the construction of facilities, procurement of goods, and purchase of services. In practice [these] agencies are often obstacles to efficient management in government. To the line manager they are important but sometimes troublesome facts of life . . . . [T]he manager's ability to respond to changing public needs and circumstances can be severely constrained . . . .[2]

Central agencies are in a position of advantage in jousts with line managers, since they have greater access to Cabinet and its committees than do officials of most other departments. This privilege allows them to invoke "ministerial interest" in support of their decision to retain authority. Departments may suspect that ministers' interests in the matter were remote, perhaps non-existent, at least until central agency officials suggested to ministers that they become involved. However, departments are poorly placed to be able to accuse central agencies of stretching the truth on such matters.

In the final analysis, there is not much incentive for central agencies to delegate to departments. Delegation may entail loss of power and prestige. If too much authority is delegated, and something goes wrong, central agency officials run the risk of being criticized by the auditor general or the media for failing to exercise appropriate control over government expenditures. Conversely, if they withhold authority and entangle departments in red tape, they are much less likely to be criticized in a direct sense. The blame will be laid on "the system".

Sorting Out Mandates

The need to attain the right balance of power between central agencies and departments is one of the most important issues of management in government. The classic central-agency stance of retaining substantial control over departments has too often led to

> ... a public service that has been overlaid by an accretion of specific poultices that reflects the intensive pursuit ... of managerial modifications [but which has not] reduced swelling or inflammation in the patient ... a surfeit of specialists, each with his attendant train of subordinate technicians ... more officials ... a plethora of regulations and procedures ... overlapping and lack of clarity in the roles assigned to the respective central agencies.[3]

In the sphere of management, as noted in chapter 2, central agencies are responsible for:

- expenditure restraint and financial propriety

- the design and operation of government financial systems

- protection of the merit principle in staffing, and of the neutrality of the civil service

- promotion of special objectives of the government, particularly in personnel management, that relate to the character of the public service (such as bilingualism or employment equity)

- execution of certain services on behalf of departments, such as pay, collective bargaining or some aspects of staffing, and

- the establishment and maintenance of administrative standards in such areas as contracting, accounting or computer systems as well as special mandates conferred upon them by the Government, such as evaluations of existing policies or programs.

Central agencies have traditionally pursued restraint through three strategies: first, by controlling the overall budgeting process of government; second, by subjecting specific expenditure proposals to rigorous case-by-case scrutiny as they move closer to implementation; and third, by setting in place a wide variety of regulations related to how work shall be conducted (affecting such matters as personnel complements, travel, contracting, staffing practices, the size of offices and the standards of furnishings, salaries and other aspects of remuneration, the classification of positions, entertainment, leave, grievances, and relocation). In the jargon of government, these regulations relate to the "inputs" of government programs. A large measure of expenditure restraint in government is achieved through input control.

Until recently, most central agencies have not seen themselves as being in the business of creating dynamic management environments in departments. A "management environment" – the context within which managers have to work – results from the sum of the regulations and procedures to which departments are subject. An appropriate management environment is one which, on the one hand, makes possible effective organizational performance and enhances motivation and, on the other, sets such controls as are essential in the interests of regularity and economy. (Canadian officials have invented the phrase, "accountability framework"; this concept is similar to "management environment" but places more emphasis on asserting control rather than empowering managers and facilitating performance.)[4]

Many central agencies' structures make it difficult for them to give effect to this role. Often responsibilities for management-related policies are divided among several agencies with no single agency accountable for monitoring the collective impact of all central agency policies, procedures and rules on departmental officials' ability to manage. No official at the centre would be able to know the cross-the-board effect of central agency policies on managers' ability to work in such areas as personnel, finance, contracting, etc. In any event, most Treasury officials view their primary task as expenditure control, which leads to a preoccupation with individual administrative and financial policy objectives, rather than the cumulative effect of such policies at the departmental level.

For example, in the U.K., the creation of management environments in departments is a responsibility that is shared between Cabinet Office and Treasury (although as of 1987 most of the responsibility appears to reside with Treasury). In the sphere of public expenditure, Treasury's principal concern is restraint. "Creating management environments" would certainly be viewed as a rather foreign notion by many Treasury officials whose training was in economics or accounting. One not unsympathetic observer has described Treasury's role as follows:

> Treasury control of public expenditures, to caricature it not wholly unfairly, consists of an annual — or sometimes more frequent — onslaught on departmental totals in a pretty crude attempt to fit them within some overall total, combined with continuous niggling throughout the year on points of often incredibly fine detail. The Treasury's concern is mainly with inputs — resources used — and to a lesser extent with outputs — the number of houses built. [Also] . . . since the abolition of the Civil Service Department in 1981 the Treasury has been responsible for one particular type of input — civil service manpower. It has been in the lead in carrying out the government's commitment drastically to cut civil service numbers, and in exercising very tight controls on any departmental activities which might actually have required more manpower.[5]

This hardly conjures up the vision of Treasury officials wondering whether a new regulation will unduly constrain managerial action, or whether a new procedure is suited to a particular department's mandate! Clearly, it is not easy to reconcile, in the same central agency, the two goals of expenditure control and improved management environments.

On the other hand, when responsibilities are split among several central agencies, other difficulties arise. After observing the division of responsibility among central departments for several years, Lord Rayner, Prime Minister Thatcher's adviser on management matters, came out in favour of greater coordination:" . . . I did not believe it sound in theory or sensible in practice to treat personnel policy, including pay, and manpower control on the one hand as if they were inherently and distinctly different from the control and planning of larger public expenditures on the other."[6]

At time of writing, in the Canadian federal government the responsibility for creating the management environment in departments is quite diffused. Staffing levels, compensation policy and collective bargaining are the responsibility of the Treasury Board Secretariat, along with expenditure control and administrative policy; financial policy and internal audit, program evaluation and some form of management policy (not clearly defined) are the responsibility of the Comptroller General; machinery of government, the responsibility of the Privy Council Office; and supervision of departmental organization, the responsibility of the Treasury Board.

In 1979, the Lambert Commission recommended a consolidation of central agency responsibilities under the supervision of a new committee of Cabinet, a Management Board[7] – a configuration along the lines adopted several years previously in the Government of Ontario. The government drew back from the idea of a Management Board, apparently concerned about the possible concentration of central agency power, and also, undoubtedly, because of the entrenched bureaucratic interests which such a proposal threatened. The Management Board concept has much to recommend it. Ideally, it should represent not just a change in name but a significant change of emphasis in the mandate of the key central agency to ensure that to the degree possible, departmental differences are recognized and managers are empowered to work in the kind of managerial context that is suited to their functions.[8]

As Lambert described it,

> The Board of Management would provide a single focus for the central management of government, consolidating the responsibilities for personnel and financial management. This consolidation would enable the establishment of clear lines of accountability for all facets of management from departments and agencies, through the Board of Management, to Parliament.[9]

Adoption of the title "Management Board" does not guarantee that the need for departmental and functional diversity has been adequately understood. In 1985, the Government of Ontario, one of the pioneers of the Management Board concept, was upbraided for its monochromatic approach to departments:

> There should be a shift by Management Board away from administrative policies and management practices which are uniformly applicable across ministries, and towards elective delegation of authority to individual deputy ministers .... [T]he delegation of authority for particular areas of managerial responsibility to each deputy minister would be tailored to the state of management capabilities in the ministry.[10]

Management Contracts

A key feature of the Management Board concept is the idea of a renewable contract between Management Board and the deputy minister of each department, setting forth the nature and conditions of delegation of authority, and making delegation subject to managerial performance. Such contracts permit a move away from the cross-the-board approach to central agency-departmental relationships which seems to have been the rule in many jurisdictions. The Government of Canada moved in this direction with its policy of increased ministerial authority and accountability (IMAA), a policy supposed to represent "a change in philosophy as much as a change in policies and practices..." governing central agency-departmental relations.

> The essence of the new regime is to provide Ministers with greater flexibility to reallocate resources and a general reduction in controls on many activities previously requiring approval by the Treasury Board, coupled with an evolving accountability regime to protect the integrity of the management process.

> The accountability regime is envisaged as consisting, to the extent possible, of: (a) an accountability framework against which plans and budgets are developed and performance is reviewed, (b) departmental control processes . . . (c) systematic performance reporting and information flow to the Treasury Board; and (d) Treasury Board periodic assessment of the performance of each department and its accountability for the authority delegated.[11]

The policy also provides for "negotiated Memoranda of Understanding between the Treasury Board and specific departments [which] will document the accountability framework and will cover various aspects of increased ministerial authority and accountability, including multi-year resource agreements, increased levels of delegation, performance reviews, etc."[12] The arrangement provides for periodic, overall reviews of the "accountability framework" of departments and a decreased emphasis upon the detailed, procedure - by-procedure type of review that previously characterized the Treasury Board Secretariat's relationship with departments.

Arrangements under a policy of this type could benefit central agency-departmental relationships. Much will depend upon how such policies are implemented and administered, and here there is cause for concern as the officials charged with this responsibility may have worked for years in the context of the classic philosophy of control. The expenditure-control frame of mind will not necessarily adjust easily to the idea that departments require "appropriate management environments" characterized by consistency in managerial policies and adequate decision-making latitude. There is a danger that in the negotiation of memoranda of understanding or management contracts with departments, Treasury officials will insist on too much detail and retain too much control, in which case the potential benefits of this change in approach will not be realized. A change in philosophy of the scope contemplated by the IMAA principles may well require a program of organizational change and realignment within the central agencies concerned if intended policy is to be translated into realized policy.

It will be a challenge for central agency and departmental officials to see how successfully management contracts can be implemented in order to create the management context appropriate to a specific department's mandate. The problem is not only to ensure suitable degrees of delegation in such areas as contracting powers, staffing, classification or organization structure but also to establish the degree to which basic policies in such areas as finance, administration and personnel should apply across all departments.

Obviously, some general policies will have to prevail. However, there are areas of management where existing common policies are not really necessary to protect the interests of the collectivity or to sustain certain fundamental features of the public service (such as the merit principle).

To some extent, central agencies are being challenged to return to first principles in this process. They are being asked which common policies are really important, and which are an accident of history or an outmoded outgrowth of the control philosophy. Management practices and policies in parliamentary democracies have evolved over the past 50 years or so on a function-by-function basis. During this process, central agencies have continued to view managerial performance primarily as a problem at the departmental level. Recently, there is some evidence of a growing awareness that managerial performance in individual departments is as much influenced by central agency attitudes and policies as it is by managerial aptitudes within departments. Contemporary central agency officials are being asked to see themselves as partners with departments, sharing responsibility for results, not just as controllers and nay-sayers.

Incentives to Manage Badly

Public servants must function within the framework of many rules and procedures designed to protect the taxpayer's money and to prevent waste and fraud. Some of these regulations, such as those related to travel or to government hospitality, are tiresome, entailing personal inconvenience and the suggestion that public servants are not to be trusted. Nonetheless, they seem to be accepted by most public servants as part of the necessary burden of working for government. However, other aspects of the regulatory framework governing civil servants have a more serious impact. They are not just tiresome: they act as a significant disincentive to good management.

One of these relates to year-end spending. Parliament traditionally approves funding from one fiscal year to the next. If resources are not spent by the end of a particular fiscal year they lapse (unless they happen to fall into a special category, such as a revolving fund in which funds may be carried forward from one year to the next). "Lapsed" funds are those for which parliamentary spending authorization has expired; they return to the government's general revenue pool.

The "loss" of lapsed funds may cause difficulties for a number of reasons. They may have been required for certain capital expenditures (e.g., in the case of a building project that was delayed). Or they may not have been spent as anticipated because of unexpected circumstances that arose in the context of running the program (e.g., the delay of an important conference for which funds were budgeted; or problems experienced by the client for a program which made it necessary to withhold resources).

In the case of capital spending, an expenditure delayed in one year is likely to reappear in the following year, when the project is back on schedule. However, if the money budgeted for this project has lapsed, it is not available to the relevant department in the following year. In jurisdictions that do not provide for carrying forward unspent capital monies, the project manager may be forced to seek special funding through supplementary estimates. This may create the impression that the project has gone over budget, and reflect poorly on the manager. Sometimes supplementary funding cannot be secured, so the project has to be stalled for months or even years; the design may have to be changed, or the construction may have to be continued but on a sub-standard basis. Managers who get caught in these circumstances are quite likely to conclude that capital projects should be over-budgeted to provide for such contingencies. Thus regulations for lapsing funds for capital projects provide an incentive for managers to pad their budgets, and add to the red tape and overhead effort involved in getting a job completed.

When an unexpected delay in requirements for operational program funding leads to unspent resources at the financial year-end, the program manager may find that his or her program is suddenly under siege. Underspending your budget in government can be like a red flag announcing, "Loose cash!" People on the lookout for extra resources – ministers wishing to finance some initiative, other managers who have overspent their budgets, or central agency officials looking to reduce a deficit – are attracted to unspent resources like bees to honey.

Whatever the reasons for underspending may have been, the bureaucracy often "decides" that because the money was not spent, it was not needed (and will not be needed in future). The program must have had too much money. It is this change in the perceptions of those outside the program that is often of greatest concern to managers. The program manager finds that the funds are transferred out of his or her budget allotment, perhaps to some other official who has run out of money because of mismanagement or overspending.

The spendthrift managers who benefit from the transferred resources may try to work the system so that the extra money can be added to the base of *their* programs. If this ploy works, the spendthrifts are rewarded by an increased budget while the manager of the original program has less money for the subsequent year (when program requirements return to normal), and has to make special application to try to get the "old" money back into the base, or to find "new" money somewhere in the system. This is time-consuming and problematic. The shrewd manager may conclude that to avoid all these difficulties, it is better to spend surplus money on goods and services of marginal value, or to provide funding to clients who are not really deserving in order to keep the base of the program intact and to avoid letting anyone else know that there might be loose funds in the system. These may be shrewd tactics, but this behaviour is not good management in a more general sense.

Another problem affecting the motivation to manage well in government relates to the retention of savings. The frugal official who economizes with a view to redeploying resources from lower to higher priorities within a program may be sadly disillusioned. Having worked hard to wring savings out of the program, the manager is told that the savings must be returned to the general revenue pool of the government to be reallocated by ministers. The program base is then correspondingly reduced. For years, the return of savings to the "centre" was a bedrock principle of financial management in government. Thus, a former secretary of the Treasury Board declared in 1971,

> It has been suggested to me by at least a few very knowledgeable people in government that ... departments concerned should be allowed to decide how to allocate funds between alternative projects and programs .... I disagree: in my view the collectivity [of ministers] is nearly always going to make these decisions ... given the nature of cabinet government.[13]

Such an approach to management in a large bureaucracy is admirably high-minded but quite impractical. It drives line managers to distraction. It makes inadequate allowance for the growth of government, perpetuating a tradition that may have been appropriate a few decades ago but was quite unrealistic even in 1971. It presumes that ministers who are members of a small committee of Cabinet, such as Canada's Treasury Board, can make intelligent judgments about how to reallocate every million or two saved, when they are trying to administer a budget in the billions. It vastly increases the degree of bureaucracy in the system.

Most serious, the channeling of savings back to the centre of government provides no real incentive for officials to generate savings, because as far as the officials are concerned, such savings are simply lost. It is entirely unrealistic to expect that an official working in the field of, say, animal diseases research, will feel strongly motivated to offer up savings from his or her program knowing that the resources may be used to finance an obscure aid program in Malawi, or the construction of a wharf in some insecure MP's riding. Even a goal such as deficit reduction tends to be remote and abstract. Moreover, every new politically-motivated boondoggle announced in the media simply reinforces the determination of civil servants to protect their budgets and programs. Who wants "their" program resources used for a project designed to purchase the re-election of the Government?

In addition, ministers like to see their programs grow bigger and better; so there are few kudos for the manager who is able to tighten operations or come in under budget. There are few incentives to economize in most public services; in effect, the philosophy that savings must return to the centre of government affirms the right of ministers to reallocate resources that will seldom be forthcoming from committed program managers.

Another problem affecting motivation to manage prudently in government is that job classifications are frequently tied to the size of the financial resources (or staff) managed by each official, not to his or her responsibilities. (This may have come about by misapplication of private-sector job evaluation techniques to the public sector.) In the private sector, a budget is a budget; one manager's financial authority is usually roughly comparable to that of another; size is the main basis for differentiating between budgets and hence between managers' authorities and classifications.

This is not true in government. The nature of spending responsibilities accorded to managers may vary widely in qualitative terms. The system tends to work as follows: the official in charge of a $10-million program, even if the program is a sensitive one involving difficult administrative judgments, will be deemed to have a less demanding and important job than the official responsible for a $20-million program which is routine to operate. In general, officials with bigger programs are more senior and get paid more. The same applies to the size of the staff involved in administering a program. The classification system is usually thought to favour those officials who supervise more persons.

The alignment of individual incentives with corporate goals is a basic element of sound organizational design. Governments wishing to economize often seem blind to the fact that personal incentives for public servants are not aligned with these objectives. The classification system typically encourages civil servants to build up their empires, not to reduce them. The official who finds ways of cutting back on his or her program, or of increasing efficiency and productivity, may be rewarded by having his or her job classification and pay diminished. These facts are not unknown in central agencies but they often seem to be ignored. Many central agency officials have shown a historic tendency to rely on policy edicts and budgetary systems to achieve restraint, and have been curiously blinkered in addressing the issue of the basic incentives that operate at the level of the individual public servant. (And when they do think about incentives, they tend to think of marginal financial supplements to base pay, rather than of the fundamental forces at work in the employment system.)

Yet another disincentive to good management arises from the government's periodic tendency to engage in cross-the-board cuts of expenditures. Right-wing governments often come in on a platform of diminishing government spending, and/or cutting the size of the public service. As it is difficult to single out one program for reduction in relation to another (because of the problem of incommensurability), and because it seems preferable to gore everyone's ox a little rather than single a few out for slaughter, the Government decides to cut everything by, say, five per cent. The frugal, economic managers are hit just as hard by this as the spendthrift managers with the fat programs.

The consequence is to disillusion and demotivate the very type of managers that the elected Government would want to encourage. The frugal managers' programs are seriously damaged, because they were operating on minimal resources anyhow. Important activities will have to be eliminated. By contrast, the spendthrift managers ride out this storm with no serious consequences. Since their programs were overstaffed by ten or 15 per cent, a five per cent reduction has no real impact on operations. The frugal managers notice that economical management has been penalized. They conclude that in future, their programs will also have a layer of fat to insulate them from the cold of the next economic freeze.

The cumulative impact of all these policies and regulations is the dilution — and sometimes, the very eradication — of the motivation to manage well. Many public servants in other jurisdictions would probably agree with those Canadian officials who stated:

> Throughout the public service, the experience of the efficient and effective manager is that he is being penalized. The very fact that he has good plans and measurement systems means that information will be used by central agencies and other critics to mount a strong criticism of his performance.

> In the Government of Canada . . . there is not enough motivation to be a good manager.
>
> Not infrequently, the manager sees the government announce 200 million worth of subsidies or grants or programs for a purpose that is widely known to be absolutely futile and unjustified. Here he is being asked to cut down on his resources by a few hundred thousand dollars while on the other hand the government is wasting literally hundreds of millions of dollars. The effect on motivation is severe. People either give up in disgust or they become completely cynical. A common reaction is, "Why should I stick around? It's four o'clock. I'm going home."
>
> [M]ore emphasis has been placed on . . . growth and expansion than on frugality. The facts show that the rewards were going to those who gave their time to developing imaginative policies and programs. And where the real rewards go, effort will follow.
>
> I can find no incentive for the manager to be efficient. I can find lots on the other side, I can find many incentives leading the manager of the public service not to be efficient.[14]

Determining the cost of such regulations is probably impossible. The problem is not readily susceptible to analysis. (For example, how would one determine the cost of the policy that savings cannot be retained by program managers?) Nonetheless, their impact on management in government is real and profound. Two researchers who conducted an analysis of constraints to management in the Canadian public service in the early 1980s concluded that:

(1)   [T]he cost of present regulations is too high. It is thought to represent no less than 20 to 30 per cent in unnecessary overhead . . . .

(2)   The origin of regulations does not lie with the managers [but with] central agencies and specialist staff groups.

(3)   Consequently, when evaluations and audits point out inefficiencies or "lack of due regard for value for money",

managers resent the implication that they are blameworthy for something in which they have no choice.

(4)   The savings that are achieved through regulations . . . may in fact be outweighed by their costs – not only the costs of developing and administering them, but also the costs of sometimes preventing quick response, flexibility and adaptation.

(5)   A thoughtful and critical evaluation should be made to determine the full costs and consequences of regulations . . . .

(6)   In any case, wherever possible, rigid rules should be avoided in favour of pliable guidelines so that managers are encouraged to exercise more discretion . . . and adaptation in specific situations.[15]

There seem to be two schools of thought on government regulations. Some officials take the view that Cabinet government cannot permit managers much flexibility. Regulations are a fact of life and the mark of the effective public servant is an ability to get things done in spite of them. "If you give me a [senior official] who, after three years on the job, tells you he can't accomplish what he needs to accomplish under the present system, give me his name because he will be dismissed on grounds of incompetence."[16] The other school of thought sees no reason to make the job of management harder than necessary. The public interest is not served by forcing managers to jump over pointless hurdles; legitimate obstacles or constraints must be separated from those that are anachronistic or counterproductive in the context of the 1990s. This school allows that there may be more than one way to operate the machinery of government, and is prepared to contemplate the possibility of change.

Fortunately, the latter school seems to be gaining ground. In Canada, the IMAA document explicitly rejected the view of previous senior Treasury Board officials and provided authority for ministers to reallocate funds within their portfolios as long as no new resources were needed. This policy proposed to change the basis of the relationship between departments and the Board in significant ways, for example, by instituting the memoranda of understanding alluded to above, by providing for major reviews of departments every three years, and by substituting periodic reviews of "significant resource requirements associated with new policy initiatives, or other urgent items" in place of "a continuous but ad hoc stream of requests for incremental resources on a weekly basis."

Another major advance, which was instituted before IMAA, was the decision to create spending "envelopes" within which ministers had to compete with each other for funds. This also represented a departure from the previous central agency gospel, which was that only the Treasury Board could be responsible for allocating government resources. Other changes have been cited elsewhere in this book.

Britain has also been taking steps toward a more flexible approach to central agency-departmental relations. Whitehall appears to have further to travel in this respect than does the Canadian government, and the pace of advance is cautious. At time of writing, Treasury had recently introduced a new regime of "running costs control", the objective of which is to give departmental managers more flexibility in program administration. It has also adopted a more flexible policy for year-end spending on capital projects, in order to address part of the problem of lapsing funds. However, possibilities such as management contracts with departments or reallocations by ministers within votes or spending envelopes do not appear to be on the horizon yet.[17]

Central Agencies as Departmental Allies

The relationship of central agencies with departments is nearly always portrayed in terms of constraints and checks on the authority of line managers. Sometimes overlooked is the key role played by central agencies in restraining ministers from engaging in ill-advised or even illegal activity, and in protecting certain institutions of democratic government.

Department heads who see their ministers trying to influence government policy in inappropriate ways, to slip party favourites into full-time positions in the public service, or to place contracts in the hands of high-priced, ill-qualified companies, often find it useful to remind ministers of the rules and restraints imposed by central agencies. Until they come to understand the traditions and institutions of government, many new ministers have difficulty accepting the requirement that they conform to these policies. However, the rules are, in the final analysis, not those of the agencies itself—they are rules approved by committees of ministers who have approved them in order to protect the collective, longer-term interests of the government as a whole.

The rules of the game thus apply to all parties. Frustrated managers tend to forget that regulations relating, for example, to the appointment of public servants, the expenditure of money, or the procedures for letting contracts were devised to prevent abuse by officials *and* ministers. Although some ministers are prone to bend or ignore the rules to advance themselves politically, they do so at their peril. The broader interests of the party in power are protected by these rules: central agency regulations have often prevented imprudent ministers from doing something that could lead to revelations in the media or the House, scandals and public embarrassment. When an inexperienced Government comes to power, the central agencies stand as a bulwark against inclinations to abuse that power. Senior public servants who previously criticized the inflexibility of these agencies may find that, from time to time, they are welcome allies in preventing ministerial excesses.

There are occasions when central agencies also permit departments to maintain more positive relationships with their client groups than would be possible if such agencies did not exist. Departments with strong clienteles, such as Canada's Department of Indian and Northern Affairs, wish to appear sympathetic to their clients even when they may not want to accede to all their demands. Often it is convenient for the department or its minister to undertake to put forward the views of the clients, while explaining that the final decision rests with some central agency.

In short, while it is true that central agencies constrain managers' flexibility and freedom to act, it must be remembered that their policies apply across both the political and administrative levels of the government. Central agencies are the institutional manifestation of certain significant conventions or traditions of government. They may allow departments to appear as advocates for their clients in certain circumstances. More important, they stand as barriers to the abuse of political power, not just administrative mismanagement.

The Changing Role of Treasury Departments

Governments are in the midst of a period of significant adjustment arising from changes in their environment and their mandates. They have long since moved beyond the role of "context-setters" to that of active participants and providers of services in the economic and social life of the country. The budgets of government organizations are far larger than they used to be, and the institutions are much bigger and more complicated. The theory of ministerial responsibility has been diluted, and it is generally recognized that greater discretion will have to be provided to departmental officials if programs are to operate efficiently. Ministers simply cannot be personally involved in, and accountable for, everything.

Two trends of strategic importance appear to be underway in central agency-departmental relationships in Canada (similar developments appear to be occurring in other jurisdictions). The first has to do with the process of expenditure management at the political level.

During the 1960s and early 1970s, the Canadian Cabinet had one committee concerned with expenditure control, the Treasury Board. The other committees of Cabinet discussed ideas "in principle," and "approved" them without worrying too greatly about costs. It was then up to the department to work out the expenditure consequences with the Board. This was, in retrospect, a bizarre method of running things: no business would think of giving "approval in principle" to major projects or initiatives while treating cost as a detail to be resolved subsequently. However, since revenues and/or the deficit were growing from year to year, there always seemed to be enough resources to finance any reasonable new idea; therefore the system worked in some sense. The control exercised by the Board during this period had to do with regularity and propriety; it was not effective in restraining the total level of expenditure.

Toward the end of the 1970s, the realization dawned that this situation could not go on indefinitely, nor could the full burden of expenditure restraint be placed in the hands of a small committee of five ministers: hence the arrival of the envelope system. This represented a major alteration in the way government worked, changing the role of Treasury Board from being the gatekeeper on all government spending. The essence of the envelope system was to divide the government's overall budget into several major clusters or "envelopes", such as the economic policy envelope or the social policy envelope. It placed the responsibility for administering the resources in each of these envelopes and for discussing the tradeoffs among different expenditure proposals where it belonged: in the hands of ministers.

Cabinet itself was clearly too unwieldy to discharge this responsibility; Treasury Board, as a committee of Cabinet, was too small and weak to hold the fort against the assaults of the spending ministers. Therefore the key role of the "functional" committees of Cabinet (economic policy, social policy, etc.,) became that of authorizing disbursements from these envelopes, and also that of managing what became known as the "policy reserve", i.e., the relatively small amounts of extra money available in each envelope to finance new programs. They also became responsible for reallocation between programs within their sphere of responsibility. In short, with the envelope system, the government put much more of the responsibility for restraint in the hands of the "line managers" at the Cabinet level – the departmental ministers. The change is so logical, it seems remarkable that it did not occur earlier.

The second major trend involves a change in relationships in the sphere of expenditure management between central agencies and departments. This change has been made possible by the envelope system. Previously, Canada's Treasury Board felt its responsibility was to impede new spending proposals. Unlike business entities, departments do not have to set the costs of their programs and policies alongside their revenues. Whereas the marketplace provides businesses with a built-in cybernetic, or feedback system, which provides an effective restraint mechanism, in government there is no equivalent. Thus political will and institutional barriers, such as Treasury Board regulations, have to take the place of the market.

In the 1960s and 1970s, the Board was the only institution that seemed to stand in the way of the "spending ministers" whose momentum seemed unstoppable. The Department of Finance was concerned with the raising of revenues and with the government's ability to pay for its schemes, but it was not intimately involved in the expenditure side of government. On the micro-economic issues, the

Board was more or less the last line of defence. Not surprisingly, the Board tended to use every means at its disposal to achieve restraint.

The development of the envelope system, which is the heart of the Policy and Expenditure Management System (PEMS), has probably eased the tremendous pressure for the enforcement of restraint by the Board. Since keeping the lid on the overall level of spending is a shared responsibility among ministers, it should be less necessary to attack individual spending proposals with the tooth-and-nail tactics of the 1970s. The challenge now facing Canada's Treasury Board Secretariat and other Treasury departments is to modify the managerial environment of the public service so that the right blend of restraint and flexibility prevails.

To do this, it will be necessary to examine the nature of the incentives at work within the bureaucracy and to consider how the motivations of line managers might be more effectively harnessed to the task of responsible management. With the adoption of the envelope concept, Canada's Treasury Board now, perhaps, has the latitude to pay more attention to its responsibilities as the Committee on Management of the government, and to address management issues above and beyond resource control and expenditure containment. Central agencies are now challenged to do what they have been telling departments to do: to look not only at the "inputs" and the costs of government, but also at the achievement of results.

Quick response, good client service and better ways to get the job done cannot readily be achieved in a government which subjects all departments to the same accountability framework or which places them all in the same management environment regardless of their functions and mandates. Research laboratories should not be subjected to the same accountability regime as air terminals, nor should hydrographic mapping officials be expected to be accountable in the same way as, say, those engaged in the review of income tax returns. Nor will effective management result if line managers feel so hemmed in with regulations designed to restrain spending, that there is no incentive for them to manage well. Treasury departments and central agencies need to recognize that it is time to forge a new alliance with departmental line managers and to provide them with both the flexibility and the accountability framework to manage well.

Footnotes:

1. Gordon Chase and Elizabeth C. Reveal, *How to Manage in the Public Sector*, (Don Mills: Addison-Wesley: 1983), p. 65. This unique and entertaining book contains a good discussion of tactics for use by line managers in dealing with "overhead agencies", as they are called in the U.S.

2. *Ibid.*, pp. 63-64.

3. Royal Commission on Financial Management and Accountability, (Lambert Commission), *Progress Report*, (Ottawa: Supply and Services Canada, 1977), pp. 3-4.

4. Treasury Board has defined accountability framework as "the full spectrum of performance for which the Minister/Deputy would be held to account." See Treasury Board of Canada, Minute No. 800978/79/80 of Meeting of 20 February 1986, "Increased Authority and Accountability for Ministers and Departments."

5. William Plowden, "What prospects for the civil service?", *Public Administration*, vol. 63 no. 4, (Winter 1985), p. 401.

6. Lord Rayner, "The Unfinished Agenda," University of London, Stamp Memorial Lecture, 1984.

7. Lambert Commission, *Final Report*, (Ottawa: Supply and Services Canada, 1979), p. 113.

8. Despite the merits of the Management Board approach, at time of writing, of 12 jurisdictions which were reviewed (10 Canadian provinces plus Whitehall and Ottawa), only Nova Scotia, Ontario and New Brunswick have chosen to adopt this title for a central agency. Sharon L. Sutherland and G. Bruce Doern, *Bureaucracy in Canada: Control and Reform*, (Toronto: University of Toronto Press, 1985), Table D-3, p. 198.

9. Lambert Commission, *Final Report*, p. 114.

10. Price Waterhouse Associates/The Canada Consulting Group, "A Study of Management and Accountability in the Government of Ontario," (Toronto, January 1985).

11. Treasury Board of Canada, Minute No. 800978/79/80 of Meeting of 20 February 1986.

12. *Ibid.*

13. A.W. Johnson, "Management theory and cabinet government," *Canadian Public Administration*, 20th anniversary ed., (1978), pp. 54-62, (first published in 1971).

14. Otto Brodtrick and Richard Paton, "Quotes: Senior Executives Talk About Management in the Public Service," (Ottawa: Auditor General of Canada, December 1982). This document contains selected quotations from about 100 interviews with civil servants conducted in 1981. They provide an excellent insight into the problems on the "firing line" of management in Ottawa.

15. *Ibid.*, pp. 28-29.

16. Quotation from a senior official cited in *Ibid., op. cit.*, p. 31.

17. Interviews with Treasury officials, June 1986. See also Supply Estimates 1986-87: Summary and Guide, Cmnd. 9742, March 1986, and *Multi-Departmental Review of Budgeting: Executive Summary*, H.M. Treasury, (March 1986), s. V. The pace and scope of change being contemplated does not seem revolutionary. In the best Treasury tradition of caution and care, one official noted, "Treasury is concerned about giving a signal that cash limits do not really matter. And departmental budgeting systems should be better before there is more delegation from Treasury. There is not enough evidence of need at the moment."

Part Three:

Managing Departments

Introduction to Part Three

Part 1 has described the institutional structure of government and the traditions and conventions that prevail in the public service in parliamentary democracies modelled on the British system of responsible government. Part 2 developed the discussion by reviewing the role of the minister and the impact of this position upon departments. It also examined the complex accountability relationships to which the head of department is subject, noting that after the ministerial relationship, the next most important relationships within the bureaucracy on managerial issues are usually with the central agencies or departments of government.

In this section, we now turn to the issue of management within the individual "line" department. This section might have been a good deal longer than it is. A comprehensive examination of management at the departmental level would have included full chapters on such issues as finance, information management, the public relations function and personnel systems. However, to address these issues would have greatly increased the length of the book. In addition, it would have turned this section into something approximating a manual or a textbook, and there are already many texts available on the above topics. Moreover, it seemed to me that it would be difficult, perhaps impossible, to discuss functions at this level of specificity without losing the generic perspective of the book: it would probably have been necessary to narrow the scope of the discussion to one particular jurisdiction, and as noted in the Introduction, it was not my intention to write a book of this nature.

Therefore, part 3 takes a different approach. It examines selected aspects of management at the departmental level. Some of the issues it considers are particular to government (e.g. the policy function), and would therefore not be found in conventional business-oriented literature on management. Other questions which it covers, such as planning and control systems, have been included because they pose special problems in an environment where there is no "bottom line." The third major topic of this section, the management of people, has been included for the simple reason that, in my view, this dimension of management is one of the most important, and it is one that has been much neglected in many government organizations.

Part 3 begins with a brief discussion of the problem of designing organizations so that they are able to perform effectively. A government department is a complex entity. I have found that many senior officials with significant managerial responsibilities have relatively little understanding of the principles of organizational design. They operate by instinct and experience, – and often do a good job on this basis. However, sometimes instinct and experience are not enough. To return to the question posed at the beginning of this book, it can be difficult to form judgments as to whether an organization is well managed without the benefit of some frame of reference or set of standards. It is all very well to conclude, as did chapter 1, that assessing managerial performance involves judgment. Upon what is that judgment to be based?

Chapter 8 takes a short excursion into the world of management theory, examining what has become known as the "fit" approach to organization design. This is a way of thinking about organizations which a number of consulting firms have employed in different variations in examining questions of organizational strategy and structure; (some readers may recall that one such model was touched on in chapter 1 of the best-seller, *In Search of Excellence*, but the model was not developed). Chapter 8 provides my own, somewhat different version of the "fit" approach, incorporating elements not

230

provided for in the *In Search of Excellence* model, and drawing on the work of a number of other authors whose contributions are acknowledged in the text. For me, this model has provided a consistently useful way of thinking about the issue of organizational performance. Chapter 8 indicates that designing the architecture of effective organizations involves much more than arraying a cluster of boxes on an "organization chart".

Chapter 9 considers the question of planning and control in organizations where there is no bottom line. It tries to reduce the jargon and complexity associated with planning systems such as PPBS, PEMS or PESC to essentials, explaining what these systems are trying (or should be trying) to accomplish at the departmental level. It also discusses the issue of strategic planning in a government context, and disposes of a number of myths and misunderstandings concerning this function. (Officials who have been confused by some of what has been going on in governments may take heart in the realization that there was a good deal of confusion in some of the early approaches to planning systems.) Chapter 9 also considers the relationship of strategic planning to the policy function in government, an important nexus which private sector texts on planning entirely overlook.

Chapter 10 carries this discussion forward by examining the policy function itself. This function is unique to government, and it therefore seemed appropriate to devote a specific chapter to it, even though as noted above, other functions have been omitted from this book.

Chapter 11 discusses the management of people. It is people who make organizations work. Governments have been afflicted with a conception of management that places too much emphasis on systems and procedures, paying too little attention to the human beings who have to make (and want to make) those systems work. It is something of a paradox that politicians, who are so concerned with the motivations of the electorate, should be relatively blind to the question of motivation when it comes to the functioning of the institutions for which they are accountable to Parliament and the public. They have paid little heed to the morale of the people who work for them, and there is increasing cause to believe that government is suffering as a result. Chapter 11 explores some of the recent evidence to this effect.

Chapter Eight:
The Architecture of
Effective Organizations

Analyzing Organizational Performance

As chapter 1 stated, management is increasingly understood to be a "situational" discipline: it recognizes that there is no single best way of managing, equally suited to all situations, and that the application of principles and concepts has to be tempered according to the nature of the organization at hand. Chapter 1 also noted that in lieu of universal principles, management literature and research provide " 'walking sticks' to guide the managers along decision-making paths about human affairs".[1]

In the absence of universal principles, deciding how to constitute or build an organization so that it can be expected to perform well – the challenge facing every manager – is much more difficult. It leaves managers facing a challenge: how to know which "walking stick" to select, or which rule or principle to apply? It leaves external auditors in a more exposed position. Once they move outside the sphere of finance into that of general management and value for money, where are their "generally accepted principles" and their audit standards? How can they be sure that their analysis of the state of management is correct, and that it will be (or should be) accepted, either by those running the organization or by other informed and objective observers? Clearly, there can be legitimate differences of view about how the task of management should be approached in different circumstances.

Does this situation mean that anything goes? that any approach to management which can be supported by a plausible argument is equally valid? The answer, of course, is no. There is a frame of reference which can help managers to determine what approach is best suited to their situation, and that frame of reference is provided by the overall priorities and strategy of the department and by what is known as the concept of "fit".

Departmental Strategy and External Relationships

Much of the literature on management today accepts the view that how an organization should be constituted and managed depends upon its strategy for relating to its external environment. In business, the theory of competitive strategy is concerned with the positioning of the enterprise in its competitive setting. The appropriately-positioned enterprise which is well managed will flourish; the poorly-positioned one will not survive over the long term. Once strategy has been determined, it provides the context within which decisions concerning the structure, systems and other aspects of institutional design must be taken.

Determining departmental strategy is probably a more difficult job than determining business strategy for reasons discussed throughout this book: incommensurability, political instability, intrusion of politics into administrative matters, incertitude regarding Governmental intentions, the need for ministers to appear to be supporting all interests, and so forth. Sometimes the turbulence of the governmental environment will suggest that the best strategy is to keep a low profile and focus on surviving. At other times, however, with the right combination of minister(s) and political circumstances, a more forthright strategy (or policy stance) should be possible for a department. A great deal, of course, will depend on how well the department head gets along with the minister, and how skillfully the department handles this key relationship.

In either event, strategy remains of central importance to questions of organizational design and management. A department's

234

ability to develop and realize a well-defined strategy (or a series of strategies or priorities appropriate to the different areas of its mandate) will largely depend upon its ability to handle its external relationships. Thus a key question in assessing the state of management in a government organization is, how well does it manage these relationships? Is it appropriately organized to do this job effectively?

Exhibit 8-1 provides an overview of the relationships of a typical government department.[2] The *ministerial* relationship is, of course, of central importance, having a powerful impact upon departmental priorities and methods of operation, as does, in some in stances, the relationship with the prime minister's office. (Both these accountabilities have already been discussed in previous chapters.) Decisions on how to handle these relationships will affect such issues as the role of the deputy minister or permanent secretary, staffing, the distribution of responsibilities among top officials, the organization of the department head's office, and the role of the policy office of the department (if it has such a unit).[3]

The quality of a department's *client* relationships tends to be a function of public perceptions of the merit and relevance of its programs. In business, the flow of revenues constitutes a way of monitoring the state of the enterprise's external relationships. Since government departments' revenues do not correlate directly with the quality or efficiency of their services, other ways must be devised to ensure that client relationships are sound and that services are relevant and responsive. Both perceptions and reality are important. From an organization design viewpoint, the central concern should be to ensure that the department is appropriately constituted and operated to be able to keep in touch with its clients and to manage relationships with them effectively. Some departments have been making increasing use of private-sector techniques such as attitudinal surveys to keep in touch with their "customers" and to provide input to the process of setting priorities. Numerous other methods of monitoring and managing client relationships can obviously be employed.

Central agency relationships affect a department's authorities, its accountability framework and its resources. For example, if relations are good with central agencies, an important contract

EXHIBIT 8 - 1
Managing in Turbulence
The External Relationships of Departments

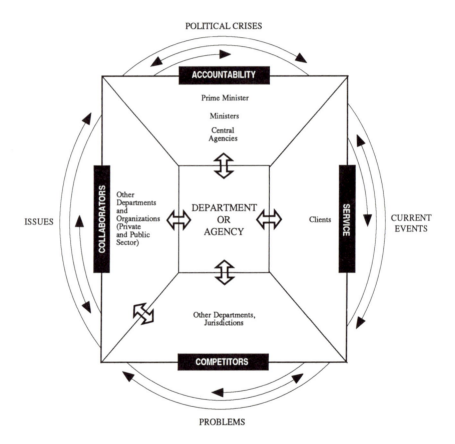

BEYOND THE BOTTOM LINE (1988)

requiring central agency co-operation is likely to be approved more easily. Extra authority over staffing required to get a new program moving or to resolve problems with an existing one might be granted, or a request for supplementary funding might make it to Cabinet more quickly. Conversely, if relations are poor, a request for special consideration is likely to be denied, ignored or even impeded. Central agency relations in the public sector are somewhat akin to the concept of goodwill on the balance sheet of the private firm: they are in themselves intangible but are nonetheless valuable in tangible ways.

Most well-run departments will manage their central agency relationships with care (an aspect of departmental management upon which central agency-inspired management guidelines tend to be silent!). As noted in chapter 7, central agencies are regarded by departments in an ambivalent light: sometimes as allies, often as opponents. Part of a department's strategy in achieving a policy goal may involve the careful orchestration of relations with central agencies, with other departments or other levels of government. Such intentions will obviously not be spelled out in documents intended for circulation outside the department, which explains why departmental plans circulated to central agencies may not always fully reflect the priorities and strategy of the organization.

Collaborative or competitive relationships are those with other levels of government or with other government organizations. In principle, different governments, and departments and agencies within a specific jurisdiction, are supposed to be working together in the common public interest. In practice, the public interest is subject to a lot of different interpretations. As a result, there are often border skirmishes, and sometimes pitched battles, between organizations and jurisdictions trying to extend their power or to achieve different policy objectives. "Good management" in government often means the ability to turn potentially competitive relationships into collaborative ones, and to fend off potential predators without incurring any loss of position or territory that is not justified in the larger public interest. A well-organized department is equipped to protect its policy interests and to manage its relationships with other government organizations effectively.

Clearly, top departmental officials must ensure that external relationships are effectively handled. They must be able to read the maze of information from external sources and derive from it a reasonably clear set of departmental priorities which can provide a frame of reference for management. This is not an easy task in the fluid and unpredictable environment of government. However, assuming that some measure of clarity surrounding strategy and priorities can be achieved, the next consideration is how to design and operate the internal architecture and machinery of the institution to realize this strategy.

The "Fit" Approach to Organizational Design

The fit concept is easy to state and difficult to apply.[4] The fundamental idea is that there must be coherence among all the different elements of an organization. (A visual representation of the model appears in Exhibit 8-2.) The idea of fit rejects the limited notion of an organization as a simple hierarchy to be operated in accordance with standard principles of management.[5] Rather, it envisages an organization as a sort of organic entity, in which the parts exist in a relationship of mutual dependency and support, with each other and, collectively, with the external environment of the organization. In such a miniature ecosystem, the components sustain and support each other, and if a serious weakness exists in one part of the system, it affects all others.

The fit concept challenges managers to think about organizations in new ways. It states that every organization is to some extent unique, and that just because one approach to, say, management control or motivation, worked in one institution, it will not necessarily be the right one to apply in another. It cautions against the wholesale importation of business methods to government, pointing out that individual business techniques or methods must be assessed in terms of their suitability to the government environment. Certain methods may be better suited to some government agencies than to others; some may not be suitable at all.

The fit concept also stresses the integral nature of organizations. That is, since all elements of the organization are linked in a symbiotic relationship, what a manager does in one part of his or her organization should be consistent with what is done in another.[6] The

EXHIBIT 8 - 2

DESIGNING EFFECTIVE ORGANIZATIONS

The "Fit" Model

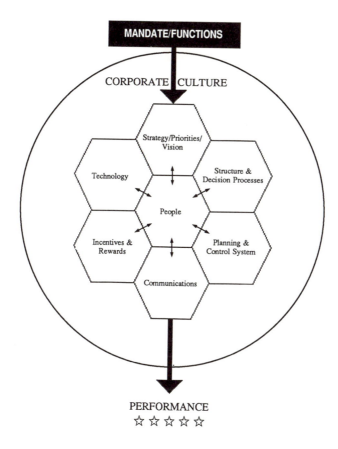

BEYOND THE BOTTOM LINE (1988)

objective, in building and managing an organization, should be to get the elements of the organization working together to increase organizational productivity. If they are not linked, they will either drag the organization off course or nullify each other's effects. (For example, if the objectives of an organization call for collaboration among staff, but the rewards and incentives motivate employees toward self-interested, parochial behaviour, the likelihood of realizing objectives is small. Similarly, if the organization's strategy calls for innovation but the staff in place have learned to behave in temperate, careful ways, the strategy will remain unrealized.)

The idea of fit also demands that managers should not simply let an organization evolve in the expectation that it will develop naturally into an efficient, productive entity. An organization is a complex web of persons, relationships, expectations, structures, processes, systems and traditions. An unplanned institution cannot be expected to develop as desired. As Peter Drucker has observed, "The only things that evolve in an organization are disorder, friction, malperformance . . . . Organization design and structure require thinking, analysis, and a systematic approach."[7] Organization design undoubtedly affects performance. "[T]he choice of structural forms makes an economic difference; that is, not all structural forms are equally effective in implementing a given strategy. Therefore [managers] should allocate the time and effort necessary to plan their organizational form, just as time and effort are allocated for the formulation of other plans."[8]

The fit approach to organizations cautions against looking for solutions to problems of organizational performance in only one or two places. In particular, it warns against relying too heavily upon structural change to achieve organizational goals. That organization structure has an impact on organizational performance is seldom in doubt. However, many managers seem excessively impressed with the ability of structural change to affect the way an organization works, and insufficiently aware of the degree to which other factors may be the cause of problems in performance. Perhaps because of the popular tendency to equate "organization" with "structure," for some managers an "organizational problem" seems to become a structural problem almost by definition. Thus "reorganizations" are invoked to fix problems that may in fact have little relationship to structure.

Clearly, there are times when structural change is necessary and desirable. However, reorganization should not be entered into lightly. When one major element of an organization changes, most of the other elements have to adapt to the change as well. The fallout from a major reorganization can last well over a year. Furthermore, it is important that the change should be managed with careful attention to the consequences for individuals.[9] In many reorganizations, difficulties arise simply because no one appreciates the importance of communicating with staff during the change, and of managing the change process itself.

Understanding the Organization

Before the fit concept can be applied, an "organization" must be understood. What exactly is an organization? The formal organization is that portrayed in organization charts and in policy and procedures manuals, often out of date. Then there is the organization as it appears to those working at different levels within it. However, employees' views are both limited and coloured by their perspective. For example, middle managers often complain that top managers do not know where they are going; yet their information is incomplete, and may be inaccurate. It may be that top managers are quite clear as to their directions, but that they have not chosen to share this information with their subordinates.

The view from the top of the organization may be similarly clouded. For example, top managers may believe that their staff are busy carrying out the directives from above, whereas in fact employees at subordinate levels may be doing quite different things. Thus what managers at both intermediate and senior levels perceive as "reality" may in fact constitute only an imperfect portion of the larger picture. Sometimes no one working in the organization has a full grasp of how it is functioning.[10]

The difficulty of coming to grips with an organization is compounded by the fact that the formal organization is overlaid with a web of networks and personal relationships, often essential to getting the work of the institution done. Chester Barnard, in his classic book, *The Functions of the Executive*, christened this overlay the "informal organization". Informal organizations are often undervalued and can be more "real" than formal ones.

> [W]hen formal organizations come into operation, they create and require informal organizations . . . . [A]n important and often indispensable part of a formal system of cooperation is informal . . . . [M]ajor executives and even entire executive organizations are often completely unaware of widespread influences, attitudes, and agitations within their organizations . . . .
>
> "Learning the organization's ropes" in most organizations is chiefly learning who's who, what's what, why's why, of its informal society.[11]

A number of years ago, I conducted an examination of the organization of a department of the Canadian government. As the study progressed, it appeared that the formal channels of authority as portrayed on the organization chart did not accurately represent the flow of information or decision-making. It soon became clear that the deputy minister was being circumvented and that the minister's office was in effect directing the day-to-day activities of one of the major departmental programs.

Effective managers know what is going on in their organizations, and have a reasonably good idea of how work is really accomplished.[12] Managers unaware of the informal networks may make decisions as if the formal policies and structures represented reality. In this event, such decisions may produce unexpected, and sometimes undesired, results. An American professor of organization design, Jay Galbraith, has suggested, "[I]nformal processes are necessary as well as inevitable, but their use can be substantially improved by designing them into the formal organization. At the very least, organizations can be designed so as not to prevent these processes from arising spontaneously, and reward systems can be designed to encourage such processes."[13]

The "Fit" Approach in Practice

A problem often confronting senior managers is how to discourage the development of separate fiefdoms where each unit of the organization tends to go its own way with little regard to the needs of the whole. How one deputy minister tried to sort this out, provides a good illustration of how the fit concept could have worked to his advantage.

Initially, the deputy tried to deal with the problem by issuing directives concerning the need for greater coordination and by instituting a new senior departmental committee to co-ordinate work in different branches. If the organization functioned according to its organization chart, this approach should have worked. The policy direction was clear; a new structure was in place to give effect to it. The deputy also set up a new planning system designed to co-ordinate branch planning. However, none of these solutions worked. Despite the efforts of the new boss, the branches continued to work in an independent manner.

The fit approach would have sought the causes of the "barony" problem in several areas, and would have led to a more broad-reaching solution. Indeed, upon investigation, the source of the difficulties proved to be subtle and deep-seated. One of the top officials was temperamentally disinclined to work with others; he ran a research operation and although he paid lip service to the deputy's injunctions, he was in fact deeply committed to the view that science should be independent of operations. The traditions and culture of the organization had for years favoured branch independence. Senior managers had developed an informal entente whereby it was tacitly agreed that proposals originating in one branch would not be criticized by the heads of other branches. Under this arrangement, each branch got more or less what it wanted. Thus, the new top management committee tended to work poorly, and the deputy found himself having to deal with branches one at a time, as they were reluctant to comment on each others' proposals. Furthermore, the minister at the time was not concerned about co-ordinating the work of the different branches and tended to deal with them directly, bypassing the deputy to some extent. Thus, the problem of baronial behaviour turned out to be rooted in organizational culture, in people, and in the informal incentive structure. It was immune to "solutions" which failed to address these elements of the organization.

In short, in building an organization capable of effectively carrying out its mandate and strategy, the "fit" of the following factors must be considered:

- people: are they right for their jobs and for the organization's strategic requirements?

- the formal structure and the decision-making processes: is the structure adapted to strategy; do necessary decisions get taken, and by the right people?

- the planning and control system(s) of the organization: are they suited to the type of organization (formal, informal); do they contribute effectively to operational co-ordination? (This issue is discussed in more depth in chapter 9.)

- methods of internal communication: are decisions adequately communicated to staff; are staff kept abreast of plans; are they consulted on decisions that affect them; does the informal organization complement the formal one?

- incentives and rewards: are officials at different levels motivated to achieve desired goals, and are they rewarded for attaining them?

- the use of technology: is it appropriate to the organization's needs?

- culture: do the values, traditions and beliefs of the organization reinforce the attainment of organizational objectives?

The Nature of the Work

In deciding on organizational architecture, senior managers have to consider the nature of the functions to be performed and their relationship to each other. One important question is that of functional homogeneity or heterogeneity. Some government agencies possess mandates which comprise closely related functions, e.g., the operation of a national library, or the administration of customs ports. Other departments, however, may be accorded several mandates, some of which may be quite distantly related. Examples would be Canada's Secretary of State Department, or Health and Welfare Canada, or Britain's Department of the Environment. In these circumstances the department head must decide whether to run the department on an integrated basis, with a "corporate" management committee that meets regularly, or as multiple organizations with several unrelated, or loosely related strategic goals, where the principal ties between major divisions of the organization are provided by common administrative services. (To use a business analogy: should the department be run like a single-product firm or a conglomerate or holding company?) Municipal governments, which may be responsible for such widely divergent activities as the delivery of social welfare and the provision of sewage and water, are examples of organizations that invite management as a conglomerate.

Another important factor affecting organization design and performance is the degree of routine inherent in the work being performed. (This issue is sometimes described in the academic literature as task diversity or uncertainty.) Routine work allows for broader spans of control and for greater reliance on devices such as manuals and training to "program" employees to respond appropriately to task demands. Thus one would expect that in some units of a department such as Canada's Supply and Services, which is responsible for a number of fairly routine functions, spans of control would be quite broad. Conversely, work characterized by a high degree of novelty or uncertainty tends to increase the need for close supervision, diminish the contribution that various methods of work standardization might make to the reduction of supervisory requirements, and thus diminish the size of work units. One would therefore expect smaller spans of control in departmental units concerned with policy development than in those engaged in more repetitive functions.[14]

A related consideration is the nature of the outputs of the work. Are the outputs tangible and quantifiable, or intangible and unquantifiable? Where the organization is dealing with tangible products, (or where the pricing mechanism assigns a value to intangible outputs such as services that can then be "counted" or quantified), the problems of organizational management are different from those of an organization with no tangible outputs. Perhaps the most important difference is that in the latter type of organizations, management control becomes *much* more complicated. Quotas or production targets become difficult or impossible to assign; accountability becomes harder to enforce and productivity improvement, harder to assess; important management information is less easily communicated through financial data; the roles of financial officials change; new functions such as program evaluation may be required. Thus the nature of the output has an impact, as the type of work, upon organizational design. Exhibit 8-3 illustrates the relationships between type of work and output upon control requirements.

Much early thinking about management was developed with reference to institutions where most functions were routine and where work involved physical goods. An increasing proportion of the institutions in Western society (including government departments) now involves work with intangible outputs: more and more organizations handle information or provide services rather than adding value to material items. This shift has progressively complicated the task of management control. Systematic approaches are less readily adaptable to the work. In general, organizations should be run in a looser, less structured manner than those concerned with routine tasks and/or tangible outputs.

Summary

This chapter has provided a short excursion through what is in fact a very considerable literature on organization design and behaviour. Clearly such a brief tour cannot do full justice to the literature; however, it may provide a point of departure for those persons interested in pursuing this topic in more depth.

The chapter proposes a way of thinking about the issue of organizational performance, and suggests that one of the key roles of departmental officials with managerial responsibilities is to develop an architecture or design which takes account of the different elements of the organization and links them into a framework of mutual support. Often it will take a manager a number of years to build his or her organization up in such a way that the desired architecture can be realized.

The architecture of a well-designed organization must take into account the major external relationships of the institution and ensure that measures exist to manage and monitor each of these well. In addition, good design takes account of the nature of the work of the organization and the type of output which it produces. Different kinds

EXHIBIT 8 - 3

THE PROBLEM OF CONTROLLING
ONE-OF-A-KIND, INTANGIBLE ACTIVITY

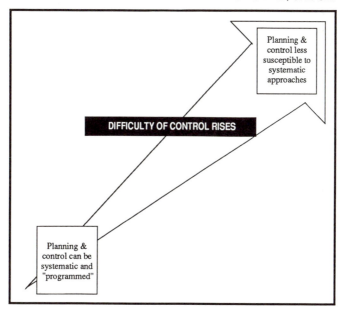

ROUTINE WORK   ORIGINAL, ONE-OFF

INTANGIBLE
OUTPUTS;
Information,
services, ideas,
etc.

Planning &
control less
susceptible to
systematic
approaches

DIFFICULTY OF CONTROL RISES

Planning &
control can be
systematic and
"programmed"

TANGIBLE
OUTPUTS;
Physical goods.

BEYOND THE BOTTOM LINE (1988)

of organization require different sorts of approaches. Finally, the well-designed organization will take into account the informal systems, relationships, conventions and networks which may play a key role in making the institution work.

Footnotes

1. Jay Lorsch, "Making Behavioural Science More Useful," *Harvard Business Review,* (March-April 1979), pp. 171-181.

2. See Michael E. Porter, *Competitive Strategy: Techniques for Analyzing Industries and Competitors,* (New York: Macmillan, 1980).

3. See Porter, *op. cit.,* p. 4, figure 1.1. Note that this diagram is an elaboration of figure 5-1, portraying the accountability relationships at the top levels of government.

4. The concept as presented here fits squarely into the contingency theory of organization design. It has drawn its inspiration from a number of models, or approaches, notably the version of the "fit" model derived by Jay Galbraith and Daniel Nathanson, *Strategy Implementation: the role of structure and process,* (St. Paul: West Publishing Company, 1978), p. 2; Henry Mintzberg, *The Structuring of Organizations,* (Englewood Cliffs: Prentice Hall, 1979), p. 64; Marvin Weisbord, *Organizational Diagnosis* (Reading, Mass.: Addison-Wesley, 1978), p. 9; McKinsey's 7-S framework described in Thomas J. Peters and Robert H. Waterman, *In Search of Excellence,* (New York: Harper & Row, 1982), p. 10; Hay consultants' "strategic issues matrix" (as described by Galbraith and Nathanson, *op. cit.,* p. 92); David Nadler and Michael Tushman, "A Model for Diagnosing Organizational Behaviour," *Organizational Dynamics,* (Autumn 1980), pp. 35-51; and Robert N. Anthony, *Planning and Control Systems: A Framework for Analysis,* (Boston: Graduate School of Business Administration, Harvard University, 1965).

5. One author has suggested that this type of limited notion provided the conceptual underpinnings to the Glassco Report on the organization of the Government of Canada which had a major impact on how the federal government was run during the 1960s and 1970s. See T.H. McLeod, "The Glassco Commission Report," *Canadian Public Administration,* vol. 6 no. 4, (Winter 1963), pp. 386-405. See also V.S. Wilson, "The influence of organizational theory in Canadian public administration," *Canadian Public Administration,* vol. 25 no. 4, (Winter 1982), pp. 545-563.

6. Galbraith and Nathanson, *op. cit.,* p. 93: "One cannot successfully change structure without making compensating and

reinforcing changes in information and budgeting systems, career systems, management development practices, and compensation policies. In organizations, everything is connected to everything else." See also Mintzberg, *op. cit.*, pp. 219-220, and Nadler and Tushman, *op. cit.*, p. 37.

7. Peter F. Drucker, *Management — Tasks, Responsibilities, Practices*, (New York: Harper and Row, 1973), p. 523.

8. Galbraith and Nathanson, *op. cit.*, p. 1.

9. See for example Noel M. Tichy and Mary Ann Devanna, *The Transformational Leader*, (Toronto: John Wiley & Sons, 1986).

10. Warren Bennis and Bert Nanus have distinguished between the "manifest" or formal organization, the "assumed" organization as perceived by staff and managers, and the "extant" organization as revealed by objective outside analysis. See *Leaders: The Strategies for Taking Charge*, (New York: Harper and Row, 1985), pp. 50-51.

11. Chester Barnard, *The Functions of the Executive*, 30th anniversary ed., (Cambridge: Harvard University Press, 1968), pp. 121-123.

12. "By having a reasonably good idea of what networks exist and who influences them, the [manager] can gain a great deal of leverage . . . ." See Noel M. Tichy and Mary Ann Devanna, *op. cit.*, pp. 199-200.

13. Jay Galbraith, *Designing Complex Organizations*, (Don Mills: Addison-Wesley, 1973), p. 47.

14. See Henry Mintzberg, *op. cit.*, pp. 134-147; Jay Galbraith, *op. cit.*, pp. 14ff.

Chapter Nine:
Planning and
Controlling Operations
The Uses and Limitations of Planning and Control Systems

Policy development was a solidly entrenched feature of government when the enchantment with strategic planning and planning systems began. Systems for planning and control were urged upon all progressive organizations, first in the private sector starting in the 1950s, and then, about a decade later, in the public sector. In Canada, the various attempts to systematize the process of government planning began with the adoption in the late 1960s of a form of PPBS (program planning and budgeting system) followed by a Cabinet Planning System, a Cabinet Evaluation System, and a Treasury Board planning system.[1] Within departments, all sorts of staff planning units were created as part of PPBS, and then, in its wake, came a modified set of program planning procedures known as PEMS (policy and expenditure management system). Britain never formally adopted any form of program budgeting, but moved in that direction with its endorsement of MINIS as well as other aspects of the Financial Management Initiative (see appendix 2). Britain also flirted with a form of central strategic planning with the creation of its high profile Central Policy Review Staff, created by Prime Minister Edward Heath in 1979.[2]

Early proponents of planning in government tended to proceed as if the function of policy development did not exist; they simply overlaid models derived from the private sector on what already existed in government. Had the nature of government and strategic planning been better understood, a number of difficulties could have been avoided.

This chapter discusses what can reasonably be expected of planning systems (and what should not be expected); it explores the relationship of evaluation, strategic planning and policy development to each other; it concludes with a discussion of new roles emerging in government in response to the need for better management of the process of planning and control in the public service.

What is a Planning and Control System?

According to one school of thought, management is a systematic, cyclical exercise in which the wheel never stops turning. Planning, one of the key elements of management, sets the wheel in motion. The next segments in the cycle are selection of a course of action, implementation, and then an evaluation of performance which feeds back into planning. At this point, the cycle starts again.

Some writers suggest that planning should begin each year with the development of a strategic plan related to the longer term; this provides the framework for the elaboration of operational objectives, shorter term in character and more closely related to day-to-day activities. Operational plans are linked with budgets specifying financial requirements for the future. To assemble all this information, a set of procedures is needed to guide the process of planning. This methodology is sometimes described as a "planning system" or, more broadly, a "planning and control system", (since the cycle of events is not complete until control has been exercised and planning is once again underway).

There is no generally accepted definition of a planning system. I define such a system to include procedures for formulating plans and designating accountabilities, formats for recording plans and submitting budgets, and a calendar of events indicating the sequence of activities and the roles of key participants such as the departmental management committee, the planning office (if there is one), the financial officials and principal line managers. Properly conceived and operated, such a system can help to organize the internal work of a government department by indicating who is expected to do what. The planning process itself can contribute to internal accountability by generating goals against which managers may be held to account. A fully developed planning *and control* system therefore provides for the collection of information related to progress against plans, that is, it includes what is sometimes called a "management information system". Without this element, the control component of the system is missing.

Planning and control are intimately linked, like two sides of the same coin. Planning provides the context for control; if there is no planning, the scope for control is reduced from substance to procedure. That is, if planning has not established substantive objectives to be attained, then it is no longer possible to ask, "Have the goals associated with your work program been achieved?" In my experience, the focus of control tends to be upon procedural or financial issues rather than substantive issues in government. There is often a lack of effective operational planning and, frequently, few sanctions associated with a failure to attain operational goals.

The Evolution of Enriched Planning and Control Systems

Planning systems in government have usually been designed around the estimates process, that is, the annual cycle for producing departmental financial estimates which are sent to central agencies and thence to Parliament. Up to the 1960s, Canada's estimates procedures, based upon the British practice, constituted a simple planning and control system for government expenditures. Each autumn, departments would prepare their expenditure plans for the forthcoming year, arranged according to categories known in the jargon of financial management as "votes."* The estimates would be

---

* In this context "vote" derives from the way Parliament approves money for departmental expenditures, by "voting" money to be spent by departments and agencies. Money is approved by Parliament either through ongoing statutory pro-

consolidated by Treasury officials into the "blue book" listing all departmental requirements; this would be presented to Parliament by the Government in about February, a month or two before the new fiscal year (April 1). Parliament would approve funds for departments by passing legislation called "appropriation acts", an activity known in the language of Parliament as the voting of "supply". Supply debates provided the Opposition with a chance to review the Government's spending priorities and objectives for the coming fiscal year.

Votes usually defined, in general terms, the purposes to which funds were to be devoted. The financial accounts maintained to report on how the money was being spent were organized according to these votes. Such accounts provided a very limited basis for the control of departmental spending: they could reveal whether overspending had occurred, but because the purposes for which money was voted were defined in such general terms, they were of little help in determining how well a department was being run or what was actually being achieved in terms of value for money.

Another shortcoming was that many government initiatives had to be planned over a number of years, although votes were concerned only with one year. Further, the process tended to project the previous year's activities into the next, without much critical analysis of whether it was appropriate to continue along the same track. An increment for the new year was simply added to compensate for inflation and to fund new ideas. The basic assumptions underlying the program were seldom queried, nor were questions asked about its continuing relevance in a changing world. This approach to planning became known as "incremental budgeting".

To cope with these limitations to the conventional estimates process, some governments decided to expand the process into a more comprehensive planning and control system for departments. PPBS—program planning and budgeting system—represented an

grams that automatically make a call upon government resources (e.g., the replenishment of commitments to international institutions), or through appropriation acts which must be approved each year. Appropriation acts, responsible for most departmental funding, are divided into "votes"—amounts of money which correspond to those programs of the government not covered through ongoing statutes.

attempt to develop departmental planning and control into an orderly, logical process and to import a philosophy of systematic planning into the public service. It divided all government activity into clumps of expenditure called programs, defined as "a package which encompasses each and every one of the agency's efforts to achieve a particular objective or set of allied objectives."3 Programs were to be devised to highlight the basic purpose of the activity – in a department concerned with economic development, for example, a program would not be described as "administering grants to industry" but rather as "promoting the level of income and employment." For each program, officials were to develop a statement of objectives defining results, or outputs, in relation to their impact on the public. This was an important development, since, as noted above, in the past, the objectives of government expenditures as articulated in parliamentary votes had usually been described only in vague terms.

The PPB concept established a longer timetable for the preparation of the estimates, dividing the cycle into planning first, then budgeting. Preliminary estimates were to be prepared some 18 months or more before the year which was the principal focus of planning. Since this got the process going earlier, there was more time for analysis. With spending intentions projected three (or, in some jurisdictions, as many as five) years into the future, it was anticipated that their longer-run implications could be assessed. Once preliminary submissions had been approved and ceilings had been set by central agency officials and ministers, departments could then develop their more detailed annual plans and budgets. Earlier preparation of preliminary estimates allowed central agencies to exercise greater control over the budgeting process, rather than getting caught, late in the day, with a flow of estimates submissions from departments which could not be financed from available resources.

Besides controlling spending proposals more effectively, the new planning systems were supposed to move the process away from incremental budgeting. PPBS called for a more rigorous scrutiny of expenditure proposals as they moved through the cycle. As part of the planning component of PPBS, analysts would examine spending proposals each year to determine if there were alternative, more cost-effective methods of delivering the program.

PPBS linked planning to control by providing for retrospective analysis of progress against plans. The operation of the system was expected to force officials to examine old methods of program delivery critically, each year. An outgrowth of PPBS was a request for the collection of performance measures, designed to report on program achievements.

One of the great advantages of the bottom line in business is that it correlates the expenditures involved in providing particular products or services to the income derived from their sale. Profitability provides a neat method of assessing performance that can be made specific to a particular product, service or organizational unit of an enterprise. It offers the manager a yardstick that measures both the efficiency of operation of the enterprise (cost of production) and public demand for what it produces. In government, income (generated primarily through taxation) does not correlate with specific services such as defence, roads or sewers. In the absence of a bottom line for public goods, it has been necessary to devise other means to assess their value to society and to determine whether they are being provided efficiently.

As the discipline of program planning has developed, it has begun to merge with a related stream of intellectual activity concerned with the evaluation of government programs. From this process, various concepts and terms have been emerging that provide a means of discussing objective-setting and the performance-monitoring in a more precise way. Gradually, these terms seem to be developing into an accepted, specialized vocabulary (or jargon) for public sector planning and control. (Most private sector managers would not be familiar with these concepts, although as a discipline for thinking, they could be useful in business as well as in government.)

First, the definition of a program.[4] According to the gospels of program planning and evaluation, a rigorously defined program encompasses several elements: (1) its objectives, (2) the human and financial resources attributed to the production of the service in question, (3) the activities of government officials required to deliver the program to the public, (4) the rationale upon which the program is based. These different elements can be summarized in the form of a program model which shows the relationships between the activities, the operational outputs which they are expected to produce, and the final outputs, to be defined according to the impact of the program on society or the specific "clients" of the program.[5]

For example, the *objective* of a program to assist the fishing industry might be to increase productivity and the incomes of fishermen by encouraging the use of new types of equipment. The *resources* of the program would include the program budget, in the form of money available for disbursement to fishermen, plus the salaries of the public servants involved, and related costs such as travel, publicity, etc., and some overhead costs. The *activities* of the program staff might involve publicity, soliciting and adjudicating grant applications, announcing decisions to successful and unsuccessful applicants, and monitoring the use of funds. The *operational* or *intermediate outputs* would include applications considered, grants processed, or money disbursed. The *final outputs* or *program effects* would be defined in terms of reduced costs per tonne of fish caught and higher returns for fisherman. Exhibit 9-1 illustrates these relationships.

The *rationale* for the program might be based upon the following assumptions or premises: (a) the fishing industry is uncompetitive because of outdated equipment, (b) fishermen cannot acquire new equipment without financial assistance, (c) grants would be used to purchase such equipment, (d) the acquisition of such equipment would enhance productivity, (e) increased productivity would not result in layoffs and unemployment because consumer demand is strong enough to absorb increases in production, as long as these are accompanied by lower prices, and (f) fishermen would pass on lower costs in the form of price reductions for fish processors who would in turn pass them on to the consumer. If any of these premises proves to be inaccurate, the program may fail to achieve its objectives; thus it is important in planning programs to ensure that the rationale is sound and clearly understood.

Efficiency would be demonstrated by various ratios, for instance, reductions in administrative costs per grant accorded, over time, or improvements in the response time for processing grant applications. Ratios are useful since they correlate the inputs of the program with the outputs. For example, it is much more helpful to know what has been happening, say, to the cost per piece of equipment provided under the program than it is to know that 200 more grants were made this

EXHIBIT 9 - 1

"PROGRAMS" CONVERT RESOURCES TO EFFECTS
A Program Model

OUTPUTS/EFFECTS

INPUTS/RESOURCES	ACTIVITIES	INTERMEDIATE	FINAL
$	for example: Research Planning Meetings	for example: -Information Programs -Applications Completed -Grants Disbursed	for example: -Jobs Created -Incomes Increased -Services Provided

PUBLIC IMPACT

BEYOND THE BOTTOM LINE (1988)

year than last. Information of the latter type is simply a statistic, not a measure of performance.

Effectiveness would be measured in terms of changes in fishermen's annual income over time, in the productivity per vessel per day at sea, or in prices for consumers. An *unintended benefit* might be a reduction in alcoholism or crime associated with a rise in employment in areas where the grants were taken up; *unintended costs* might be new, unanticipated maintenance charges for keeping the new equipment in sound operating condition.

Obviously there is an intimate relationship between program objectives and program outputs. Objectives in fact may be expressed in several ways. Some departments express objectives simply in terms of activities to be performed: "our objective is to operate the fisheries assistance program." Objectives expressed in this manner are not very useful, since they are usually a restatement of responsibilities which already appear in job descriptions, and they say nothing about what is to be achieved or attained, or about the purposes of the program.

A more useful approach is to state objectives in terms of efficiency — to process all grant applications in a maximum of four weeks, to lower the cost of record-keeping through computerization — or in terms of effectiveness — to raise fishermen's average annual income to X amount, to lower the cost per tonne of fish landed to Y. Objectives expressed in terms of efficiency are sometimes alluded to as *"operational objectives"*, since they tend to be more closely associated with the day-to-day activities involved in running the program; objectives expressed in terms of effectiveness are sometimes called *"final objectives"*, as they are the ultimate goals which the program seeks to achieve. Both types of objectives are useful, the former for day-to-day management control, and the latter for control at a more basic or strategic level.

There are probably no pure PPB systems of the sort originally envisaged by PPBS left, but different jurisdictions and departments have adopted a variety of approaches to planning, budgeting and control, all built around the simple estimates process. Such systems constitute an "enriched" form of planning and control system, as compared with the bare-bones, original process.

Defining the Program Structure

A key element in the improvement of planning and control is the program structure. Departments often have trouble defining it: some go looking for programs as if they had somehow always been there, and are frustrated when they cannot find them. It may take them a long time to realize, as Aaron Wildavsky has noted, that "programs are not made in heaven. There is nothing out there just waiting to be found. Programs are not natural to the world; they must be imposed on it by men.... There are as many ways to conceive of programs as there are ways of organizing activity...."6

A specific illustration will demonstrate the difficulties involved in determining a program structure. (The following example is very loosely based on the Canadian Correctional Service, but has been simplified and modified for the purposes of this discussion. It should not be construed as an accurate representation of the Service.)

The organization is responsible for maximum, medium and minimum-security prisons, each with different policies and procedures, scattered throughout the country. Accordingly, it is organized by region at the top, with the wardens of each prison reporting to a senior regional official. For purposes of this example, we will assume that funding for the prison network is provided through two parliamentary votes which fund other parts of the criminal justice system as well. Thus in this model, the vote structure does not correspond with the departmental structure. We will also assume that each prison carries out only four very basic services: ensuring security, providing food and housekeeping, processing arriving and departing prisoners ("reception services") and providing vocational training to prisoners.

In order to define the program structure for this organization, senior departmental officials might wish to consider a number of alternative ways of conceiving of the purposes and activities of the organization. One obvious option is to base the program structure upon the organization structure. Since the basic organizational unit in this department is each individual prison, financial and operational records would be maintained for each one. Officials could decide that each institution was running a "program". If the program structure were designed in this manner, the organization structure and the program structure would be identical.

However, the prison service is not only managing institutions. Senior management might decide that the four major activities within each prison — housekeeping, security services, reception services and vocational training — should be managed as "functional programs" of the department. If so, objectives would have to be established for each of the programs and record-keeping systems developed to track performance. New financial procedures would be necessary to monitor the costs of each functional program at the institutional level.

So far, our planning and control system has been designed around two conceptions of the role of the department: (a) running institutions and (b) running functional programs. Another equally valid perspective is to see the department as being in the business of rehabilitation for different categories of prisoners (male, female, young and repeat offenders, etc.) and the prevention of recidivism (the reincarceration of released prisoners). In this interpretation, the department is seen to be operating a young offenders' program, a female offenders' program, a drug offenders' program, etc. To monitor performance would require the collection of data about inmates as they moved through the prison system and after they left.

In this case, all the ways cited of interpreting this department's mandate are legitimate, all are potentially useful, none is more "right" than another (see exhibit 9-2). The design of a planning and control system at this level is clearly more than a matter of financial management. It involves judgments about how the business of the organization should be viewed, about just what things have to be "managed," and about the types of information needed to support the management process. To establish interconnected management information systems so that each of these conceptions of the business of the department could be controlled is a very complicated job.

For each department, there is somewhere a point of diminishing returns, where the time and effort involved in developing and maintaining information systems for purposes of planning and control can no longer be justified. Top officials must determine how the business of the department needs to be conceived and when that point of diminishing returns has been reached. In making judgments about how the department's activities and achievements are to be monitored, senior officials will have to make decisions about what types of information should be collected routinely (and with what

EXHIBIT 9 - 2

PROGRAMS CAN BE DEFINED MANY DIFFERENT WAYS

Alternative Conceptions of Programs in a Prison Service

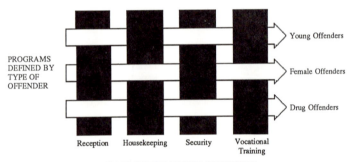

PROGRAMS
DEFINED BY
TYPE OF
OFFENDER

Young Offenders

Female Offenders

Drug Offenders

Reception Housekeeping Security Vocational Training

PROGRAMS DEFINED BY TYPE OF FUNCTION

BEYOND THE BOTTOM LINE (1988)

frequency), and what types should be collected periodically, e.g., through periodic special surveys or studies. Devising an appropriate approach to management control in a government department which is practical, cost-effective and relevant to both the operational and more strategic requirements of decision-making can be a very difficult task. Many departments underestimate the difficulties and as a result rely upon methods that are either excessively simple (e.g., producing purely financial data only), or hopelessly complicated, resulting in reams of computer printouts that are ignored by most managers.

My own view, somewhat at odds with that of the originators of PPBS,[7] is that in establishing a framework for planning and control, it is advisable for departments to walk before they try to run. In this view, programs are not the logical point of departure — the organization structure is. In any government agency, people's jobs are defined, and they are held to account within the context of this structure. Information systems should first of all be designed to monitor costs and performance according to units of the organization. Once efficient systems have been developed for operational planning and control at this level, the challenge of developing information systems for the purpose of monitoring programs, however conceived, can then be tackled. My belief is that programs should constitute an overlay to this basic framework.

In general, there is no formula as to how a planning and control system should be configured — around organization structure, or around programs, defined in various possible ways. Requirements will vary from department to department. However, the temptation to overcomplicate the management process by trying to set objectives in too many ways and to collect information routinely about too many things must be avoided. In management, simplicity and clarity are cardinal virtues.

Evaluating Government Programs

As experience with planning and control systems grew during the late 1960s and 1970s, it became increasingly evident that government programs could not be evaluated solely through the kind of annual review that was supposed to occur in the planning cycle. In both

Britain and Canada, more thorough and systematic methods of evaluation were thought to be required.

In the U.K., PAR—program analysis and review—came into being early in the 1970s. It involved the systematic analysis of the performance of major clumps (programs) of government expenditure to determine the goals of the program, the amount and use of resources, and alternative ways of achieving program goals. PAR studies were to proceed under the watchful eye of a high-level committee (PARC) made up of Treasury and departmental officials, as well as other central agency officers. Ministers were by and large excluded, apparently because "ministers might have foreclosed the analysis by ruling out options that ought to have been considered."[8] The PAR process was launched with considerable enthusiasm in Whitehall, attracting attention from other jurisdictions intrigued by this British experiment.

The enthusiasm soon waned. The process became excessively bureaucratic and over-formalized, with a lack of methodology that resulted, too often, in "an essay with little evidence of rigorous appraisal or of prescriptions for action." Apparently the expertise to conduct the required analysis was not always available at the time in Whitehall. According to some observers, the studies themselves had no clear client; there was no established basis for the selection of topics for study, and often what was chosen by departments was unsuitable. PAR constituted

> an approach rather than a clear methodology . . . [leading to] the irregular production of a mixed bag of studies with an uncertain fate . . . [which] seemed neither to fit ministerial timetables nor to correspond . . . to ministerial interest. . . . It was wound up in 1979 as one of the initial acts of Mrs. Thatcher's administration . . . . [M]inisters did not find PARs helpful in making political judgments . . . . [M]inisters preferred superficiality . . . . [T]he PAR experience stands as a warning . . . of efforts that produce small scale results for large scale commitments.[9]

Evaluations tend to make enemies rather than friends, especially if they ask really hard questions. As one British official commented, "Socrates was the first to do a PAR. He did it on Athens going round asking fundamental questions. Athens put him to death. That's why I don't want to do any more PARs."[10]

A former Treasury official assessed PAR as follows:

To the extent that the PAR system was designed to take a radical look at policies and not merely at methods of carrying them out, there was a lack of reality about the idea that the whole organic process of policy formation could somehow be subordinated to a mechanical review procedure. Spending Ministers and their Departments simply did not put the crucial policy issues in their fields on the PAR list . . . .

[P]rogrammes and policies are reviewed and changed when the pressure of events makes itself felt, rather than at the behest of some theory of administration.[11]

In Canada, a somewhat more rigorous approach, known as program evaluation, was adopted in 1977, drawing upon intellectual roots in social psychology, sociology and economics and upon previous efforts in effectiveness evaluation in the U.S.[12] A new Treasury Board policy instructed departments to carry out a series of revolving reviews of all their programs on a five-year cycle. ("Program" was initially not defined; later instructions described a program, for purposes of this policy, to be a "program component," colloquially, if rather vaguely, defined by central agency officials as a "chewable chunk" of departmental activity.) Departments were told to set up internal program evaluation units, reporting directly to the deputy minister; Treasury Board issued guidelines and principles to departments on methodology, how the evaluation should work, and who should be involved in studies. Official Ottawa began to become familiar with a new vocabulary: formative evaluations, summative evaluations, program modeling, evaluation assessment, longitudinal studies, control groups, and the like.

Progress in implementing this structured, rather rigid, system was rocky. Departments were understandably confused by the fact that Treasury Board was defining program one way for purposes of budgeting (program in this context was usually a large clump of expenditures) and in another, disaggregated way for evaluation purposes. Deputy ministers did not rush to realign their priorities to provide time to direct this new function; ministers were largely outside the process, which was conceived as an internal regimen of the bureaucracy; and many evaluation units languished for lack of direction or interest. The policy called for a revolving program of reviews, but there simply were not enough people with the requisite skills, either inside departments or on contract, to institute an initiative on this scale.

Many programs could not be readily evaluated according to the policy's requirements. Sometimes there were no relevant data available, and to assemble the required information was too costly or impractical. For some programs, the objectives had never been specified, either because of bureaucratic oversight, or because everyone knew that the real objectives were implicit and political, but no one (least of all the responsible minister) was prepared to set them down on paper. In still other cases, the objectives were clear, but they were unquantifiable, and difficult to assess even through qualitative methods. (For example, how might one assess the performance of a program of support to interest groups representing native peoples in Canada, the purpose of which was to help preserve the culture of these peoples and to enhance their capacity to assume responsibility for the direction of their own affairs?)

But the more fundamental problem was that, as in the PAR exercise in the U.K., ministers were largely uninterested. Also, as in the U.K., the really important evaluations tended to take place outside the context of the program evaluation routine, often influenced by political considerations which weighed more heavily than did the guidelines promulgated by central agencies. Many studies died before the implementation stage, and program evaluation developed a reputation in the bureaucracy as a sort of backwater rather than a lively, policy-relevant place to work.

Despite these hurdles, the evaluation efforts forged ahead, making progressive concessions to practicality as experience accumulated. Less emphasis was placed on the requirement that evaluation units report directly to the deputy minister or that they had to be organizationally separate from departmental policy units; from time to time it was envisaged that they might conduct special studies directed to political priorities such as staff reductions. Central agency officials also conceded that once every five years was unrealistic, and that political pressures had to be taken into account in scheduling sensitive studies.

By the mid-1980s, much of the rigidity of the initial policy had been abandoned; the Office of the Comptroller General reported that some 250 evaluations had been completed, one fifth of the total number of "program components" in the federal government. Although the goal of reviewing all programs every five years had not been attained, progress of a sort was certainly being made. Studies, said the Office, "are, in fact, being used"; the results of some evaluation studies were reportedly finding their way into policy documents and memoranda to Cabinet.[13]

Is program evaluation in Ottawa "working"? Evaluation is like chastity: people support it in principle, but in practice they prefer if it is mandatory for others and optional for them. Although the OCG's assessment may be coloured somewhat by the fact that evaluation is a mainstay of the Office's mandate, it is clear that some useful work is being done. However, the results are a good deal less than what was originally hoped for: evaluation has not, at time of writing, become a key element in the resource allocation process, and major studies still tend to take place outside the system. In the mid-1980s, five deputy ministers, questioned on the usefulness of the program evaluation system, agreed that there should be more rigorous reviews of program performance, but their assessment of the system in place at that time was broadly consistent: "The jury is out."[14]

Problems with Planning and Control Systems

Implementation. When PPBS was first introduced, the system was overly ambitious, and officials had difficulty grasping that its main purpose was to establish a better basis for accountability in departments. In Canada, because the exercise was dominated by the financial officials in departments, PPBS seemed to be an accounting exercise, even to some departmental officials leading the process. The method of introduction of program budgeting tended to translate the undertaking into a tiresome mechanical process, roundly resented by line officials who felt they had more important matters to attend to than writing tedious descriptions of their activities.

As noted in chapter 7, PPBS, although never officially abandoned, was gradually amended, adjusted and embellished, and the system now in place is known as PEMS (Policy and Expenditure Management System). PEMS retains a number of the features of PPBS, such as multi-year planning, but it has introduced some significant and practical alterations. These include the "envelope system" alluded to previously which provides for ministerial supervision of "envelopes" of expenditures, the better linking of policy decisions and financial resources, the abandonment of the unrealistic PPBS idea that every program should be analyzed in depth every year, and also the disavowal of the make-work notion that a "strategic plan" should be produced every year for every department (see below on the difference between corporate and strategic planning). PEMS attempts to encourage ministers to look for the resources to finance new expenditures out of their existing budgets, rather than constantly coming back to the public trough for fresh money, as had occurred under PPBS.[15]

In many U.S. jurisdictions, PPBS flagged, and only a few years after its introduction at the federal level in 1965, PPBS was officially abandoned by Washington.[16] Officials felt that the creation of program structures took too much time, and raised too many questions for which there were no clear answers. People got bogged down in philosophic discussions around objectives and entangled in meandering debates on cost attribution. Many programs which at first seemed to be good candidates for performance measurement proved upon closer examination to be difficult to adapt to this discipline.

Inability to produce strategic plans. Although in theory PPBS was supposed to serve as a strategic planning exercise, it seemed unable to yield plans that were truly strategic in nature. The plans that emerged from PPB-type systems continued to be rooted in existing assumptions about program effects and reflected previous patterns of expenditure.

Incommensurability. The new planning systems did not remove the basic difficulties involved in comparing programs. Although central agency guidelines claimed that planning systems would facilitate the "rational" reallocation of resources and setting of priorities, after the programs had all been defined and costed, it was still just as difficult to try to conduct a "rational analysis" of say, culture in relation to defence, of airports to the environment, or prisons to education. Even within single departments, judgments about priorities remained intractable. Improved information about performance did not help in deciding where to allocate new resources, or how to assign lower and higher priorities to various activities, because such issues involved questions of value.

For example, in a national library was it "better" to build up the book collection through new acquisitions, to invest in conserving the collection already available, or to devote resources to making it more accessible to the public? In international development, was it "better" to put more resources into the hopelessly impoverished countries or those with a foot already on the ladder of economic growth? In the field of health, was it "better" to finance research into disease or to provide capital equipment for hospitals? Neither PPBS and its derivatives, nor methodologies such as program evaluation provided any conceptual breakthroughs that could help officials or ministers with judgments of this kind. As in the past, such decisions continued to be made incrementally, on the basis of history, the values of decision-makers and political pressure. Incremental budgeting turned out to be a sort of institutional cockroach, immune to extermination through administrative innovations.

Lack of policy impact. The new planning and evaluation systems did not result in wholesale reorientations of policies and programs. Ministers remained loath to kill programs; they showed little intention of using the power of the new systems to reallocate resources from one program to another. Reflecting the priorities of their constituents, their general attitude remained, "More is better." They concentrated on securing new resources to expand programs rather than husbanding or "rationalizing" the resources already available. Program planning and control systems seemed overdesigned for this purpose—the traditional estimates process served equally well to dip new resources out of the cistern. There was little motivation for officials to develop and maintain resource control systems when new resources always seemed to be available. The really big issues remained outside the dictates of the planning system, and the elaborate structures of planning and control remained somewhat disconnected from political realities.

Lack of suitability to some functions. Although planning systems adapted well to the routine and repetitive functions of departments, they were less helpful in the case of unique, non-routine activities, especially those which were qualitative in nature. They proved difficult to apply to such functions as maintaining relations or adjudication, where tangible operational goals could not be specified. In Canada, when PPBS was first instituted, Treasury Board officials tended to make little distinction between departments or functions; officials who tried to point out the problems involved in adapting the new systems to their activities were treated as foot-dragging recalcitrants. Since the planning system did little or nothing to facilitate the task of management in such functions, an attitude of resentment to "management reform" grew among some departmental officials.

Operational Planning and Control

The notion that all planning for an organization takes place at a certain time of year, or that planning should proceed in an orderly fashion from the strategic to the operational level, with the cycle repeating itself each year, is an oversimplification of how planning really works — or can be expected to work — in most big organizations. The reality is that planning goes on at different levels and in different spheres of large organizations all the time. An organization is like a plate of spaghetti in which, at any juncture, many planning initiatives are entangled: some strategic, some operational, some short-run, some long-run.[17] The idea of a single governing planning system for an organization suggests that somehow all these strands can be disentangled and laid out end to end, like a project flow chart. In practice, organizations do not slow down long enough, and their functions and issues are too complex and interrelated for this to be possible or desirable.

To illustrate: in a government department, during the course of any given week, several planning initiatives may be going on at various levels: planning in response to a new thrust in government policy; planning related to the recruitment of staff over the next few years; updating the operational work plans for the forthcoming quarter of the current fiscal year; changing the method of delivery of a departmental service; determining the kind of computer system the department will need next year; deciding what to do in response to a disappointing evaluation of the effectiveness of a departmental program.

Most of these plans will be connected to each other; each is at a different stage of evolution — some just starting up, others nearing completion. The point which some of the pundits of integrated planning systems seem to have missed is that the main job of any manager is to plan; and that this is an ongoing responsibility, not one that occurs only at a particular time of year. The principal vehicle for integrating and co-ordinating plans is the *organization itself*. Different initiatives are co-ordinated and integrated through the everyday activity of running the institution: through the meetings of the top management committee, the functioning of subordinate co-ordinating committees and task forces, the observance of agreed standards and policies, the effective communication of intentions and decisions to employees, the repartition of responsibilities, the formal decision-making processes and the informal networks that complement the formal organization structure. In short, the organization that plans and controls its activities well is the organization that is well-designed (see chapter 8) and effectively led.

Within an organization, there may be a number of different planning systems — an information technology planning system, a project planning system, a human resource planning system, and a particularly important one, an expenditure planning and control system, which all departments must have, since without it they cannot secure financing. The preparation of information to feed an expenditure planning system does not involve "all" the planning in the department. Rather, this system sweeps together information about future resource needs derived from the many other planning initiatives and projects underway within the department: the policy work, the capital projects, the program activities, the evaluations, the preparations for a new minister, and so forth, in order to communicate the aggregate resource requirements to the elected Government through central agencies.

An expenditure planning and control system of this type may be enriched or embellished to become an *operational planning and control system*. The difference between a simple expenditure planning system and an operational planning and control system is that the latter requires managers to specify operational objectives and related work programs intended to attain those objectives, whereas the former simply requires managers to state their financial (and perhaps, person-year) needs without tying these to substantive objectives. The latter monitors whether operational goals are being achieved, whereas the former monitors financial commitments and expenditures against budget, but does not keep track of the actual achievements of the organization. An operational planning and control system usually embraces all the activities and resources of the department with different sections of the department (such as the personnel and financial units) co-ordinating the various aspects. In this sense it is a "corporate" planning and control system (but not, as discussed below, a "strategic" planning system.)

Both the utility and the design of operational planning and control systems will vary from department to department, depending upon the nature of the activities of the organization. By requiring employees to formulate and record intentions for the forthcoming year or two, such a system can improve accountability within the organization. It will be especially useful for organizations with routine, ongoing operations, for those where outputs are measurable and to some degree comparable from one year to the next, or for those which function in a stable environment.

It is important that the level of detail required by such a system be tailored to the character of the organization's work and to its environment. In circumstances where priorities are externally dictated (for example, certain policy units), it is pointless to require the development of detailed operational plans, for such plans will go out of date rapidly and will be useless as a vehicle to promote accountability. In these circumstances, a general statement of intentions should suffice; the planning system should not insist upon detail for its own sake.

An operational planning system may help to *co-ordinate* plans in an organization (for example, by encouraging senior managers to communicate their intentions to subordinate levels) but it will not necessarily *integrate* the various initiatives of an organization. As discussed elsewhere in this book, it takes a cohesive overall strategy and vision for an organization to provide the glue that will truly integrate the efforts of discrete units of an institution carrying out related functions.

In summary, a planning and control system in some organizations may serve primarily financial purposes. In others, it may serve wider goals. However, such a system should not be expected to produce strategic plans or to handle major decisions. The decisions taken in the context of such a system are likely to be incremental. (This does not mean they are unhelpful; a great deal of the best work that is done in organizations involves building gradually on what was there previously.) The objectives of such a system should be: to provide a context within which to establish operational goals and work plans; to compile a statement of aggregate resource needs of a department; to monitor and adjust (in minor ways) the consumption of resources during the course of each year, in light of operational developments; to help co-ordinate activity across organizational units; and finally, to strengthen the accountability process in departments.

Planning Systems, Strategic Planning and Major Policy Development

An operational planning and control system cannot be turned into an effective vehicle for strategic planning simply by tagging certain types of analysis on to the front. Strategic planning is here defined to mean the development of big, important plans that may question past assumptions or involve significant departures from past practices. In government, strategic planning is (or should be) a synonym for a "major policy development initiative", since this is where the "big, important" planning occurs in the public sector. The process of strategic planning cannot generally be made to conform to a cycle or a predetermined timetable of events. Rather, it is a customized activity that evolves according to the nature of the issue. It may loosely follow a logical sequence (see chapter 10), but it tends to develop in an unpredictable manner, often doubling back on itself or taking off in unexpected directions.

A useful analogy is to think of strategic planning (or major policy formulation) in terms of the formation of a rain cloud. Over time, as a result of some change in the environment, moisture collects. Initially, no one can say just how long it will take to form a cloud, nor what shape the cloud will assume. Sometimes the cloud may drift away, with no consequences for the terrain below. Sometimes it may take months or even years to mature. When the process is sufficiently advanced, the strategic planning cloud rains on the routine activities of the organization. The overall directions emerging from strategic planning will become progressively incorporated into operational planning. Sometimes it may not rain for a long time — there may be no cause for major adjustments to existing activities and priorities, and the business of the organization may proceed satisfactorily from year to year with only minor adjustments. In other circumstances, there may be a chain of strategic changes called for over a short period. Sometimes an organization may be involved in several strategic planning exercises (or policy reviews) touching different parts of its activities at the same time.

The beginning of the cycle of operational planning each year can provide a routinely scheduled opportunity to scan the environment of a department and to revisit some of the assumptions inherent in existing policies. Such a review anticipates what issues are likely to arise during the forthcoming year or two and helps set the policy agenda for the department for the planning period. It can also provide an opportunity to tell staff about forthcoming priorities; this will provide an updated context within which operational planning can take place. Thus, the beginning or front end of the operational planning cycle can be used to revisit, and to keep current, an existing strategic plan.

However, if fundamental change seems necessary on any front, a separate strategic planning initiative will have to be set in motion. This activity will almost certainly break free of the routine of the operational planning cycle and will assume a life of its own in which approach, timing and methodology are all dependent upon the issue(s) at hand. Unlike operational planning and budgeting, which have to cover the whole organization, strategic planning will not necessarily encompass the full range of an organization's activities.[18]

As noted above, PPBS confused operational planning and strategic planning by calling for annual strategic reviews of every program's performance against its objectives and for an examination of alternative, more cost-effective modes of program delivery. A large department simply cannot, every year, routinely consider fundamental changes to its objectives and operations. Departments in Ottawa that set up planning units in the 1970s to undertake this type of work soon found themselves dismantling them or changing the units' mandates.

Moreover, PPBS was politically naive to assume that government programs could be treated in an "objective", rational manner. It ignored the problem posed by differences in values leading to different interpretations of what might be "rational". Almost every government program has associated with it a set of vested interests. For example, the implementation of a program involves considerations such as the location of capital facilities and the creation of jobs. Programs delivered in one community or region cannot be simply uprooted and transplanted to another locale, or delivered in a new way, without significant political consequences.[19] Contrary to PPBS' premises, how a program is delivered can be a question of policy to some voters, even if, in the eyes of a "rational" policy analyst, it may seem to be simply a matter of administration (see the introduction to part 2).

After detaching the ill-advised notion of an annual strategic plan from the original premises of PPBS, (recognizing that strategic planning (or a major policy review) is going to take place *outside* the framework of the planning system), one is left with something that looks very much like an operational planning and control system. This is really what the present version of PEMS is in Ottawa. The goals of such systems are less ambitious than those of PPBS, but their great advantage is that, if sensibly designed and managed, they may actually work.

Staffing the Planning and Control Process

During the period when governments were growing and the stock of resources seemed almost endless, control was not a matter of great concern. Planning was essentially a matter of assembling ideas for starting new programs or expanding old ones, and of developing the estimates for presentation to central agencies. The responsibility for co-ordinating this process rested comfortably with the chief financial officer in most departments. This activity had little impact upon departmental operations; financial officials were more or less to record decisions taken by the minister, the deputy minister and line managers, and to ensure that central agency regulations were followed.

Times have changed. The processes of planning and control in departments are becoming more complex. It has become crucial that the overall approach to planning and control be determined at the top of the organization. The example set by the head of the department will set the standards that will prevail elsewhere; if the top official is not committed to strengthening the process of operational planning and control, efforts at subordinate levels to improve the process will be of little avail. (Commitment in this context means being prepared (and being able) to spend the time to ensure that the process is effectively designed, to enforce the discipline inherent in the system, and to recommend to the minister any difficult decisions that may flow from the operation of the system.)

Not all deputy ministers will pay much attention to their departments' corporate planning needs. Political realities, as well as the culture and the incentives of the public service, continue to direct department heads' attention toward coping with strategic issues of policy, managing the sensitive external relationships of the department, and devising new, politically attractive initiatives with which the minister's name can be associated. Because deputy ministers are so strongly pulled toward these priorities, they need associates upon whom they can depend to assist with resource management issues – individuals with specialized knowledge of the elements of resource management that extends beyond the expertise associated with the limited, classic financial management function in government.

In the public sector, the finance function does not usually attract the high flyers. Despite the Canadian Auditor General's laments at the quality of financial management in the late 1970s, and his call for improvements, there remains a real lack of substance in the traditional financial role at the departmental level. In a business firm, the senior financial officer is usually an important member of the top management team, responsible for issues related to the evaluation and financing of major investments, the maintenance of corporate liquidity and a healthy balance sheet. This is a far cry from the accounting responsibilities of a departmental financial officer in government, for in the public service, the most interesting and demanding financial functions are centralized: they are managed on behalf of the "collectivity". Departments such as Canada's Finance department or Britain's Treasury keep for themselves the major financial responsibilities equivalent to those of a private sector comptroller or treasurer.

Line departments are left with much more routine and bureaucratic responsibilities, such as assembling the annual budget, contract administration and accounting. As a result, the financial management area in departments does not tend to attract the best and the brightest in the public service. Those who are looking for the best route to the position of deputy minister or permanent secretary tend to gravitate toward policy development roles in departments or to central agencies.

Many government departments are realizing that someone in the organization should be accountable for making the operational planning and control system work. Likewise, some person has to be responsible for either executing periodic evaluations of existing policies, or seeing that they are done by others. (Line managers are usually thought to be too close to operations for this purpose.) Someone should be supporting the department head in asking the tough policy-related questions about whether programs have been responsibly planned, or whether the financial implications of new initiatives have been adequately assessed. Similarly, if there is to be some basis other than the political process for determining whether programs are meeting their goals, someone must be responsible for improving management information in departments and introducing, where appropriate, performance indicators. Although some officials suggest that the logical home for these responsibilities is in finance, these activities are beyond the scope and experience of many departmental financial officials. Where in the department should these responsibilities be situated?

Britain, Canada and other jurisdictions are wrestling with this problem. In the U.K., when interviews for this book were conducted, efforts were being made to add some limited responsibilities for planning, better management information and program performance to the role of the principal finance officer. In Canada, in 1983, a somewhat more intrusive and ambitious role was proposed for the senior financial officer of departments by the then Comptroller General, Harry Rogers.[20] Following a line of thinking initially advanced by the Auditor General, Rogers suggested that the position of departmental comptroller be established, which would include responsibility for the planning process and the co-ordination of management information, in addition to the traditional accounting and regularity functions. Rogers also suggested the institution of a "challenge function" whereby the financial officer would have the prerogative "to subject departmental proposals to a systematic, independent, impartial review and analysis before they are submitted for approval external to the department."* This latter function, which included a private sector type of responsibility for "rationalizing the final resource allocation proposal for the department", was pregnant with possibilities for conflict between financial and line officials.

During the 1980s, there has been some movement toward the acceptance of such a comptrollership function in Ottawa, but the challenge function has encountered heavy weather. All these proposals imply a cultural shift in the public service, which could lead to a fairly substantial transfer of power to financial officials. However, they tend to run counter to political forces. Non-financial officials are dubious about the capacity of traditional finance units to discharge such responsibilities effectively. They raise questions about the relationship between the financial section of the department and other organizational units with responsibilities for policy formulation. Line managers tend to perceive in them another fetter on their ability to move proposals through a system already larded with rules, regulations and requirements for consultation.

Clearly there are variations on the comptrollership proposal which are possible; and its adaptability to any specific department will depend in great measure upon the capacities of the staff in place. In Ottawa, some departments have divided staff responsibilities

---

* Specifically, this role would include the responsibility "to appraise all major resource proposals that are to be considered by the deputy head and the departmental executive committee . . . [and] certification to the deputy head and line managers that the financial and personnel resources requested are consistent with the assumptions and forecasts of what the program is expected to accomplish . . . ."

related to the planning system and different types of control. Some have established small operational planning and control offices separate from the finance function, reporting to the deputy minister, whose basic responsibility is to develop and maintain the process and to co-ordinate the development of performance measures. Some departments have established a program evaluation office in a policy branch with cross-departmental responsibilities; others have created a combined departmental audit and evaluation unit, reporting to the deputy minister. Some departments have clustered different mixes of planning- and evaluation-related responsibilities under a senior official variously called a departmental comptroller, an Assistant Deputy Minister (ADM) Corporate Management, an ADM Policy and Planning, or something similar.

The task of planning and control in the public sector has become a good deal more complicated in the last 20 years or so. Schools of public administration and professional institutes may find it useful to develop a specialized definition of the financial management role in a public sector context, one which recognizes the evolving requirements of this function in government. They may need to reorient some aspects of their educational programs to prepare new graduates to cope with the particular challenges of management in the public sector.

Conclusion

The practice of management has been afflicted by two misconceptions related to planning—the notion that organizations need a "strategic planning system" to produce a new strategic plan each year according to a programmed annual cycle; and the belief that the quality of planning in a large, complex organization is primarily dependent upon the functioning of a planning system.

Strategic planning is a synonym for major policy development work. Such planning is inherently unsystematic; hence planning systems that represent themselves as "strategic" (whether in the public or the private sector) will frequently be found to be little more than operational planning systems dressed up in impressive verbiage. Such systems are unlikely to produce truly strategic change.

BEYOND THE BOTTOM LINE

A distinction has been drawn between "strategic planning", defined as important planning that questions basic assumptions, and "operational planning", defined as planning which accepts the fundamental premises upon which existing activities and programs have been based, which does not contemplate dramatic change, and which seeks to identify tangible and specific objectives to be attained within a relatively short period (one or two years). Strategic planning is issue-specific, responsive to political direction and custom-designed. Operational planning is more concerned with the ongoing administration of existing programs; it is corporate in scope and can be made to function in a systematic and orderly manner.

Planning is an intrinsic part of all managers' jobs. It is an ongoing function, not one that is turned on and off at different points in the year. The quality of planning and decision-making in any organization is primarily determined by the quality of leadership and by the overall design of the institution—its structure, methods of communication, committees, decision-making processes, delegation of authority, etc.

An operational planning and control system is one element in this overall design. Such a system can help to co-ordinate work in different parts of the organization; it can provide a context within which individuals may be formally held to account for past performance; and it can help to link financial needs to operational requirements. In a large organization, such a system is typically not "the" planning system, but rather one among several systems designed to serve a variety of planning-related purposes.

Governments have devised a number of concepts and methodologies to help with the problem of managing in the absence of a bottom line. Surrogates for the bottom line have been developed in the form of output measures of various types. Attempts have also been made to devise methods for systematically evaluating government programs through periodic, in-depth examinations of their efficiency and effectiveness. Evaluation, like planning, has to take account of political realities. The evaluation of smaller, less politically sensitive programs can take place in response to an administratively-determined timetable; however the bigger, or more sensitive, evaluation initiatives will probably always have to be custom-designed, timed to accord with the elected Government's political agenda.

Increased emphasis on the management of resources in departments has brought new functions to the surface, to do with the design and operation of the operational planning and control system, with the development of performance measures and management information and with evaluation of existing programs. The roles of senior officials are evolving to accommodate these responsibilities; in future, the top jobs in departments may increasingly require expertise in concepts and methodologies related to planning and control of a type unique to the public sector.

Footnotes:

1. See Richard D. French, *How Ottawa Decides*, (Toronto: James Lorimer and Co., 1980).

2. See Peter Hennessy, Susan Morrison, and Richard Townsend, "Routine punctuated by orgies: the Central Policy Review Staff, 1970-1983," Strathclyde Papers on Government and Politics, no. 31, Jeremy Moon ed., (Glasgow: University of Strathclyde); also William Plowden, "The British Central Policy Review Staff," in Peter R. Baehr, and Bjorn Wittrock, *Policy Analysis and Policy Innovation*, (London: Sage Publications, 1981), pp. 1-89.

3. Samuel M. Greenhouse, "The PPB-System: Rationale, Language, and Idea-Relationships," *Public Administration Review*, vol. 26, (December 1966), p. 273.

4. See Robert N. Anthony and Regina E. Herzlinger, *Management Control in Non-Profit Organizations*, (Homewood, Ill.: Richard D. Irwin Inc., 1975), chapters 8 and 9 for a detailed and insightful discussion of program definition and analysis.

5. See for example, Leonard Rutman, ed., *Evaluation Research Methods: A Basic Guide*, (Beverly Hills: Sage Publications, 1977), ch. 1, "Planning an evaluation study".

6. Aaron Wildavsky, "The Political Economy of Efficiency: Cost Benefit Analysis, Systems Analysis and Program Budgeting," *Public Administration Review*, vol. 26, (December 1966), pp. 302-303.

7. Greenhouse, *loc. cit.* "A program which mirrors a given agency's established organization structure will be a rarity, unless the agency happens to have only one program." Officials received somewhat confusing advice from Treasury Board on PPBS: the Planning Programming and Budgeting Guide told them that the focus for program planning should be "independent of the organization structure used to execute it," while the Guide on Financial Administration told them that "a program should be ... capable of assignment as far as possible to a specific person who can be held accountable for achieving its purpose," an injunction that suggested that the organization structure and the program structure should coincide. See Treasury Board, *Guide on Financial Administration*, (September 1973), part II, 4.4.

8. Andrew Gray and Bill Jenkins, "Policy Analysis in British Central Government: The Experience of PAR," *Public Administration*, vol. 60, (Winter 1982), pp. 435-437.

9. Andrew Gray and Bill Jenkins, "Policy Evaluation in British Government: The Search for Efficiency," paper prepared for a workshop at the European Consortium for Political Research, (Barcelona, Spain, 25-30 March 1985). See also, by the same authors "Policy Analysis in British Central Government, *loc. cit.*, pp. 429-450.

10. From H.H. Heclo and A. Wildavsky, *The Private Government Of Public Money*, 2nd ed., (London: Macmillan, 1981). Cited in Gray and Jenkins, *loc. cit.*, p. 446.

11. Leo Pliatzky, *Getting and Spending: Public Expenditure, Employment and Inflation*, rev. ed., (Oxford: Blackwell, 1984), pp. 98-99.

12. Rodney Dobell and David Zussman, "An evaluation system for government: If politics is theatre, then evaluation is (mostly) art," *Canadian Public Administration*, vol. 24 no. 3, (Fall 1981), p. 405.

13. Office of the Comptroller General, Program Evaluation Branch, Treasury Board of Canada, "Program Evaluation Newsletter" no. 11, (October 1984); see also no. 14, (August 1985). These reports stated that, based on a sample which the Office had investigated, about 15 per cent of studies were contributing to savings, while 10 per cent had contributed to expansion decisions. About one third of the studies had generated recommendations for "significant changes to program design," while 20 per cent simply reconfirmed the wisdom of existing policies.

14. Author's interviews.

15. Ian D. Clark, "Recent changes in the cabinet decision-making system in Ottawa," *Canadian Public Administration*, vol. 28 no. 2, (Summer 1985), pp. 185-201.

16. Herman R. van Gunsteren, *The Quest for Control: a critique of the rational-central-rule approach in public affairs*, (London: John Wiley & Sons, 1976), p. 48.

17. See H.I. Ansoff, "Toward a Strategic Theory of the Firm," in *Business Strategy*, Ansoff, ed., (Harmondsworth: Penguin, 1969), pp. 11-40. Ansoff points out that several different kinds of decisions, described in his terminology as "logistical," "administrative" and "strategic," are all competing for top management time. There is no pre-ordained degree of attention that top managers should be addressing to strategic issues at any given point: what is appropriate will depend upon the circumstances of the firm.

18. Robert N. Anthony, *Planning and Control Systems: A Framework for Analysis*, (Boston: Graduate School of Business Administration, Harvard University, 1965), especially chapter 2. This little-known book is a lucid and rigorous guide to the concepts of strategic planning and management control. In the present book, "operational planning and control" is used synonymously with Anthony's "management control" as I believe Anthony's usage is potentially confusing, (it suggests strategic planning lies outside the sphere of management). Anthony points out that, contrary to popular belief, strategic planning is typically not directed to the whole of an organization, but only some aspect of it; it is difficult, irregular, unstructured, tailor-made for the problem, and it tends to take a long time (longer than the budget cycle, for example) to complete. See p.67.

19. van Gunsteren, *op. cit.*, pp. 58-59. "[M]any PPB proposals ignore or deny the rationality of politics, and thereby throw away one of the very few known ways – if not the only one – to ... deal with interdependence and plurality."

20. H.G. Rogers, "Comptrollership in departments and agencies of the federal government," *Optimum*, vol. 14 no. 3, (1983). See also a later version of this document: "Comptrollership in departments and agencies of the federal government: a restructured role for the Senior Financial Officer," Office of the Comptroller General, Policy Development Branch, 16 January 1984.

Chapter Ten:
The Policy Function

One of the biggest differences between business and government is the presence in government of a function called policy development. This is the function that is most difficult to explain to people who do not understand government. It looks quite a lot like the strategic planning function in business, and a number of the techniques employed by policy analysts, particularly in the sphere of financial analysis, are similar to those which might be employed by a strategic planning office in the private sector.

However, it is not the same. The focus of the policy function in government is different; the considerations that have to be taken into account are more diverse; the objectives being pursued are broader and more variable; there are fewer certitudes or reliable reference points to provide a context for new initiatives than in business; and the cast of characters whose interests have to be taken into account in moving a proposal from conception to implementation is much bigger. All this makes policy development a more complicated and time-consuming process than that of business planning. It can also be more difficult, more subtle . . . and at times, a good deal more exasperating.

Just as marketing, finance, production, and, more recently, human resource management, corporate planning and corporate affairs might be said to constitute the core functions of business administration, policy development is a core function in government. This chapter discusses the two aspects of the function. The first section of the chapter discusses the substantive side of policy development, by defining what it is, how it has been approached in the past and some more recent ideas about how it should be conducted. The second explores the process side of policy work: the skills required of a policy analyst, the function of a policy "manager" in government, and some techniques that have been known to help in moving policy proposals through the decision-making process.

Defining the Problem

Within the public service, the need for policy development emerges in response to an "issue," a catch-all word, often used in government to describe some divergence between the present state of affairs (real or perceived) and a desired state of affairs—in short, a problem. In business, most issues of corporate strategy (or policy) have to do with the positioning of the business enterprise in the marketplace. However, in government, policy issues are concerned with the socio-economic context: such questions as the functioning of the economy, foreign affairs, the social welfare system, national sovereignty, pollution, education, scientific research, and so forth. A government "policy" may mean anything from a full-blown plan of action involving extensive expenditures, regulations, legislation, press conferences, etc., to something much more mundane, such as the position which a minister might take if asked about a matter in a public forum ("our policy is that while we share the concerns of the Honourable Member about the decreasing size of the caribou herds, the matter lies outside the jurisdiction of this Government.")

Whether the issue is big or small, the analytical aspect of the process of policy development often proceeds through a number of steps, but not necessarily in a logical sequence. Defining a policy issue is often a matter of ranging around intellectually, looking for the heart of the matter. If the issue is complicated, the steps are not readily "programmable", (i.e., susceptible to being arrayed in logical order with defined time frames for their completion) since it is almost impossible to say how long each will take. Frequently, even though one step seems to have been completed, it proves necessary to return and do it over again. The process is typically iterative. Progress is not linear and the best way to move forward may sometimes be to go backward (e.g., to first principles). This applies particularly in the early stages of policy development, when the following questions are being addressed:

1.   *Is there really an issue? What is its nature?*

A recent opinion poll indicates rising concern about pollution. Is one poll a reliable indicator of public concern on such a matter? Were the findings statistically significant? How important was this issue relative to others revealed by this or other polls? What kind of pollution: acid rain? nuclear waste? noise pollution? municipal garbage? industrial effluent? Who is causing this pollution? What are its consequences? How did the constituencies concerned vote in the last election? How important are they to the Government's position in the House?

Until the particulars of the issue are better understood, it is impossible to know what might reasonably be done.

2.   *Is it something government should address? Who are the stakeholders and what are their interests?*

Perhaps there is an issue here. Should government get involved or should the problem be left to voluntary action or to market forces? If left alone will it go away? What are the likely consequences of involvement? If government gets involved, will this constitute a precedent that could lead to pressure for it to become involved in other issues it wishes to avoid? Should government play the role of catalyst, or should it assume a direct leadership role? What are its options? What can be expected of the private sector? If business is made to pay the costs of cleaning up pollution, what impact will this have upon competitiveness and employment? What are other jurisdictions' roles and policies with respect to pollution? What is the history of their involvement in this issue?

Some questions will have a high political content. For example, what interest groups are involved in this issue and how much political clout do they possess? What are the opportunities for the accumulation of political capital presented by this issue? To what extent might involvement in this issue permit the Government to achieve political advantage and to portray its party and its ministers in a favourable light, without necessarily having to expend a lot of time or resources? Does this issue present opportunities for media exposure?

3. *Is it urgent?*

Will a much worse situation develop if action is not taken quickly? What will the substantive or political consequences be of delaying action? What might be the consequences of rapid response?

4. *What are the forces or developments that gave rise to the issue? Can these be ascertained? To what extent is the issue susceptible to technical or scientific analysis?*

Why is pollution increasing? Is the problem due to primary industry or to secondary manufacturing? Or is it due to inadequate municipal treatment of effluent? Perhaps waste is being treated, but the problem lies in the standards, which are set too low. Then again, existing standards may be adequate, but the problem may relate to new pollutants for which standards have not been developed. Or, it may be that pollution is coming from other jurisdictions; the problem is not a matter for domestic scientists or industry to address, but one for the diplomats and politicians to negotiate. Obviously, different views as to the causes of the problem will suggest very different responses. But can the causes be ascertained, and can their relationship to each other be apprehended?

These initial questions all have to do with defining the problem. Geoffrey Vickers says the first step in policy development is an assessment of the prevailing reality. It involves "the capacity to comprehend and analyse a complex situation extended in time, to assess the outcome of multiple, causal interactions, to apply appropriate time scales, to comprehend uncertainties, most of all perhaps to simplify without distorting by excluding the inessential.... Its basic use is to supply a predictive picture of what is going to happen next."[1]

Defining the problem and its causes can be the most difficult part of policy formation. A group of senior U.K. civil servants who briefed the Fulton Committee said, "[P]olicy-making is a matter of combining in new ways points of view and sources of knowledge which have not previously been usefully related to each other."[2] It is an attempt to understand what may be a very complex chain of social and economic interactions. As a senior Canadian policy ADM indicated, "Half the problem is identifying the problem that has to be solved. It's a bit like going to the doctor – the symptoms may be in one place but the problem may be somewhere else. The key is to be analyzing the right issue."[3]

Sometimes the causes of a problem can lie deep in the past, in conditions about which nothing can be done now. At other times, the sources of the problem may be more recent, but it still may be impossible to untangle the skein of causes and effects leading up to the present situation. Officials may find themselves embroiled in chicken-and-egg controversies to which there is no clear answer.

Meanwhile, outside the borders of the department, on any major policy issue, there is usually no shortage of self-styled experts ready and willing to tell the responsible minister what the problem is and what type of action is needed – now – to address it. "Fine the companies responsible for polluting!" "Ban all insecticides!" "Give grants to municipalities!" "Jail the senior executives!" "Jail the pollution protestors!" Hire more scientists!" "Leave pollution cleanup to market forces: industry will solve the problem." "Talk tough to the Americans!" How to tell who is right?

Thinking through the Issues

Some people seem to be more adept than others at thinking through policy questions and identifying the core of an issue, but we know remarkably little about how they do it. The process of thinking about practical problems has been tackled by several authors, among whom is Edward De Bono, best known for coining the phrase, "lateral thinking", which has now passed into common usage.

De Bono points out that achieving insights into a problem we do not initially understand involves restating, in progressively specific terms, what we believe to be the cause of the problem.[4] In the early stages of analysis, vague terms such as "a thing" or "a force" serve as useful "porridge words" — conceptual coat hooks upon which meaning can be hung until a more precise formulation of the problem can be made (usually based upon new information, or perhaps simply new insight arising from cogitation). This process frequently goes on in meetings held to discuss problems, without many of the participants being aware of what they are doing.

> Thinking often proceeds as drift and waffle and reaction to what turns up from moment to moment. There is a background sense of purpose, but this is never spelled out either as an overall objective or as sub-objectives. Suggestions, judgement, criticism, information and plain emotion are all mixed together in a sort of thinking stew. It seems to be a matter of messing around until a thinker stumbles on some tried approach which seems to achieve what is desired .... There is also the assumption that the thinking will be moulded by past experience and present constraints in such a way that an outcome "evolves" and is purified by criticism ....[5]

De Bono observes there is no such thing as a policy which is right or wrong in an absolute sense, and that being right or wrong is a matter of values, prejudices or preconception. Even "logical" thinking is simply an array of linked ideas that can often be "refuted" by another set of linked ideas. In view of the often-noted need for officials to maintain a balanced point of view when engaged in policy development and to avoid commitment to existing policies and programs, De Bono's observations have a special relevance for the public servant.[6]

De Bono argues that thinking is too often conducted in accordance with traditional and conventional methods of problem definition, with insufficient attention given to the contributions that humour, insight and creativity can provide in expanding intellectual horizons. Most of what passes for training in thinking in our academic institutions is, in fact, training in criticism. "It is always claimed that the word *criticism* covers an honest appraisal of both positive and negative aspects. In practice, however, the verb *to criticize* implies the pointing out of what is wrong ...."[7]

What is required in a policy shop is an atmosphere conducive to creative, innovative thinking. This issue is pursued later in this chapter (see "Managing a Policy Shop").

Objectives and Strategies

Once the problem has been sufficiently well defined, its solution usually begins to come into focus. As the problem becomes clearer, it becomes possible to set objectives in progressively specific terms. For example, taking the example of pollution cited above, the initial objective might have been to diminish the incidence of pollution; once it becomes evident that, say, the main cause of increased pollution has been lack of regulations and inadequate international agreements, the objectives become more precise: to increase regulation and improve standards; to negotiate stronger treaties with offending neighbours.

In determining what the objectives should be and what policies to recommend to ministers, the government policy officer faces a more complex range of options than does the planning officer in a business corporation. Often there are many different stakeholders affected by the policy and a large number of institutional and jurisdictional interests to be taken into account. The problem of what to do becomes inextricably entangled with who should do what, with the jockeying for power that may be going on and with the different values held by the groups or individuals involved.

The Rational Model of Planning and Policy Development

A great deal of the thinking about the development of policy and strategic planning has been influenced by what has sometimes been called the "rational" model. This model, which was probably derived from the military, suggests that there is one correct way to plan in organizations. According to this model, planning is a top-down process, proceeding from the general to the specific in a logical, structured fashion. It involves the articulation of overall, comprehensive aims by the top officials of the organization; these are in turn disaggregated into more specific objectives that are susceptible to measurement and time-bounded. ("The objective is to secure 15 per cent of the widget market by 1990.")[8]

The rational model portrays planning as a process that moves from problem definition through identification of alternatives to decision. Different strategies for attaining a particular objective are to be developed, costed and analyzed for effectiveness. The optimal strategy is then selected, perhaps with the assistance of some of the mathematical tools of what is known as "decision analysis". The organization unable to demonstrate that it has a planning process of this type is presumed to be planning poorly.[9]

This view of planning has a seductive simplicity. Making planning work, according to this model, is in large measure a procedural problem. Methods have to be developed for scanning the environment, for setting objectives and analyzing strategies. Activities have to be scheduled in the proper sequence. In business, this line of thinking led to the establishment of corporate planning departments and structured planning systems. In government, it found expression in new approaches to budgeting, of which the best known was undoubtedly the program planning and budgeting system (PPBS). As discussed in chapter 9, PPBS constituted a codified, organized method of putting the precepts of rational planning into effect into large government organizations.

The problem with this reasonable, logical, top-down approach to planning was that it often did not work. Some students of business administration began to question why, with all the investment in planning systems and analysis, business still seemed to be having trouble with planning. Was it reasonable to take a complex process dependent upon the personalities of the planners, upon intuition and upon chance, and program it into a logical sequence of events? How important was analysis in the making of important decisions? What happened when there was not enough time to analyze all the alternatives? One writer has argued, "As corporate planning has become increasingly popular and sophisticated, its methods have become increasingly divergent from corporate reality."[10]

The Donaldson-Lorsch study of decision-making in U.S. corporations which has been cited previously in this book noted that in reality, things do not work the way some "experts" said they did. Top executives do not analyze every alternative. The "right" decision, even in the private sector, is often difficult to identify and dependent upon the interests of several different parties. Finding the course of action is not simply a matter of accepting the analysis of highly educated planning staff. The study found that business executives typically advance in an exploratory, tentative way that relied a lot upon intuition, personal beliefs and perceptions of the interests of various stakeholders or constituencies, not just "rational" analysis.[11]

As the bloom wore off the rose of rational planning in business, a parallel development occurred in government. One aspect of this was the decline of PPBS. In Canada, during the early 1970s, in addition to PPBS, several other efforts were mounted by central agencies to create rational, structured systems to facilitate the analysis of programs and the setting of priorities.[12] The best-known version, and the one that enjoyed the greatest measure of central agency and political support, was a PCO-sponsored initiative called the Cabinet Planning System. This system sought to attach priorities to every aspect of government activity, and to create some kind of logical construct within which to decide whether the government should be assigning higher priority (whatever that meant) to, say, constitutional reform, national sovereignty, social welfare or environmental protection.

A former principal secretary to the then Prime Minister, Pierre Trudeau, joined with a former official of the PCO to ask if this system worked. They concluded, "The answer is 'no,' although it is a qualified 'no.'"[13] Richard French, who also worked in PCO from 1974 to 1977, described the system as a failure with little qualification.[14] A deputy minister, looking back on the era of Trudeau and his ex Cabinet Secretary, Michael Pitfield, made the pungent comment, "It seemed as though the philosophy of the time was, 'That might work in practice, but what about in theory?'"[15] Another deputy minister who climbed to the top of the public service ladder during the 1970s said of the system, "it was completely rational but deeply impractical. It was based on a belief that you could construct a system and then force not only people but events to fit themselves into it. It required a breed of supermen and a universe unfolding as it should. Instead, it produced an administrative nightmare."[16]

New Ideas about Planning: Alternative Models

In the face of widespread concern about the legitimacy of the rational, or systematic, approaches to planning, a number of writers began to reexamine the original premises of planning and policy development. Some suggested that it advanced in a more organic and unpredictable manner than originally thought. Others pointed out that strategic planning in business often did not involve the entire enterprise, and counselled against too much emphasis on "comprehensive" approaches to planning.[17] One experienced observer of business executives pointed out that good managers seldom took policy decisions in the textbook manner, as a result of a systematic process and clinical analysis. He described a process that sounded much like a politician testing a new idea. "Rather than produce a full-blown decision tree, [successful executives] start with a twig, help it grow, and ease themselves out on the limbs only after they have tested to see how much weight the limbs can stand."[18]

Charles Lindblom, the distinguished American professor of public policy, stated, "[Policy-making is not] a relatively orderly, rationalistic process, like writing a term paper with a beginning, a middle, and an end, with each part tied logically to each succeeding part . . . . [It is] . . . an extremely complex process without beginning or end . . . whose boundaries remain most uncertain."[19] He noted that policy decisions tend to be resolved by "muddling through" rather than a rigorous, staged methodology of analysis. Such decisions typically involve questions of values. Values cannot be reconciled by analysis and systems, but only through interaction – that is, the political process. Policy development involved "a never ending process in which continual nibbling substitutes for the good bite that may never be offered."

Policy often emerges as a result of the efforts of a "policy entrepreneur", an individual buried deep within an organization, a long way from the top where policy was supposed to originate. In other cases, policy seems to advance by chance or serendipity, not because of a well-organized process. Henry Mintzberg, as noted in the introduction to part 2 of this book, pointed out that a lot of policy is "emergent", popping up like "weeds in a garden" rather than as a result of planned, systematic direction from the top of the organization.[20]

Mintzberg concluded that there is more than one type of strategy that an organization may legitimately adopt.* The rational model (christened the "hothouse model" of strategy) is not invalid but is suited only to certain circumstances. Specifically, it best fits a stable situation where the organization responsible for the policy has a high degree of control over policy development and implementation: for example, a military organization.

Where the conditions of stability and control do not obtain, an "umbrella" strategy might be more appropriate. Umbrella strategies are those where leaders have only partial control over what shall be done; they set general guidelines or broad objectives within which others manoeuvre. Such policies are suited to circumstances where those who have the vision do not control its realization, or where multiple interests have to be brought together to develop and then implement the policy.

In government, the rational approach to planning is often impaired by the constitutional necessity of involving other levels of government or other jurisdictions. For example, in Canada, delivery of educational programs involves both municipal and provincial authorities. Certain types of economic development policy are conceived at the federal level but must be integrated with provincial policy in the same field. In Britain, local authorities are deeply involved in many aspects of Whitehall's policies, transportation, education, housing, and health being cases in point. These are fields where a loose umbrella approach to policy and its development may be in place already; such a strategy is likely to be more suitable than a structured approach.

Another type of strategy (or policy) identified by Mintzberg and Waters is a "process" strategy, suitable in an unpredictable or uncontrollable environment when, for example, information is best gathered and processed at the local level. Here, leaders control the process of strategy development while leaving the content to others. It would work particularly well in organizations which do not require a great deal of co-ordination between local units — organizations

---

* In the discussion which follows, the words "policy" and "strategy" are used interchangeably.

engaged in heterogeneous, unrelated operations, or where each local office is, to a large degree, a separate enterprise.

A process strategy assumes that the right process will produce the right results. For example, a firm with highly decentralized operations might simply specify a very broad financial goal that each local unit was to attain, and a planning process which each was to follow. The local units would not be expected to fit their plans into detailed objectives outlined by head office, but simply to use the approved process to develop their policies within the broader framework of financial targets. Process strategy says, "Follow the rules, and the right result will emerge." In some circumstances, such a strategy is appropriate; in others it clearly is not.

Process strategy has particular relevance to any field of government activity where the concept of due process applies. This includes courts and regulatory tribunals and commissions of various sorts. Organizations that are essentially adjudicative in nature do not need a structured plan featuring a hierarchy of objectives, but do need a well-framed process strategy. That is, they are responsible for ensuring that the adjudicative process to which they submit applicants is robust. In such organizations, the overall objective is not to get somewhere or arrive at some specific, time-bounded goal, but rather to ensure that appropriate procedures exist so that due process is observed in the treatment of applicants.

Different types of policy may be employed to attain the same ends. For example, in the field of economic policy, some countries have opted for a state-controlled, centralized, dirigiste policy (structured or planned policy). Others have chosen a more laissez-faire approach (umbrella policy) which tries to create the conditions to promote industrial growth by relying more upon the free play of market forces than a state-imposed industrial strategy. Yet so pervasive is the structured, rational model of planning, in countries where the latter approach has been adopted, the government is often accused of not having an industrial policy, simply because the approach they have chosen does not conform to the rational model.

Policy officers must determine which generic type of policy (or combination of types) is best suited to the policy field within which they are working. For example, the Canada Council, Canada's equivalent of the Arts Council of Great Britain, employs a combination of umbrella and process policies in providing grants to organizations and individuals in the arts. The Council has some broad umbrella strategies related to the development of individual disciplines (such as providing support to professional organizations only), but it does not dictate how each will evolve in detail, nor does it try to run arts organizations in the country. To decide which organizations to fund, the Council applies general criteria through a complex process of adjudication known as peer assessment, a form of process strategy. It is thought that this approach will permit the development of culture in an atmosphere of artistic freedom.

There are times when, in the formation of policy, the option of doing *nothing* should be seriously considered. Edward Wrapp notes how experienced senior managers often hold back on decisions, waiting for what he calls the "corridors of comparative indifference " to open up so that, at the right time, the decision may be pushed along a little further without encountering hostile forces.[21] They are well aware of the importance of timing, and that sometimes the best option is to wait. Not entirely tongue in cheek, another author has argued the virtues of "masterly inactivity" and "disciplined inaction", noting that there are certain issues (for example, race relations) that are sometimes best left alone, and that solutions "might just as legitimately be alterations of perceptions as changes to the actual state of affairs."[22]

In summary, a fundamental step in determining the right course of action for an important policy issue is to choose the appropriate strategy, bearing in mind the roles of different levels of government, the character of the institution(s) affected, and the relationships that should prevail between governors and governed in a democratic society. Policy officers must also consider what instrument(s) to use. Here again, government officials will have more difficulty than would their business counterparts, because of the number of tools they have to consider — legislation, regulations, expenditures (direct and indirect), taxation (or tax credits), income transfers, moral suasion, or various combinations of these options. Assessing the advantages, disadvantages and adaptability of each of these instruments to a particular issue is often a major part of the policy development exercise.

Course-Holding: A Different Kind of Objective

Policy officers must also choose the objectives appropriate to the problem at hand. The popularity of the rational model in planning literature has promoted the view that objectives must be specific, preferably quantified and time-bounded. Wrapp points out that, in his experience, (which coincides with my own), senior management does not usually work in this way.

> The successful manager . . . seldom makes a forthright statement of policy. The management textbooks contend that well-defined policies are the sine qua non of a well-managed company. My research does not bear out this contention.
>
> The "management by objectives" school . . . suggests that detailed objectives be spelled out at all levels in the corporation. This method is feasible at lower levels of management, but it becomes unworkable at the upper levels. The top manager must think out objectives in detail, but ordinarily some of the objectives must be withheld, or at least communicated to the organization in modest doses. A conditioning process which may stretch over months or years is necessary in order to prepare the organization for radical departures from what it is currently striving to attain.[23]

Similarly, Geoffrey Vickers proposes that, particularly in the field of public policy, it may sometimes be more useful to think of policy-making in terms of holding to a course, or maintaining a set of relationships, rather than arriving at a destination. (The suitability of this approach to policy is immediately apparent in such spheres as external affairs or federal-provincial relations.) "I believe that great confusion results from the common assumption that all course-holding can be reduced to the pursuit of an endless succession of goals."* Much policy-making is really about the establishment of relations and the preservation of certain norms rather than the achievement of the

---

* "Problems of policy-making . . . involve judgments of value made by processes and according to criteria that cannot be specified . . . . For the policy maker . . . the executive problem is not given; it is for him to decide what it shall be. [Policy making

tangible, quantifiable goals promoted in some of the business planning literature.

In summary, there is no single "best" or "correct" approach to the development of policy; different types of strategies (such as structured, umbrella or process strategies) will be suited to different contexts. The suitability of the approach will depend to a great extent upon the institutional relationships affected by different policy options and the politics of the situation.

The Skills of the Policy Analyst

No matter how intractable a policy issue, once expectations have been aroused, the government must usually do something. The job of the policy officer is to do the staff work for ministers and top officials to help frame a course of action. One permanent secretary who was leading a policy department looked for the following qualities in his best officials:

- a capacity to deal with the minister

- steadfastness of personality

- experience

- humanity

- ability to simplify

- a capacity to see the heart of an issue

- good drafting skills and an understanding of the power of language.[24]

A top official from the Department of Health and Social Security, which has to work closely with Britain's huge National Health Service, placed a somewhat different emphasis on the attributes of a good policy officer, arguing that of key importance were qualities such

---

involves] the evaluation and modification of the course, the norm, the standard, the governing relation which is inherent in every policy and the selection and ascertainment of the facts relevant to it." See Vickers, *op. cit.*, pp. 39-41.

as an ability to listen to staff, to consult with those involved in the direct delivery of operational programs, and to make people feel they are not just cogs in a big machine.[25] Certainly intelligence is an attribute any senior official would look for, and indeed, it is a quality also appreciated by ministers (as a former provincial treasurer from Ontario has observed, "[B]right people are usually easier to appoint than elect!"[26])

It used to be thought (and continues to be thought in many quarters) that the best form of training for policy work was a good general education, preferably in the liberal arts or classics. More recently, however, this view has been displaced in some quarters by the concept of the "policy analyst", a practitioner of a new discipline known as policy analysis, largely emanating from the U.S. Charles Wolf, Dean of the Rand Graduate Institute in California, has defined policy analysis as "the application of scientific methods to problems of public policy, choice and implementation in domestic, international and national security affairs. Its successful pursuit depends on familiarity with the social sciences, economics, and the physical sciences, competence in a number of analytical techniques, and the ability and confidence to move across disciplinary lines . . . ."[27]

During the late 1960s and the 1970s, it became fashionable in some quarters to believe that officials were not qualified to develop policy unless they possessed skills in quantitative, or "hard-edged", methods of analysis. More recently, in the wake of disappointing experiences with the application of systematic methods of analysis to policy development, questions have been raised about the investment of large amounts of time and money in quantitative analysis. In the U.S., Wolf himself has noted the "sad and sorry condition of the public policy domain" arising from a "combination of good intentions with perverse outcomes." A British civil servant observed that in Whitehall, "both cost-benefit and operational research were among the forms of analysis which developed in the British public service in the sixties. But neither made the impact that some expected of them."[28] An observer of the Canadian scene during the 1970s concluded that the "rationalists" were "discredited by events," and that public policy-making had moved "from system to serendipity."[29]

The present academic thinking on public policy seems to be anti-rational and away from analytic methods. However, much of the criticism of rationalism fails to define what is meant by the term; we are invited to reject rational, or analytic, approaches to policy making but it is seldom made clear what is to replace them. (An irrational one?) What seems legitimate in the anti-rational movement is the criticism of attempts to impose simplistic systematic solutions on complex problems, to treat institutions as if they were mechanical rather than human enterprises, and to overrate the ability of analysis to cope with certain public policy issues. However, recognition of these limitations should not lead to the conclusion that the only legitimate approach to policy development is instinctive or emotional. Nor does it mean that mastery of Virgil's Aeneid (even in the original Latin), is sufficient grounding for analyzing the causes of urban blight or for determining the impact of highway construction on sensitive ecology.

The tendency to equate the term "policy analysis" with quantitative modeling has caused a lot of confusion. Quantitative methods are just one of a variety of techniques that may usefully be applied to the analysis of public policy problems. They are not universally helpful; nor do they supplant the need for other forms of technical knowledge specifically related to the policy field in question (economics, agriculture, geology, sociology, etc.) To suggest that "analysis" is taking place only when hard-edged quantitative tools are being applied, and to divorce such tools from the disciplines within which they are employed, confuses the definition of analysis. It is possible to analyze many problems without using statistical or other numerical techniques!

The complexity of many public issues today can only be addressed by a blend of skills and technologies. Policy work requires professional knowledge of the relevant discipline (as well as, at times, certain skills of quantitative analysis), combined with the more traditional policy capabilities: direct experience in the relevant policy field: political savvy; writing skills; a sensitivity to the human and administrative consequences of policy options; knowledge of the machinery and procedures of government; and that elusive but all-important quality, judgment (see chapter 5).

Business people may wonder why writing skills rate so highly among public sector officials. Government generally has much more affinity for the written word than does business because of the legislative, regulatory and adjudicative functions of government, and in its public accountability. Businesses, unencumbered by the degree of scrutiny to which public institutions are subject, can often afford to be more casual in the conduct of their affairs.

If a new business initiative is not entirely right the first time round, there will often be opportunities to fix it in future. By contrast, the government program which gets off to a bad start may be pilloried in the press, leading to embarrassment for the minister and the government. The program acquires a bad reputation and cannot be fixed later on. In passing legislation, the government is often entering into a sort of contract to deliver services to members of the electorate; a mistake in wording can cost a lot of money. Similarly, the choice of the wrong phrase in an act of Parliament or a regulation can have unexpected, and sometimes distressing, results. As in a business contract, powerful consequences may hang upon a single word.

An American writer has illustrated this with reference to the problem of providing benefits to impoverished blind people. While there may be general agreement on the objective of supporting such persons, what does "blind" mean in the context determining eligibility for a multi-million dollar government program?

> The answer might seem obvious: someone who cannot see. But what if an individual can "see" – that is, perceive light, shadow, and even shape – but not well enough to work? The proper answer might still seem clear enough: include such people in the blind category too. But are we speaking of the ability to see with or without corrective lenses? With corrective lenses, of course.

> We are not done yet. Precisely how weak must a person's corrected vision be before we say that he or she is blind? What instructions shall we give to the government worker who is determining eligibility? . . . What if an individual has tunnel vision . . . .?

The author points out the different kinds of "blindness" and the different degrees of visual impairment; these must be dealt with in the regulations through detailed, specific language. He then goes on to list the complications involved in the definition of "poor". This necessitates determining a person's income.

From all sources? Well, yes. Alimony? Yes. Inheritance? Yes ... from all sources, earned or not. What if the blind person is a college student with a scholarship? Are the scholarship proceeds counted as income? Well, no, not if the scholarship is for payment of tuition and fees. Only the excess above that needed for tuition and fees should be treated as income. What if the blind person is a child living with parents who work? Income in such cases shall mean the parents' income. What if the parents are poor and there are brothers and sisters? Make exceptions for those situations ....

[Thus] a seemingly straightforward term such as "poor" [or "blind"] is translated into thickets of words that appear impenetrable to the uninitiated. They conceal choices with enormous social, budgetary and political consequences, however.[30]

Government policies and program regulations are framed in language where each word may carry huge implications. Moreover, the intentions underlying policy may have to be communicated to persons whom the policy officer has never met, and never will. The written word continues to be the principal vehicle of communication in large bureaucracies. Individuals who understand its power and are able to control it are invaluable to the process of policy formation and implementation.

The Policy Process

It will be apparent by now that, while analysis can be an important component of policy formation, there is a good deal more to the exercise. As one senior official observed, "Rational analysis is a very important part of the game, but you're always a bit disappointed that it doesn't play more of a role."[31] In the framing of policy, many different interests may have to be consulted, and conflicting points of view reconciled. As noted previously, there is no analytic procedure that can cope with the problem of incommensurability, or with issues where differences in values must be reconciled. Recognition of the limitations of analytic methods has directed attention to the other aspect of policy development, the process side.

Some public servants believe that "process" skills are as important, perhaps even more important than analytic capabilities in policy work. Public servants with policy responsibilities must learn the formal process of policymaking: for example, they must understand the roles of relevant central agencies, know how the Cabinet document system works and when an issue ought to be brought to the minister's attention, be able to draft white papers or legislation, understand relevant Treasury regulations and procedures, and so forth. However, they also should become proficient at what one official has called the "invisible process". This is the process outside the formal procedures of policy development which really determines outcomes in many instances. "This 'invisible process' is an arcane field to most planners and innovators, who are at a loss to understand why some perfectly sound proposals lie still-born in a file drawer, while other, apparently less worthy, proposals are accepted and implemented . . . ."[32]

Form and Substance

Developing policy requires an ability to combine substantive analysis with the cosmetic and the political dimensions of the issue. The policy analyst must deal with the objective problem, as revealed by some type of scientific or other investigation, as well as the *perceived* problem, quite different but just as important to resolve. Sometimes it may be even more important. For example, when people in a community do not believe that a flood is imminent and refuse to be evacuated, but the officials *know* the flood is about to engulf them, it is the residents' perception that will determine their behaviour, not reality. Policy analysts have to develop the capacity to deal with both the perceived and the real issue — with both the substance and the form.

> The interrelationship of form and substance is something that, until you've been in it for a while, you're not aware of. The really successful policy people are good at reading both sides of the issue and getting at the root of the problem . . . . You may have to handle both the cosmetic and the substantive sides of the problem concurrently. Sometimes you have to appear to be treating one problem

while actually getting at another. There's a lot of that. Both perceived and actual problems are reality.[33]

Consulting with the Stakeholders

The process of policy development will often involve external consultations with interested parties. There is no formula as to when this should occur: sometimes it is better to consult early, at other times it is preferable to develop some specific proposals for action, and perhaps to circulate a "green paper" or some similar document in order to generate public debate.[34]

A good strategy starts from analysis of the environment, i.e., an investigation of the forces playing on the policy issue and of the interests that different stakeholders may have in the outcome of a policy. The stakeholders include those both outside and inside the bureaucracy. As the policy ideas mature, the objective may be to sell a particular viewpoint, rather than just to gather opinions. Some officials speak of the need to "market" an emerging policy or viewpoint.

> The best policy isn't worth anything unless you market it well, outside the government. To market a policy, you've got to have all the answers. You've got to appear credible. This is because government is not engineering. What works is what the public can feel satisfied with, and if they do, in many ways the policy will work. You've got to have credibility, glibness, and so on to give the public a sense of confidence.[35]

The external consultative strategy for any important new policy idea will have to be developed in close consultation with the minister. The experienced policy officer will engage the minister's interest in, and commitment to, the policy exercise, and will seek opportunities where the minister can be made to look good while engaging the public in discussions or promoting a particular policy stance. Often an extensive program of consultations may be required. (In developing a new set of proposals for agricultural funding in the early 1980s, a former Canadian Minister of Agriculture, Eugene Whelan, was said to have participated in nearly 300 public meetings over the course of one and a half years.[36])

For lesser policy initiatives, officials will have to develop their own consultative strategies, being careful on the one hand to collect the required information and to determine what courses of action are likely to be well received by the public, while on the other hand avoiding any appearance of upstaging the minister. With the increasing size of government, many officials find they have to keep their own networks to the public in good order. External consultation by public servants raises a number of questions of both principle and tactics; as argued later in this book, in my view this function has not enjoyed the priority that it deserves in public management (see chapter 12).

Inside government, there are also many interests to be taken into account. Sometimes moving a new initiative through the bureaucracy can appear more difficult than the process of public consultation. Some proposals should not be committed to paper too early. "It's important to figure out the best way of pushing the issue forward: should it be on paper or off paper? When in doubt, involve more people, not less. You really have to get the coalitions on side."[37] This can be done in all kinds of ways—over lunch, on the phone, at a squash game, or in more formal settings. The effective leader of a policy unit has a capacity to sense the currents of both electoral and bureaucratic politics, and an ability to steer proposals through the interdepartmental channels and the minister's office while maintaining momentum. Building and maintaining networks—with interest groups, with other groups in the same department, with the minister's staff, with central agencies, with other departments—is a key part of the policy manager's job. The actual analysis of the issue is often left largely to subordinates.

Attention to Detail

Nonetheless, part of the process is to make sure that the analysis is good and that the documents for interdepartmental meetings are well crafted. One senior official, asked what advice he would give to a new head of a policy unit, replied, "Get an analytically sound team together so that your paper is beyond challenge. (You might even learn something from analysis, though often you do not!) You have to cover off that base—know your stuff, or have people working for you that know theirs." It's also important to see what ideas have been developed previously. "Almost anything that's plausible has been proposed before in some variation. Make sure you are not reinventing the wheel. Talk to people who have been around; look at the files. Don't assume that you're the smartest person around."38

Attention to detail is important. Another official indicated, "Whatever you put on paper has to be very high quality. Remember that when you send a letter or an interdepartmental memo, it is likely to be copied a couple of hundred times. If it has two spelling mistakes it affects the whole aura of what you want to do." Difficult arguments that will be raised in interdepartmental meetings have to be anticipated. "Around the town, you have to be on your toes."39

Detail is important for another reason. One official pointed out that it is often not the big policy issues that get an elected Government into trouble, but the little questions.

> An atomic energy plant can slip through [Parliament] easily. A rug in the mayor's office — an issue everyone can understand — can tie up a [municipal] council for ages.
>
> The risk is asymmetric. In government, what gets you into a hassle is seldom the huge decisions that were clearly wrong, it's the little things that often are trivial by comparison. You can make big mistakes and paradoxically they won't catch up with you. An example would be Canada's economic policy in 1973-75, which led to the Anti-Inflation Board and all that. But the Government survived it. Whereas [former Finance Minister John] Crosbie made a tiny mistake — 18 cents on gas — and that killed him . . . .
>
> You can in some sense make huge errors because if it's big enough, people have trouble comprehending it. But the public can understand little mistakes. Therefore to do good public policy, to do the big stuff, you can't afford to screw up on the little stuff. You have to . . . take the extra 48 hours to think through the ramifications.40

Timing

Equally critical is timing. One of the skills of the seasoned executive in the private sector is to know when to move with an issue, and when to hold off. It is the same in government. Effective policy officials will not try to advance a pet project according to some schedule set forth in a departmental planning manual. Rather, they will scout the situation and determine when it is propitious to push the proposal into the stream of events. Sometimes a proposal has to move quickly to catch an unexpected surge in the current. On other occasions, for example, when there are other larger and more important vessels occupying the main channel, it may be prudent to moor a proposal to the banks of the stream and leave it there until the traffic clears. Another tactic may be to attach a line to a larger proposal and allow it to tow a smaller initiative along in its wake.

An experienced official spoke of the need to look for "policy windows."

> Be prepared. Wait for the right time — the right window. You may have to wait one year or a year and a half. Then when the window opens, you have to move fast. There are times when it's in vogue to build things up and there are times when it's in vogue to tear things down . . . .
>
> If you're too early, people forget; they say, that's very nice, but what are you going to do for me today? If you're just right, you get the credit. If you're too late, you'll get criticized . . . . Don't put it in too early. That's hard, and it requires real discipline . . . . You have to take account of things like the electoral cycle, caucus, and the mood of the House . . . .[41]

Other Tactics

At Health and Welfare Canada, approval for a new $17 million program to promote fitness and amateur sport was secured by the use of a number of tactics: ensuring that the proposal was timely (i.e., fashionable); securing support for the proposal from individuals known to have influence with the prime minister; solid staff analysis; using a marketing consultant to help with the promotion of the idea and the preparation of an attractive report on the issue; marshalling support from a national council outside the public service; timing the proposal to coincide with a forthcoming election campaign; and creating a certain amount of pizzazz and publicity through a national conference featuring high-ranking speakers (including the Governor General who, at the time, was himself a fitness enthusiast).[42]

Managing a Policy Shop

Of course not all policy is developed in specialized policy units; many program areas help to form policy affecting their own activities. Although the following discussion focuses on specialized units, it is equally relevant to individuals in staff planning units attached to line operations, or to persons in other parts of a department who are involved in policy development.

Running a policy unit is not always easy; and the maxims of management from the classical school — provide clear objectives, set measurable goals, assign tasks that do not overlap, ensure that position descriptions and functions are clearly understood — are not much help. The management of professional work is a special challenge.[43]

Policy unit tasks are generally unique and non-routine in nature. The responsibilities of staff ebb and flow in response to constantly shifting political priorities. Frequently, who works on what issue has to be adjusted in light of individuals' experience, training, temperament, abilities and availability. Officers' responsibilities are often as difficult to define as the issues which have been assigned to them; and they change as the issues change.

Big units, engaged in a wide range of issues, are difficult to manage. Most experienced policy officials I have known perceive an inverse correlation between the size of a policy unit and its effectiveness, once it gets over a sort of minimum critical mass (which will vary depending on the kinds of issues involved). Issues overlap; it becomes almost impossible to keep on top of the work; and it is hard (but important) to maintain an atmosphere of collegiality when there are so many opportunities for co-workers to tread in each other's (ill-defined) territory.

The leader of a policy shop has to be able to foster creative thinking and to encourage the ability to set aside what currently exists. Geoffrey Vickers describes creativity as "the power to rearrange in imagination the constituents of some familiar object of attention, so as to see them in a changed relationship and another context . . . . [I]t comprises also the ability to envisage the possibility of organizational and social change."[44] Arthur Koestler defines creativity in science as "the putting together of two and two to make five . . . an apparent bit of magic" which consists in "combining previously unrelated domains of knowledge in such a way that you get more out of the emergent whole than you have put in."[45] Other writers speak of the need to "make the familiar strange . . . to distort, invert, or transpose the everyday ways of looking and responding which render the world a secure and familiar place." Analogy is often a powerful tool in this connection.[46] De Bono cites the need to be explicitly provocative: creativity arises "from the logic of asymmetrical patterning systems . . . . We can sit around and wait for provocations or we can set out to produce them deliberately . . . . The ability to use provocation is an essential part of lateral thinking."[47] So, it seems, is the capacity to synthesize: "Creativity requires the ability to reach out to widely separated components, and to synthesize them."[48]

Directing a policy unit appears similar to the private-sector job of managing research or product innovation. One study of business practices found that "[e]ffective managers of innovation . . . administer primarily by setting goals, selecting key people, and establishing a few critical limits and points for intervention rather than by implementing elaborate planning or control systems." This study also stressed that "innovative companies find special ways to reward innovators."[49]

Other studies of innovation in industry cite the importance of establishing an atmosphere of freedom, and of withholding premature judgment regarding new ideas, recognizing that young ideas usually look anemic. According to an innovator with established credentials: "Not a single one of the 75 patents that have been granted to me came as a result of top management's direction. They all came, however, as a result of top management's patience and encouragement." New methods of thinking or provoking the mind are not treated as gimmickry: "The skills of brainstorming, matrix analysis . . . and the like, should be mastered and understood as well as the normal skills that scientists and engineers are expected to possess. Creativity favours the prepared mind."

As for the organizational setting, "simple organizational problems can be terribly discouraging to the innovator . . . ." Specific barriers to innovation are overplanning, rigid control and a failure to give credit to workers who produce good results. "Most truly major developments defy the 'planned approach' . . . ." The majority of big corporations, this innovator suggests, manage creativity poorly, seeming to "take pride in keeping their creative people anonymous, giving most of the credit for the inventive genius to what they call 'our research staff'."[50]

Contrary to the common belief that creativity "just happens", and that one cannot "manage" it or encourage it in a conscious way, there is, in fact, a body of evidence to suggest that processes can be engendered within organizations which increase the likelihood of creative insight. Such processes often call upon humour, emotion, intuition, a sense of fun, and other attributes sometimes considered to be out of place in a "serious" workplace.

Authors who have studied the process of creative thinking suggest that problem-solving should not be approached as if it were a conventional administrative task. Some suggest that institutions need consciously to encourage such thinking in addition to subjecting ideas (such as new policy initiatives) to the discipline of criticism. They have tried to make people more conscious of alternative ways of thinking through problems and of the kinds of norms and institutional arrangements that tend to foster inventive thought.[51]

Those people responsible for managing creativity have to learn to make the change from doing (i.e., direct personal involvement in creative or conceptual work) to creating the conditions that will make it possible for others to achieve. Herbert Simon argues that managing creative activity involves "a major shift from problem solving to facilitating the work of others."[52]

In interviews, experienced policy unit managers in government echoed some of the conclusions about managing innovation in business. They stressed the importance of encouraging policy officials through such little gestures as leaving their names on memoranda to the minister, rather than treating them as anonymous workers, and of encouraging officials to have direct contact with the minister through attending meetings where the issue is discussed. "It helps a lot if the minister thanks them."* In the public service, anonymity is required in relation to the outside world, but this does not preclude celebrating the work of an effective individual or policy team inside the department.

Some underlined the importance of maintaining an open, collegial atmosphere, of keeping associates briefed, and of sharing information even when this might involve risks. They allowed as how not everyone would agree with them. A top central agency official had this advice for new policy unit heads:

> Be open about the objective and the courses of action as much as possible. It's a matter of personal style, but I find it useful to have frequent management meetings, lots of copying of memos, frequent debriefings after external meetings. Some people have a greater need to know than others, but in general everyone on a project has a right to know what others are doing. With a little effort a manager can engender this open attitude.

> Where information is power, if one can remove the cancerous presumption that colleagues are keeping information back to gain power, or to embarrass others, that's very important. [As a policy manager,] you don't always know what's relevant. Only the person in charge of a dossier really knows that. This is costly in terms of time and photocopying, and it increases the possibility of leaks and embarrassment dramatically, but it's worth it.... Touch wood!

A top official in another department took a similar viewpoint: "You have to get the politics down to [your subordinates'] level, and the substance up to the political level." He agreed with the business managers on the importance of intellectual freedom: "I think you have to give your people scope. Other people tend to be a lot more dirigiste than I. Being dirigiste leads to high turnover." Equally important is defending the work of subordinates.

_____

* Unless otherwise indicated, the quotations in the balance of this section are from interviews and discussions with senior public servants conducted by the author, principally in the period February to April 1987.

A key task of the policy manager is finding good people to work in the unit. If the people are poor, the manager has to spend too much time on analysis and cannot devote the required attention to the process side of policy – to building networks and devising strategies. One deputy secretary said that in general, when seeking staff, he looked for,

> the "sense of residual responsibility" – the responsibility to just stay there until the thing gets done, whatever it may be. There's only one in five or ten people who have that sense to the degree required.

> You have to find someone (or you have to do it yourself) who can produce on time – agendas for meetings, letters for the DM's signature, Cabinet documents, etc. You need a second-in-command who has the commitment to do what's necessary – someone other than yourself to deliver the "process" goods. It may require bending the rules . . ., but you have to have the "system smarts" to get the people you need.

Both attracting and motivating the kind of people needed for policy work seems to depend in great measure upon the content of the work itself. Providing staff the chance to work on timely, relevant issues may well be the most important incentive. The policy manager must try to ensure that staff get to work on issues that are high on the minister's agenda and likely to result in political action and implementation. "Good professionals thrive 90 per cent on being able to make an impact on the process of government. If a guy isn't in it for the pleasure of doing a good job, you probably don't want him around."

Finding the right balance between long-term, general issues – intrinsically important but probably low on the minister's agenda – and short-term fire-fighting is a particularly difficult problem. Many policy officers complain about getting too far toward one or other end of this spectrum. Constant involvement in long-term issues is a recipe for irrelevance. The unit acquires a reputation as an ivory tower. As one official said, "The trouble with long-term work is that if you get too caught up in that stuff, when cuts come along, your unit is the first to go." Many talented policy officers become dissatisfied if, as the months pass, they perceive that their work is having little effect upon key, current departmental decisions. They seem to prefer to leave to academics the pleasure of exploring ideas for their own sake.

On the other hand, excessive involvement in policy fire-fighting — responding to urgent, sometimes relatively unimportant issues that surface continually in most departments — creates other problems. Such issues may not fit conveniently within the mandate of other units in the department, or they may cut across the responsibilities of several other branches or divisions. (Typical examples are drafting ministerial speeches, replies to questions in the House, or ministerial correspondence.) Policy fire-fighting can be a source of influence, and it undoubtedly helps in the development of networks, but it can also lead to the impression that the policy unit is little more than a sort of organizational catchall. Swamped with urgent but less important duties, it will not be able to participate in more significant policy development work in the department. In such circumstances, the good staff officers will soon get fed up and leave.

In short, each end of this spectrum may represent its own form of irrelevance. The challenge facing the policy manager is to position the unit somewhere in the middle, close enough to the current issues to be "plugged in" to the day-to-day action in the department, but far enough away from the trivia so that the unit can work on questions of higher intrinsic significance.[53] The "right" place on this spectrum will depend upon the temperament and interests of both the minister and the deputy. Some ministers are concerned with long-term issues, and some are not. Some DMs use policy units effectively, treating them as an extension of their office; others pay little attention to them. A new DM can rapidly change what used to be an organizational backwater into a dynamic, influential place to work — and vice versa.

I have worked with officials in policy development units, in professional firms, and in scientific research establishments. Although the three types of organizations are not identical, there are similarities. None are easily led. Professionals tend to be quirky, irreverent, strong-minded and allergic to systems, routine, or top-down direction. Most seem to work best in an atmosphere that is relaxed, collegial, relatively unstructured and open.

According to one study, creativity in professional organizations is enhanced when:

- Open channels of communication are maintained.

- Contacts with outside sources are encouraged.

- Non-specialists are assigned to problems.

- Ideas are evaluated on their merits rather than on the status of their originator.

- Management encourages experiments with new ideas rather than making "rational" prejudgments.

- Decentralization is practised.

- Much autonomy is allowed professional employees.

- Management is tolerant of risk-taking.

- The organization is not run tightly or rigidly.

- Participative decision-making is encouraged.

- Employees have fun.[54]

Professionals are generally not reputed to be good managers. They often have difficulty making the transition from hands-on activity to managing the work of others. In government, a chronic complaint about officials who have "graduated" from policy work to managerial responsibilities is that they are unable to keep out of detail. Accuracy and attention to detail in policy work is, as noted previously, very important, but policy shop leaders have to strike the right balance between legitimate quality control and nit-picking. They have to learn to rely upon others, for there is obviously a limit to how much they can control personally.

Some policy directors have difficulty creating an open managerial environment: although they valued intellectual freedom when they were themselves at the working level, they forget this as they move up the hierarchy. They carry with them a passion for accuracy that often turns management committee meetings into group drafting sessions where their associates pore endlessly over the wording of policy documents (and are thereby reduced to stupefaction). Some officials continue to "manage" in this fashion as they move well up the management ladder; I have known at least one deputy minister who was unable to leave his job as draftsman behind him.

One final point relates to the need for intellectual leadership. This is an ephemeral quality, and its importance is difficult to gauge, but it may have a bearing on which units secure the reputation within the bureaucracy of being "good places to work" — which in turn attracts the good staff. Many policy units are largely responsive, taking each issue as it comes, doing the analysis and developing the necessary documents. However, some seem to go beyond mere responsiveness. They function within the context of a larger frame of reference which the effective leader is able to throw around their work. One official, who used to work in Ottawa's now defunct Ministry of State for Economic Development, described this in the following terms:

> I personally need a framework to work within — a touchstone. In MSERD it took three or four months to develop an initial point of view, which in the end was applied micro-economic theory. The policy leader has to provide that framework, related to the business that the department is in. You have to identify what the best minds have decided is "right" before you apply the political overlay to it. You need a broad framework to retain your sanity, because the political issues can very quickly drive you off course.

In summary, policy development managers need strong analytic and process skills, the ability to find and attract able professional staff, and the initiative to identify and run with the right mix of issues. They must provide intellectual leadership combined with the human sensitivity to motivate and control high-powered staff members.

Policy managers must ensure that the work done by their unit is accurate and reliable, while avoiding the creation of stifling controls. They have to learn to keep out of detail — but not always. The art of being an effective manager, contrary to some popular notions about management, is not to be oblivious to detail, but rather to know when to get involved, and when to stand back. (Although on a day-to-day basis, attention to detail is perhaps more important in government than in the private sector, even in business, general managers do not leave all the details to subordinates.)55

In certain respects, the job of the senior policy manager resembles that of the general manager in business. Networks are extremely important. So is a sense of timing, an ability to judge the flow of events and to spot unexpected opportunities to advance an issue. The formal systems for getting things done often seem to be less important than the informal ones.56

Conclusion

The function of policy development has received little attention in the literature of management. Policy analysis requires a combination of "classic" policy capabilities and more contemporary skills of investigation and analysis. One of the key attributes is knowing what questions to ask. Policy development often proceeds in a tentative and exploratory manner as officials try to understand the scope and implications of each issue. Defining the problem properly can frequently take the analyst half way or more toward a solution.

Policy analysts should be aware of the pitfalls inherent in the rational model of planning, which is legitimate in certain circumstances, but by no means universally appropriate. Sometimes other strategies, such as loose umbrella strategies, or process strategies, may be more suitable. It may be more advisable to create a management environment that is conducive to the evolution of emergent strategies or policies than it is to try to develop all policy in a top-down manner.

Objectives need not always be framed in the textbook manner, with defined time frames and specific goals. This can be useful in planning certain kinds of work, but for other circumstances or policy issues, it may be more helpful to think of objectives in terms of "course-holding" or maintaining certain kinds of relationships, rather than arriving at a specific goal.

In the development of policy, the political process should serve to reconcile differences of values, making provision for all legitimate voices to be heard. Public servants must devise effective methods of external consultation to test and refine policy ideas, and to help ministers sell the results. The shrewd policy manager will also pay attention to the internal process, maintaining the right networks to guide policies through the course of interdepartmental meetings and central agency hurdles.

The more senior the policy manager, the more engaged he or she will tend to become in the process (and political) aspects of policy. A well-staffed and well-led policy shop will provide the necessary analytic back-up. Nonetheless, policy managers must stay reasonably close to the details of policy proposals, for it is often the small mistakes rather than the massive errors that dump the Government into hot water. Quality control must be an ongoing concern; yet the degree and type of control must be appropriate to a professional organization, otherwise creative ideas will be stifled and good people will leave.

Footnotes:

1. Sir Geoffrey Vickers, *The Art of Judgment*, (London: Chapman and Hall, 1965), pp. 73-75.

2. *Submission of the Association of First Division Civil Servants to the Fulton Committee*, "The Civil Service and Government Policy," (London: April 1967), p. 23.

3. Author's interview, February 1987.

4. See also Charles H. Kepner and Benjamin B. Tregoe, *The Rational Manager: A Systematic Approach to Problem Solving and Decision-making.* (Toronto: McGraw-Hill, 1965). This book, though simplistic in approach and attuned to the business environment, contains useful insights. It also presents a (somewhat dated) summary of other authors' work in the field of "problem-solving."

5. Edward De Bono, *Six Thinking Hats.* (Toronto: Key Porter Books, 1985), pp. 171-172.

6. Edward De Bono, *Practical Thinking*, (Harmondsworth: Penguin Books, 1971).

7. *Ibid.*

8. See, for example, Charles H. Granger, "The Hierarchy of Objectives," *Harvard Business Review*, (May-June 1964).

9. A good example of the school of rational problem-solving is Charles H. Kepner and Benjamin B. Tregoe, *The New Rational Manager*, (Princeton Research Press, 1981).

10. Robert H. Schaffer, "Putting action into planning," *Harvard Business Review*, (November-December 1967), pp. 158-164. See also Robert Hayes, "Strategic planning — forward in reverse?" *Harvard Business Review*, (November-December 1985), pp. 111-119; also Thomas J. Peters and Robert H. Waterman, *In Search of Excellence*, (New York: Harper & Row, 1982), pp. 30-31: "The rational approach to management misses a lot.... What we are against is wrong-headed analysis that is too complex to be useful and too unwieldy to be flexible, analysis that strives to be precise . . . about the inherently

unknowable ... and especially analysis that is done to line operators by control-oriented, hands-off staffs."

11. Gordon Donaldson and Jay W. Lorsch, *Decision Making At The Top — The Shaping of Strategic Direction*, (New York: Basic Books, Inc., 1983), p. 201: "Lindblom has labeled the [top-down, comprehensive, rational] method advocated by strategic planning experts the 'root' method. What he has called the 'branch' approach is clearly closer to the reality we have found. It recognizes that ends and means are interconnected; that the real test of a decision is that the decision makers agree that it is the right policy; and that, necessarily, certain outcomes and alternatives are not fully explored."

12. See, for example, Richard J. Van Loon and Michael S. Whittington, *The Canadian Political System — Environment, Structure and Process*. 3rd ed., (Toronto: McGraw-Hill Ryerson, 1981); Richard D. French, *How Ottawa Decides: Planning and Industrial Policy-making 1968-80*, (Toronto: James Lorimer and Company, 1980).

13. M.J.L. Kirby and H.V. Kroeker, "The Politics of Crisis Management in Government: Does Planning Make Any Difference?", in C.F. Smart, and W.T. Stanbury, eds., *Studies in Crisis Management*. (Montreal: Institute for Research on Public Policy, 1978), pp. 179-195.

14. French, *op. cit.*, p. 157.

15. Author's interview, March 1986.

16. Quoted by Christina McCall-Newman, in "Michael Pitfield and the Politics of Mismanagement," *Saturday Night*, (October 1982).

17. Robert Anthony, *Planning and Control Systems — A Framework for Analysis*, (Boston: Graduate School of Business Administration, Harvard University, 1965); see also Donaldson and Lorsch, *op. cit.*, p. 201.

18. H. Edward Wrapp, "Good Managers Don't Make Policy Decisions," *Harvard Business Review - On Management*, (New York: Harper and Row, 1975), p. 14. Originally published in HBR, (September-October 1967).

19. Charles Lindblom, *The Policy-Making Process*, 2nd ed., (Englewood Cliffs: Prentice Hall, 1980), p. 4; also pp. 34-40.

20. Henry Mintzberg and Jan Jorgensen, "Emergent strategy for public policy," *Canadian Public Administration*, vol. 30 no. 2, (Summer 1987), pp. 214-229. See also Mintzberg and James A.Waters, "Of Strategies, Deliberate and Emergent," *Strategic Management Journal*, vol. 6, (1985), pp. 257-272.

21. Wrapp, *loc. cit.*, pp. 5-18.

22. See David S. Sawicki, "On the Virtues of the Policy of Doing Nothing," *Journal of Policy Analysis and Management*, vol. 2 no. 3, (1983), pp. 454-457.

23. Wrapp, *loc. cit.*, p. 11.

24. Author's interview, May 1985.

25. Author's interview, May 1985. See also Hugo Young and Anne Sloman, *No, Minister*, (London: British Broadcasting Corporation, 1982), pp. 46-48.

26. W. Darcy McKeough, "The relations of ministers and civil servants," *Canadian Public Administration*, vol. 12 no. 1, (Spring 1969), p. 4.

27. Charles Wolf, "Policy Analysis and Public Management," *Journal of Policy Analysis and Public Management*, vol. 1 no. 4, (Summer 1982), pp. 546-551. For an alternative, somewhat broader definition of policy analysis, see Yehezkel Dror, "Policy Analysts: A New Professional Role in Government Service," *Public Administration Review*, vol. 27 no. 3, (September 1967), pp. 197-203.

28. Desmond Keeling, *Management in Government*, (London: George Allen and Unwin Ltd., 1972), pp. 183-193. See also Andrew Gray, and Bill Jenkins, "Retreat or Tactical Redeployment? The Fate of Policy Analysis and Evaluation in Government," in Gray and Jenkins, eds., *Policy Analysis and Evaluation in British Government*. (London: Royal Institute of Public Administration, 1983), pp. 77-80.

29. A. Paul Pross, "From system to serendipity: the practice and study of public policy in the Trudeau years," Kenneth

Kernaghan, ed., in *Canadian Public Administration: Discipline and Profession*, (Toronto: Butterworth and Co. (Canada), 1983), pp. 79-102.

30. Lawrence E. Lynn, Jr., *Managing the Public's Business: The Job of the Government Executive.* (New York: Basic Books Inc., 1981), pp. 26-29.

31. Author's interview, February 1987.

32. Hubert Laframboise, "Moving a proposal to a positive decision: A case history of the invisible process," *Optimum*, vol. 4 no. 3, (1973).

33. Author's interview, February 1987.

34. See Audrey Doerr, "The role of coloured papers," *Canadian Public Administration*, vol. 25 no. 3, (Fall 1982), pp. 366-379.

35. Author's interview, February 1987.

36. Author's interview, March 1987.

37. Author's interview, February 1987.

38. *Ibid.*

39. Author's interview, February 1987.

40. Author's interview, February 1987.

41. Author's interview, February 1987. See also Charles H. Levine, "Where Policy Comes From: Ideas, Innovation, and Agenda Choices," *Public Administration Review*, (January-February 1985), pp. 255-258.

42. Laframboise, *loc. cit.*

43. See Albert Shapero, *Managing Professional People — Understanding Creative Performance*, (New York: The Free Press (Macmillan), 1985), p. xv.

44. Geoffrey Vickers, *op. cit.*, chapter on Innovation.

45. Arthur Koestler, *Bricks to Babel*, (London: Hutchinson and Co., 1980), p. 345.

46. William J.J. Gordon, *Synectics — The Development of Creative Capacity*, (Toronto: Collier-Macmillan Canada, 1968), p. 37.

47. De Bono, *Six Thinking Hats, op. cit.*, p. 149.

48. Shapero, *op. cit.* p. 194.

49. James Brian Quinn, "Managing innovation: controlled chaos," *Harvard Business Review*, (May-June 1985), pp. 73-84. See also Peter E. Drucker, "The discipline of innovation," *Harvard Business Review*, (May-June 1985), pp. 67-72.

50. John A. Bridges, "An Innovator's Perspective," in James K. Brown, and Lita M. Elvers, eds., *Research and Development: Key Issues for Management*, (New York: The Conference Board, 1983), pp. 76-78.

51. See for example Gordon, *op. cit.*; also Allen F. Harrison and Robert M. Bramson, *Styles of Thinking.* (New York: Doubleday, 1982), p. 1: "Most people, most of the time, think about things in only one way.... When we approach problems or decisions, we employ a set of specific strategies, whether we know it or not.... We seldom take the trouble to learn new ways of thinking."

52. Herbert Simon, "How managers express their creativity," *Across the Board*, (March 1986), pp. 11-16.

53. See Organization Policy Group, Personnel Policy Branch, "Organization for Policy Development — The Role of Central Policy Branches — Factors Promoting or Constraining Success," Treasury Board Secretariat, (July 1984): an unpublished report based on interviews with senior executives in 17 Canadian departments.

54. Shapero, *op. cit.*, pp. 205-206.

55. John P. Kotter, *The General Managers*, (New York: The Free Press, 1982), p. 8.

56. *Ibid.*

Chapter Eleven:
People in the Public Service

The New Civil Service

The civil service in many jurisdictions has passed through profound changes in the last century. In 1870,

> The scope of the liberal state . . . was still relatively small, and the tasks of civil servants were still largely clerical. . . . By 1970 the state had expanded fantastically in both size and task. Real public expenditure had increased twentyfold to thirtyfold in ten decades. The gross national product was also growing, but the share spent by the state was rising several times faster. The inevitable concomitant was an explosion in the size of the government bureaucracy.[1]

Despite these massive changes in the size of government and the range of its activities, the image of the civil servant as a discreet, intelligent, classically educated confidant of ministers working with a small cadre of elite colleagues has continued to colour popular perceptions.[2] Public administration took some time to recognize that there had been a huge in-filling of staff between the top policy advisors to ministers and the clerical jobs at the base of the public service. Large numbers of officials had appeared in the system with extensive supervisory responsibilities.

The "new" civil service in many countries is large and often extensively decentralized. The majority of civil servants no longer live in national capitals such as London or Ottawa. They may never see a minister except on television, and they are more preoccupied with trying to deliver existing services efficiently than with formulating new policies for ministers. As managers, more and more public servants face the same problem as their private-sector counterparts: how to motivate and provide leadership to a large, diverse staff.

Lee Iacocca reminds us that management is first and foremost about people.

> [M]anagement is nothing more than motivating other people .... When it comes to making the place run, motivation is everything. You might be able to do the work of two people, but you can't be two people. Instead, you have to inspire the next guy down the line and get him to inspire his people.[3]

A top British industrialist, the Chairman of ICI, has put it in similar terms: "Management is essentially about people, about the organization of people, about obtaining their commitment to worthwhile commonly shared values and objectives ....[4]

During the 1960s and 1970s, management reforms in Canada, Britain and other jurisdictions tended to emphasize systems, procedures and controls. People have not been a central concern. Governments tend to be poor managers of people, treating individuals like factors of production and approaching personnel management in a procedural manner. It is not without significance that in a 1983 booklet describing the role of the branch of Canada's Treasury Board Secretariat responsible for personnel policy across government, the words "morale" and "motivation" do not even appear; all the emphasis is on policy, programs and systems.[5] In the world of government personnel managers, the goal of achieving a motivated work force often gets lost in the continuing preoccupation with mechanics — performance appraisal systems, grievance procedures, staffing systems, human resource information systems, classification and grading systems, and so forth.

Morale in the U.K.

Much of the evidence with respect to civil service attitudes to their work and their employers tends to be anecdotal. With respect to the situation in Britain, such evidence gives cause for concern. One observer has said of the 1970s, "[T]here is no doubt that the Civil Service at all levels has been deplorably treated in this decade to the point where its morale and in some ways its effectiveness has been wantonly damaged."6 The main theme of a House of Lords debate in December 1984 was the "discouraging" state of morale in the civil service.7 At the same time, an article entitled "The Attack on the Civil Service," cited the pessimism of the higher civil service and how its members "have become the subject of savage outside criticism."8

The Director General of the Royal Institute of Public Administration wrote in 1985, "My impression is that there are indeed signs of a developing problem of morale in and around the civil service," and as evidence pointed to the following signs of malaise:

> the failure in the last three years to fill all the vacancies for administrative trainees . . . an unprecedented wastage higher up, whether in the form of young principals leaving the Treasury for the City or their seniors retiring prematurely at 55 . . . the prevalence of leaks . . . [and] numerous anecdotes current about officials who believe that if they offer uncongenial advice to Ministers they will be at best ignored, at worst, penalised . . . . I fear that many civil servants . . . believe . . . that their organisation has no commitment to them.9

The Canadian Situation

In Canada, the talk in the corridors of power in Ottawa in the mid-1980s was of cutbacks and reductions, of difficult relations between the elected Government and the public service, and of interference by officials of the Prime Minister's Office in departmental administration. A study of the demography of the federal public service documented the fact that channels for promotion were closing off in a shrinking bureaucracy, and that there was "nowhere to go" for ambitious, promising performers.10 A "golden handshake" program offering early retirement for senior public servants was welcomed by many people looking for a way out. Day-to-day contact with many public servants seemed to indicate a growing malaise, and a feeling among many officials that the government was a less happy place to work than it had been a decade or two previously. But were such impressions accurate?

Fortunately, in Canada, we do not need to rely on anecdote or conjecture concerning the state of human resource management in the federal government. An exhaustive study of the Canadian government by David Zussman and Jak Jabes, conducted concurrently with the writing of this book, provides what may be one of the first scientific analyses of managerial attitudes in government and business in a parliamentary democracy.[11] The study included 2,000 civil servants in 20 departments and 1,300 managers and executives from 13 large business enterprises.

Unlike many other studies of public services, the Zussman initiative probed well below the level of the senior mandarins who are frequently equated with the "civil service", to examine the views of middle-level officials closer to the delivery of services. The purpose of the study was to compare the perceptions of managers in the public and private sectors in the areas of attitudes to their work and their organization, morale, corporate culture, leadership and job satisfaction.

When the survey results first began to emerge, they sent something of a shock wave through the top ranks of the Canadian public service. What had previously been conjecture was now documented fact; what had been privately suspected by many public servants was now about to become public knowledge. The agreement of top officials of the civil service to have a survey of this type conducted on the basis that results would be made public was unusual in itself. It can be difficult to secure information about the inner workings of government due to the tradition of anonymity and public servants' desire to protect ministers from embarrassment, and this can sometimes discourage fresh thinking about internal management practices. The Zussman/Jabes survey provides the basis for a constructive discussion of "people management" in the public service. Central agency officials showed commendable fortitude in supporting this initiative.

The most important discovery was the existence of a big gap between middle-level managers in business and their public sector counterparts. In almost every case, business middle managers indicated a more positive attitude to the job, a stronger sense of identity with, and commitment to, organizational goals, and a greater appreciation for the leadership of the person at the top. Very broadly speaking, on most variables, at lower levels of management the responses of managers in government came out 15 to 30 per cent less positive than those of their business counterparts.

On the whole, top managers in business and government tended to respond in parallel and positive terms. However, in business, a positive attitude at the top management level was usually reflected by similar sentiments three, four and five levels down from the CEO. If top management was "up" (which it almost always was), then middle management was also "up" (perhaps not to the same degree as the top managers, but still reasonably high).

Not so in government. In addition to the gap between middle-level managers in government and business, the survey revealed a second gulf, between middle-level government managers and their senior colleagues in the public service. The difference is so pronounced that the authors concluded that managers four and five levels down from the deputy minister simply do not share the same perceptions or assessments of the current management environment as do their more senior associates. The data suggest that they belong to what the authors call "a separate management culture". Of those at the top, in close contact with the deputy and the minister, between 80 and 90 per cent usually indicated that they felt committed, part of the action, and generally pleased with their situation. However, the pattern changed very noticeably at middle-management level; often as few as 50 per cent of subordinate managers responded positively, and sometimes even less.

The public service response was by no means universally negative; in fact, in a few areas — sense of accomplishment on the job, degree of job independence and the challenge of the work — public sector respondents were particularly positive in their replies. However, in most areas, the survey results imply that respondents did not constitute an enthusiastic, "turned on" workforce:

- With respect to *morale,* on average only 13 per cent in business noted the existence of morale problems in their firm, compared with 40 per cent of government employees; those at lower levels in government were most negative. Compared with business, almost twice as many government managers indicated that they had contemplated leaving their job.

- In terms of attitudes to their *organization,* almost 90 percent of business managers indicated satisfaction with their organization, compared with about 55 per cent of government managers; once again, whereas high levels of satisfaction prevailed right down the line in the private sector, in government, attitudes to the organization became more negative at lower levels — only 50 per cent of the lowest level of management indicated satisfaction compared with well over 80 per cent in business.*

- Similarly, at the lowest level of management, almost 90 per cent of business managers felt that there was a strong commitment of senior management to their organization's development, as compared with less than half (42 per cent) who felt this way in government.

- Concerning *leadership,* the differences were striking. Almost 85 per cent of private sector respondents, regardless of level, thought their CEO provided leadership, whereas in government the sense of leadership, even among top managers, was less pronounced. In addition, there were dramatic differences between government managers at senior and intermediate levels: 70 per cent of managers one down from the top thought the DM provided leadership, whereas five levels down from the DM, only 30 per cent thought this was true. A similar pattern

---

* This formed an interesting contrast with attitudes to their jobs. Asked if they agreed with the statement, "In general, I am satisfied with my job," 86 per cent of business respondents indicated agreement. The public service average was lower (76 per cent) but still quite high as compared with their attitudes toward their organization. The authors of the study caution that job satisfaction is not a unitary concept. Rather, it is a complex mix of a number of factors related to one's job.

was evident in replies to queries related to participation in decision-making and involvement in long-term planning.

- Not surprisingly, there was quite a divergence between the sense of loyalty to the CEO/DM in the two sectors. While there was strong loyalty to the top person among the most senior officials in both sectors, at lower levels of management, roughly 60 per cent of those in business professed loyalty to the top person, compared with only 40 per cent in government.

- Managers' responses to questions on the *values* and *orientations* of their organizations revealed some interesting differences. Business managers said their firms were committed to the provision of good service to customers, to growth, sales, profits and innovation; they felt that their firm cared for its employees and attributed importance to its human resources. Efficiency per se was not cited as a major value; the broader concept of excellence in performance was.

- Government managers indicated that their departments believed in providing good service to clients but, beyond that, their organizations were said to be committed to the somewhat arid virtues of efficiency, effectiveness and value for money. There was noticeably less assurance that respondents felt valued as people by their employer. Furthermore, innovation was thought not to be valued. (Conversely, civil servants will not be surprised to learn that public sector respondents expressed a loyalty to "the Canadian public" that was almost twice as strong as that of their private sector counterparts.)

Two particular factors were consistently and strongly associated with the existence of positive attitudes among managers. These were, first, managers' perceptions of the quality of leadership of their organization, and second, the degree to which employees felt that they were personally valued by their organization. As noted, in both these areas, government departments scored consistently (and in some cases quite dramatically) lower than business. Even the government organizations with the most positive profiles tended to score lower than the most negative business entity.

Another very interesting finding of the survey relates to differences among departments within government. Because departments are so varied, and because many execute a mix of functions (some routine, some highly unpredictable and unique), it is difficult to generalize about the state of morale in many departments. Particularly in large departments, it may be high in one part of the organization and low in another. However, in the survey results, some rough patterns can be detected. The replies indicate that on the whole, morale tends to be higher in central agencies than in line departments. Morale seems higher too, in departments that appear reasonably clear as to their mandate and priorities, than in departments afflicted with vague, changing or conflicting mandates.

These are only highlights from a most intriguing and revealing survey. It is, of course, not possible to apply the survey's findings to other public services, but they do appear consistent with anecdotal evidence concerning the situation in the U.K. such as that cited above. The findings of the survey reinforce the premises of the "fit" approach (see chapter 8) which states that leadership and strategic direction are critical to organizational health; they provide the focal point around which the other aspects of the organization—the people, structure, incentives, planning and control systems, technology, methods of communication and culture—can be aligned and integrated. Indifferent leadership and unclear direction lead to problems in the organization in other areas. As argued earlier in this book, lack of clarity in strategy and direction is an all-too-common problem in the public service context. So is the preoccupation with policy and the disinterest, especially at the top, in what are viewed as the "mechanics" of administration (and the associated issues of motivation and people management).

The results of any survey must be read in context. This one constitutes a snapshot of perceptions at a particular time (1986). In the absence of previous benchmarks, it is not possible to know whether the data represent stable or changing views. The survey was conducted during an extended period of cutbacks and staff reductions within the public service, and during a general swing to the right in party politics which made it increasingly fashionable to criticize governments and public servants. As well, many public servants undoubtedly were influenced by the considerable difficulties and tensions in the relationship between the Government of Prime Minister Brian Mulroney elected in 1984 and the public service, arising from this new Government's suspicion of the public service, its determination to seek policy guidance from political rather than administrative sources, and its publicly proclaimed intention to abolish "unnecessary" programs across the government.

These factors will have had some bearing upon the state of morale at the time of the survey. However, the responses suggest that the problems cannot be entirely attributed to the then-current political context, and that many of the difficulties identified by the survey are rooted in the traditions, management practices, values and general environment of the public service. The survey should have the effect of placing a number of important issues related to the management of the public service squarely on the table.

In summary, in both Ottawa and Whitehall, there is troubling evidence that the public service is viewed more and more as a difficult, sometimes dispiriting, environment in which to work. The problem is not, apparently, confined to Canada and Britain. In the United States, for example, an official of the American Society for Public Administration wrote to a governmental task force on morale in 1984, saying

> neither morale nor productivity in the government workforce will be high so long as it is denigrated by people running for office who blame the implementors of congressional or executive policy for society's ills. It is grossly unfair, irresponsible and unthinking to publicly impugn the characters and competence of able civil servants . . . .[12]

Increasingly, many public servants believe that public censure by politicians or the media is as likely as not to be the reward for a career of service. When a program is attacked by the opposition or the press, public servants are learning not to anticipate a spirited defence in the House by a minister squarely behind the department's policies and mission. Many politicians hasten to dissociate themselves from "administrative errors" or from initiatives that could be seen to have contributed to growth of the public service. They imply that the main cause of growth in the public service arises not from new programs and increased expenditures which they fought for on behalf of their constituents (and approved with legislation), but from creeping bureaucracy and officials' desire for self-aggrandizement. When things go wrong, the size of the service makes it easier for a politician to plead ignorance of managerial problems; but when things go well, the tradition that credit goes to the responsible minister remains unimpaired.

Moreover, the coincidence of changes in management practices with extensive cuts has led some public servants to conclude that "management reform" is not intended to make the workplace more pleasant and productive, but rather something unpleasant that happens when there is a change of Government or a policy of expenditure restraint. As a result, they want as little as possible to do with it. There is some glimmering evidence that Governments are gradually coming to realize that it is impossible publicly to denounce the foibles of the public service and to engage in widespread, often somewhat arbitrary reductions without severely depressing the morale of the service. Awareness may be growing that, particularly in a government department heavily dependent on people to execute its programs, morale and productivity are intimately related. As one observer has written in connection with Britain's initiatives of the period 1979-1984, "[I]nstitutional arrangements, or systems ... predominate in the quest for efficiency and effectiveness. There is need for more attention to the *human* side of management, such as leadership, morale, the importance of good supervision, and other factors...."[13]

What Affects Employees' Attitudes to Work?

Employees' attitudes to their jobs and their organizations result from many influences. Job content—that is, the intrinsic interest which the work itself holds for the employee—is one important consideration. Relations with the boss is another. How an immediate superior sets goals, clarifies expectations, praises achievement, confers authority, responds to complaints, accepts responsibility for errors, carries through on commitments, appraises performance, manages external relationships and communicates information to staff, all set the tone of the workplace. A good boss can make an apparently indifferent job come alive; a poor boss will render a potentially fascinating job deadly.

Incentives are another factor: employers seek to influence employees' attitudes to their jobs and their organization through salary, benefits, and other material rewards such as special forms of performance-related compensation. (Although objective research does not always establish strong correlations between these factors and behaviour on the job, some "human resource management experts" seem to think that these are the main levers for improving productivity through people.) Other less direct incentives include opportunities for personal growth and advancement through training and other forms of career development such as job rotation and secondments. Employers also confer status, prestige, power and other intangible rewards upon deserving employees.

All these factors may have a bearing upon employees' attitudes and motivation. However, the impact of the larger organizational context upon managerial and employee attitudes is often overlooked. Its importance should not be underestimated. Employees' attitudes can be strongly affected by the degree to which the organization is able to support them in doing their jobs. Organizations have a responsibility to provide an environment which permits those at subordinate levels to get on with their work. This environment is determined to a considerable degree by the delegation of authority, which as far as possible should be commensurate with the responsibilities of each job. Government employees' attitudes to their work are also affected by less apparent factors such as the department's (and the minister's) ability to take decisions, and by senior managers' capacity to co-ordinate work in different parts of the organization. Nothing can be more dispiriting for employees than to see their work wasted because of incompetence or mishandling once it is out of their hands. Bonuses and incentives will do little to compensate employees who feel their work is not valued, for by extension, such employees will tend to feel that they are not important to their employer, either.

Departmental employees' attitudes can also be profoundly affected by the larger environment within which they are working. This was well illustrated by the official cited in chapter 7, who commented upon the impact which government profligacy had upon public service attitudes.* My experience over the years has persistently reinforced the view that the problem of improving motivation and managerial attitudes is not solely related to those aspects of the organization that touch the individual in a direct and immediate way. It is also essential to consider the general environment within which the employee is working. This is well illustrated by the story told by a public servant who had previously worked for the Canadian Post Office.

> When I joined the Post Office, I was determined to approach it with an open mind. I found a lot of good people working there, trying to resolve a lot of very difficult problems. I liked my colleagues. But after a while the atmosphere began to get to me. You kept seeing the criticism of the Post Office in the papers. The organization always seemed to be having problems, and relations with the unions were really difficult. Operational decisions on matters like closing local postal stations couldn't be taken because of political sensitivity. You like to work for a place you can be proud of; but frankly, after a while, when I went to a party and people asked me, "Where do you work?" I'd say "In the government." Finally, it got to be too much, and when a chance to join another organization came along, I jumped at it.[14]

Many employees seem to relate to their organizations through a sort of unwritten contract which states, "I'm prepared to work hard for you, if you treat me as if I am valued, as if my work is valued, and if I can take pride in this organization's performance and leadership." It is a relationship of mutual support. The impact upon morale of such problems as vacillation, lack of vision, indecision, lack of clarity on matters of policy, failure to provide consistent backing to programs considered valuable by the employee, or political expediency cannot be overlooked. Everything in organizations is connected to everything else.

---

* "Not infrequently, the manager is . . . asked to cut down on his resources by a few hundred thousand dollars while on the other hand the government is wasting literally millions of dollars . . . . A common reaction is, 'Why should I stick around? I'm going home.'"

A broadly-based review of attitudes to work published in 1983 in the U.S. reinforces these conclusions. A national study of the American workplace noted that in more and more jobs, the key to productivity is not simply a matter of ensuring that employees carry out a set of predefined tasks, but rather to encourage them to release "discretionary effort", defined as "the difference between the maximum amount of effort and care an individual could bring to his or her job, and the minimum amount of effort required to avoid being fired or penalized: in short, the portion of one's effort over which the job-holder has the greatest control." The study argued that American enterprise was suffering from a widespread "commitment gap", whereby "many high-discretion job-holders are, by their own admission, holding back effort from their jobs, giving less than they are capable of giving, and less than they are, in principle, willing to give."[15]

Contrary to some popular rhetoric, the study does not attribute the commitment gap to a decline of the work ethic, but rather to managerial ineptitude. "The actions of many managers blunt rather than stimulate or encourage the work ethic." Among the major causes of this situation, the study cites a tendency of employers to be too concerned with factors affecting job satisfaction — e.g., lack of stress, good location, relationships, and benefits — which may have little to do with productivity, rather than those factors which cause people to work more effectively. The release of discretionary effort was found to be much more dependent upon such considerations as opportunities for advancement, challenging work, a chance to develop individual abilities, tying remuneration to performance, sharing productivity gains with staff, and giving "public and tangible recognition to people who keep standards of quality and effort that exceed average satisfactory job performance."

In this study, a group of employees in one community were asked to identify those job-related values most important to them. The respondents replied:

- "working with people who treat me with respect"

- "interesting work"

- "recognition for good work"

- "working for people who listen if you have ideas about how to do things better"

- "having a chance to think for myself"

- "seeing the end results of my efforts"

- "working for efficient managers"

- "a job that is not too easy" (note: they said "not too easy," not "an easy job"!)

- "feeling well informed about what is going on."[16]

In summary, the public service is one of the most people-intensive industries. The key to the performance of people lies in closing the "commitment gap" and in creating work environments where public servants feel motivated to contribute discretionary effort. Evidence in Britain, Canada, the U.S. and elsewhere suggests that this is not being done very well at present. What must be changed? This is the subject of part 4.

Footnotes:

1. See Joel D. Aberbach *et al*, *Bureaucrats and Politicians in Western Democracies*, (Cambridge: Harvard University Press, 1981), p. 2.

2. John Garrett, *The Management of Government*, (Harmondsworth: Penguin, 1972).

3. Lee Iacocca with William Novak, *Iacocca: An Autobiography*, (New York: Bantam Books, 1984), pp. 53-56.

4. J. H. Harvey-Jones, "The development of management as an art in the private sector," *Royal Society of Arts Journal*, (May 1984), pp. 380-389.

5. "Role of the Treasury Board Secretariat and the Office of the Comptroller General," (Ottawa: Treasury Board, March 1983).

6. Garrett, *op. cit.*, pp. 1-2.

7. Hansard, *House of Lords Official Report*, vol. 457 no. 15, 5 December 1984.

8. Geoffrey Fry, *Parliamentary Affairs*, vol. 37 no. 4, (Autumn 1984), pp. 353-363.

9. William Plowden, "What prospects for the civil service?", lecture to the Royal Society of Arts in February 1985, published in *Public Administration*, vol. 63 no. 4, (Winter 1985), pp.393-414.

10. Nicole S. Morgan, *Nowhere To Go*, (Montreal: Institute for Research on Public Policy, 1981).

11. David Zussman and Jak Jabes, *Survey of Managerial Attitudes: Preliminary Findings*, (Ottawa: Institute for Research on Public Policy Working Paper, 1987). The respondents were from one to five levels below that of the chief executive officer or deputy minister. The response rate was remarkable: in excess of 70 per cent in private and public sectors. Detailed analysis of the Zussman/Jabes findings is to be published by the Institute for Research on Public Policy in 1988.

12. Charles W. Washington, "To the Morale Officer," *The Bureaucrat*, (Summer 1984), p. 18.

13. Rosamunde M. Thomas, "The Politics of Efficiency and Effectiveness in the British Public Service," *International Review of Administrative Sciences*, vol. L no. 3, (1984).

14. Conversation with the author, June 1987.

15. Daniel Yankelovich and John Immerwahr, *Putting the Work Ethic to Work*, (New York: Public Agenda Foundation, 1983), pp. 1-7.

16. *Ibid.*, p. 23. These findings were derived from a local study of 500 workers in the Puget Sound area of Washington, but the study authors indicate the findings were consistent with more general studies of employee attitudes across the U.S.

Part Four:

An Agenda for Public Management

Introduction to Part Four

The Differences between Government and Business

The discussion so far in this book will, I hope, have made it clear that government is a very different enterprise from business. Although there is certainly room for the adoption of some private sector practices in the public sector, government is not, as some persons seem to think, simply a sort of mismanaged business corporation.

Too often, the problem of getting things done in government is approached as if politics were a minor inconvenience and politicians, a footnote to the process of administration. In reality, the nature of the political process profoundly affects the context for management in the public service.

Businesses can be made more efficient than government because in the final analysis, their goals are simpler and their authority structures less cluttered than in government. The conventions of decision-taking in business tend to lay less stress upon consultation than in government, and more emphasis upon getting on with the job (although there does appear to be some evidence of a trend toward greater participation by business employees in decision-making and risk-taking). Compared to government, the advantage of the business form of organization is that it focuses power and accountability in the interests of facilitating the exercise of power. This is a luxury we can afford because in a pluralist society, the power of business can be checked. There are external power centres, such as the courts and the government, which can be used to hold business enterprises to account in cases of abuse of trust, and there are legally-sanctioned ways of changing the management in cases of incompetence. In government, however, since there is no external arbiter, checks have to be woven into the very fabric of the system. Sound management must therefore be sought within a framework of certain practices and structures which discourage efficiency as conventionally understood.

Democratic government diffuses power and accommodates a diversity of influences upon decision-taking in order to prevent the abuse of power. It is, as Plato said, "a charming form of government, full of variety and disorder . . . ." It has also been aptly described as the worst form of government . . . with the possible exception of all the others. Democracy creates conventions, systems and structures which impede action, complicate accountability, increase the number of people and interests involved in taking decisions, and silt up the flow of business. The question of administrative reform or management improvement in government cannot be divorced from the need to protect the fabric of responsible government. It would be imprudent, to say the least, to try to change all the factors which complicate managerial life in government simply in the interest of promoting administrative efficiency.[1]

On the other hand, in my view, it would be facile and wrong to conclude that the institutions and conventions of government are untouchable, and that the appropriate motto for the public service is: "as it was in the beginning, is now and ever shall be." We need to separate those aspects of government which cannot or should not be altered from those which have outlived their utility, which are simply accidents of history, or which are outright errors.

Below, a number of the impediments to management which have been mentioned in the preceding chapters are summarized. This list comprises those which "go with the territory" of government and which appear unlikely to change.

INTRODUCTION TO PART FOUR

A. Problems arising from the political process or context.

Elections. These administrative inconveniences lead to periods of indecision sometimes followed by changes of direction; even if directions do not change, there may be months, or even years, of uncertainty until the priorities and values of the new Government become apparent.

The tradition of Cabinet solidarity. This generates a need for a great deal of consultation before decisions are taken. Regrettably, such consultation tends to retard decision-taking, dull initiative and cause bold new ideas to fade into bland and unexciting policies. Also, too many cooks tend to spoil the broth; programs that attempt to meet too many goals may meet no one's.

Ministerial interference in administration. Some ministers (or members of their staff) get involved in the details of departmental operations. While ministers have the right to direct many aspects of administration if they so desire, most are inexperienced in the management of big organizations. Their influence can be demoralizing or even damaging when they intercede in ways that confuse the hierarchy of command or are calculated to gain partisan advantage. Such interventions run counter to most public servants' views of what constitutes responsible administration.

The need for consistency in the delivery of programs. This requirement exists in government to a degree unknown in business (since business has no obligation to treat different members of the public even-handedly); it leads to a more complex bureaucracy and more reliance upon procedural manuals and written instructions than in business.*

---

* "Bureaucracy grows because of pressure to have every transaction, and the steps leading up to it, conform to someone's expectations of how they should be performed .... An effective way to ensure that expectations are fulfilled is to specify the procedures to be followed in designing and conducting the transactions." See Lawrence E. Lynn, Jr., *Managing the Public's Business: The Job of the Government Executive*, (New York: Basic Books Inc., 1981), pp. 36-37.

The need for attention to detail. There is a need in government to support the minister in dealing with the House of Commons and the public on matters of detail that would never pass through the executive suite in business. This leads to persistent difficulties in ordering one's time or agenda, especially at senior levels of the public service. (As one American public servant expressed it: "It is not possible to set your own schedule. You can try, but you have to be ready to junk your whole schedule and go to whatever the crisis is.")[2]

The need to protect the minister from embarrassment. This creates disincentives to innovate or to take risks.

Difference of time frame between political and administrative levels. Ministers have an understandable bias toward decisions which provide tangible and visible evidence of results prior to the next election. Civil servants have no vested interests in the re-election of the Government and may therefore be more inclined to look for policies which show benefit in the longer term.

Neutrality. This tradition, particularly important at senior levels of the public service, requires officials to maintain a certain objectivity about programs and policies. It tends to discourage the type of passionate commitment to programs that would be an asset in the private sector (as noted in chapter 5, the department head "must try to develop a feeling of participation in policy formulation, without invoking a sense of paternity for ideas.")

Two-ended program delivery. Because ministers like to be seen to be personally and visibly involved in government programs, programs are "delivered" from the top (through the minister's office) as well as through the bottom of departments. This increases the need for special assistants and other help to move the volume of paper up and down the hierarchy, and it can clog decision-making channels with relatively unimportant, but urgent correspondence.

B. Problems arising from the inherent nature of governmental activity.

Multiplicity of goals, and the lack of any clear distinction between means and ends. This complicates the process of administration greatly. Related to this is the not uncommon problem of politicians' unwillingness (or inability) to specify their objectives.

The lack of any clear basis for measuring performance of many activities. This leads to unique difficulties in the planning and control of government operations. Related to this is the following problem.

Incommensurability of different government activities and programs. In the absence of a common yardstick for measuring the contribution or value of different programs, governments are forced to rely upon much more vague and contentious standards in taking difficult decisions about the allocation of resources or the setting of priorities. No amount of system improvements or structural adjustments will change this situation.

Intractable problems for which "solutions" are demanded by the media and the public. Problems such as unemployment or the alienation of youth are ones for which there is no obvious answer, for which, as one commentator has put it, the required "technology" simply does not exist.[3] Nonetheless, officials are expected to resolve them, often in the glare of critical or even adverse publicity which can be damaging to departmental morale. The not-infrequent public expectation that there must be "quick fixes" available for complex problems, and the pressure upon ministers to provide simple "answers" that can fit in a ten-second television clip only exacerbates this problem.

C. Problems arising from the institutional context of government.

Multiple accountabilities: to the minister, to central agencies and to the prime minister. Some business persons upon learning the type of environment within which department heads and senior officials must function are amazed at their ability to cope with such fluidity.

Public visibility of government institutions. The requirement to be publicly answerable and constantly under scrutiny by the media and by parliamentary committees, not only for what is achieved but also for how programs are delivered, creates great stresses in management. For example, a business CEO administering a program of incentive pay can make quite arbitrary decisions about who gets how much bonus; if required to justify decisions, he or she will usually face a relatively sympathetic board of directors predisposed to accept the CEO's judgment. A senior government official has to be prepared to defend this sort of administrative decision, and many others, in front of outsiders who may be unsympathetic, suspicious, and even hostile.

Multiplicity of stakeholders. Relative to the private sector, government has to spend far more time taking many stakeholders' and interest groups' views into account.

Institutional complexity. This arises from the size of government, the special traditions of the public service such as the merit principle, the diffusion of power among different organizations, and the many accountabilities mentioned above. For the public servant newly recruited from university, or the business executive brought in from outside, just learning how to navigate the system takes a lot longer than it does in most business organizations.

Collective as well as departmental responsibility. Civil servants have to function both as members of their departments and also as members of the collectivity of the public service. This can create uncertainty about priorities and diminish commitment to departmental goals. In addition, it blurs accountability and makes it less common for individuals to be acclaimed for producing outstanding results.

As an observer of the U.S. government has suggested, the difference between government and business "is a difference in degree so great as to be a difference in kind.... If government and business are in crucial aspects dissimilar ... applying business management concepts may be futile or even counterproductive .... "4

The Scope of Part Four

If these are the factors that cannot or should not be changed, what remains? This section of the book examines those issues which, in my view, constitute the key challenges facing public management in the next few years. They are presented as an agenda for change, and they fall into the following general categories.

1. *Better political linkages*: the need to improve the links between the political and the administrative levels of government.

2. *Customized accountability*: the evolution of "accountability frameworks" for government institutions which are tailored to their particular mandates and functions, in place of the generalized approach to administrative and financial policies which has tended to characterize central agency-departmental relations in the past. Initiatives in this area should include a careful review of what types of functions are best suited to the public service environment, and what types may be better suited to other accountability arrangements, such as those provided by contracting, Crown corporations or quangos, and other alternatives.

3. *Increasing the "public" content in public policy*: building better bridges between the public and the process of public policy formation, in recognition of the poor regard in which many government organizations are held and the inadequacy of the electoral process to provide all the necessary public input to policy development.

4. *Achieving performance through people*: the adoption of policies within the public sector which accord more recognition to the fact that people are the key to performance, and which are founded upon the realization that it is necessary to build institutions in government which value the individuals who work within them.

The first three of these issues are discussed in chapter 12; suggestions with respect to the better management of people in the public service are considered in the final chapter.

Footnotes:

1. Les Metcalfe and Sue Richards, "The Impact of the Efficiency Strategy," *Public Administration*, 62, (Winter 1983), pp. 445-446: "That there is scope for improving governmental performance through better public management is widely accepted. What is less frequently recognized is the extent to which progress depends on overhauling the framework of democratic control and public accountability."

2. Cited in Lawrence E. Lynn, Jr., *Managing the Public's Business: The Job of the Government Executive*, (New York: Basic Books Inc., 1981), p. 130.

3. *Ibid.*

4. *Ibid.*, p. 115, p. 104.

Chapter Twelve:
Relationships and Accountabilities

Although the pace and areas of change vary from one jurisdiction to another, some notable advances have been made in the sphere of public management in the last two decades, and some important lessons have been learned. Probably the greatest progress has been made in the development of procedures for expenditure management. Whereas 25 years ago, governments could be run on the basis of relatively simply budgeting processes, it was becoming apparent by the 1960s that these were no longer adequate to an era of big government.

Systems such as PPBS, PESC and PEMS have evolved during this period (as well as other approaches such as ZBB, which for reasons of space have not been reviewed in this publication). These developments have helped to make public administrators more conscious of the importance of managing expenditures with an eye to the results or impacts being achieved through those expenditures. More effort has been devoted to relating costs to programs; analytic techniques have been developed which help to trace how expenditures affect the economy and society. Financial officials have backed off some of the over-ambitious and overly complex systems that were first devised during the 1960s. The quality of financial information being made available to parliaments and ministers is substantially better than it was two decades ago. Better contextual data are available to ministers concerning the resources available for planning, and more attention is devoted to anticipating the longer term expenditure consequences of today's decisions. The public and members of Parliament also have better information about expenditure intentions thanks to documents such as the Autumn Statement which Whitehall publishes each fall before its estimates are presented to Parliament.

A particularly important advance, in my own view, has been the institution of the envelope system adopted in Canada. As noted earlier in this book, this system had the effect of linking policy proposals more explicitly to planned expenditures, and of placing more responsibility for tradeoffs among related programs in the hands of the politicians. It changed the sociology of the expenditure management process: instead of one institution, the Treasury Board and its Secretariat, trying to fend off or coordinate all the new proposals being advanced by other departments and ministers, the public purse was divided into envelopes — each under the jurisdiction of the committees of Cabinet responsible for different policy fields such as economic and regional development, foreign policy and defence, or social policy.[1]

The designers of expenditure management systems have also, I suspect, become more realistic in what they believe such systems can provide. It has become clearer that "rationality" is a somewhat elusive concept when it comes to government spending, and that difficult decisions depend upon values as much as "logic". Expenditure management systems should allow differences in values to become explicit; but there is no single outcome that is more "rational" or "correct" than all the others.

Another lesson learned during the past two or three decades is that the most elegant system is no match for political will. If ministers want to spend, and the prime minister is prepared to let them do so, no system will hold them in check. On the other hand, good information developed in the context of systems like PEMS or PESC can certainly facilitate decision-taking and provide better perspective on the consequences of alternative courses of action. There is no "perfect" system for budgeting and planning; different approaches have different characteristics, and the advantages of one are likely to be the disadvantages of another, and vice versa.

While those responsible for the machinery of public expenditure management will no doubt continue to refine their systems, and while continuing efforts will be required to improve the quality of information available for decision-making, my own belief is that, in view of the progress made in this sphere, more attention should be devoted to other aspects of the machinery of government. The following pages suggest where some of these priorities for the next few years might lie. The present chapter deals with relationships at the centre of government and with different accountabilities to which the public service is subject; the following, and final, chapter considers issues associated with the motivation of people responsible for making the public service run effectively.

Cooperation with Parliamentary Committees

A recurring theme in this book is that the impact of the political centre of government — Parliament, caucus, Cabinet, elections and the like — upon the administrative level cannot be ignored. It is, after all, from the political level of government that the leadership for the administrative level is drawn. The political level likewise defines the priorities to be pursued by the bureaucracy. In short, how the political level works has an important bearing upon how well the administrative level is able to function. Most informed observers of government seem to agree that the optimal situation is one in which there are effective relationships between the neutral civil service and the political centre.

In general, political institutions are outside the focus of this book. Existing traditions and practices have been taken as given. However, there are two areas where the political and administrative levels touch which, in the light of developments over the past 25 years, require some observations. One of these has to do with the relationship between parliamentary committees and the public service, an area in which there have been changes in both Britain and Canada during the last few years.

No serious observer of government can fail to be struck by the relative unimportance accorded to elected members of Parliament.

Ministers are close to the levers of power, and may have great influence if they are competent. However, without good luck, the likelihood of an MP being appointed a minister is often not great. Many members stuck on the back benches of the House of Commons (i.e. not part of Cabinet, or the Ministry in the U.K.) do not find their jobs very rewarding.

In Canada, former Liberal Prime Minister Pierre Trudeau characterized members of Parliament as "nobodies" once they left Parliament Hill in Ottawa. A former backbench MP, Gordon Aiken, wrote in 1974 that politics is "physically and mentally exhausting. Constant travel, foul-ups, criticism, bad news, tense situations and long hours leave many Members worn out in a very short time." Opposition backbenchers were "stifled by their lack of influence" and yet they were in reality "far ahead of [Government members] who had ... recently backed a massive majority." An MP unable to attain Cabinet rank was characterized as little more than a trained seal.[2]

Addressing a Special Committee on Parliamentary Reform established in Ottawa in 1984, one MP stated,

> I am absolutely amazed at how little input private members have into the formulation of legislation, policies and/or regulations .... [M]ost of the time we are told what a minister will be announcing in 48 hours and we do not have access, any means to study or contribute or change the finished product. But members must go to their constituencies to explain and support the decision of the government. Sometimes this is extremely difficult.[3]

Another commented, "[S]ince I have come to Ottawa ... there is this incredible frustration. What ought to be the pinnacle of exchange of ideas is in fact the black hole in which nobody listens to anybody."[4] The Committee itself concluded, "In recent years the influence of the private member in the legislative process has been seriously reduced." In addition, party members were too often being required to submerge their principles or beliefs under the weight of the party system.[5]

A democracy where the representatives of the people find their jobs unrewarding and lacking in substance has cause for concern. Private citizens who might be admirably suited to public office and able to make a real contribution to the process of government will certainly think twice about whether to offer their candidacy. Good people who do get elected will be unlikely to stay in office for long unless they can secure a seat at the Cabinet table (a problem specifically identified by Aiken.)[6]

In 1979, Britain adjusted its structure of parliamentary committees with a view to enhancing MPs' roles. Previously, so-called "Select" Committees had been kept small, and their mandates had been confined to specific issues such as parliamentary procedure, financial estimates and nationalized industries. The new approach to the role of these committees was described by Douglas Wass, a former Permanent Secretary to the Treasury and Joint Head of the Home Civil Service, as "one of the most important and exciting of recent developments."[7]

Organized so that their mandates more or less conformed to those of government departments, they opened up a new relationship between MPs and civil servants, for they provided the opportunity for MPs to call officials before the committees to explain what departments were doing and why. They provided a vehicle for greater continuity and a sharper focus on specific departments and areas of policy than did the Public Accounts Committee, whose mandate had extended across the full sweep of government activities and institutions. They also provided the chance, if MPs cared to seize it, for members to influence government policy and/or the procedures of the executive.

Not surprisingly, the advent of these committees was greeted with considerable suspicion in the civil service. Douglas Wass stated,

> [M]any civil servants, including, I regret to say, myself, viewed the development with concern, because we expected the committees to delve into matters which, for apparently good reasons, had been kept confidential, and because, too, we were apprehensive that officials under public examination would become politically exposed . . . .

> In the event, most of these fears have not been realized. The anxiety that civil servants would become identified in public with ministerial policies has been allayed by the committees' separation of policy questions . . . from questions of fact and analysis . . . . There have been few breaches of the convention that officials' advice to Ministers on policy is privileged and confidential.[8]

The committees in the U.K. have not been an unalloyed success. Wass' view was that their examination of witnesses tended to be superficial; committee members were often ill-prepared; committees did not focus on many questions of long term importance. On the other hand, "The existence of the committees has . . . had a number of what I regard as beneficial effects on policy-making." These included: more care by ministers and officials in policy development, knowing that there could be detailed scrutiny at some point; more publication of information about policy, expectations and judgment; more exposure of questionable ministerial decisions. Wass' conclusion was, "The Select Committees have an immensely valuable part to play in getting at the facts and the analysis which underlie policy, and they have the potential to perform well in the reviews of the actions and policies of Ministers and departments, provided these are not the subject of acute party controversy."[9]

Although the development was little noted in the media, a restructuring of Canada's committees of Parliament along similar lines was instituted in the mid-1980s, in the wake of the report of the Committee on Parliamentary Reform cited above (also known as the McGrath Report after its chairman, MP James McGrath). Making these committees a constructive part of the policy and accountability process in government is an important challenge for public administration. It will require the committees themselves to determine whether they serve the public interest better by taking partisan, short-term attitudes toward matters of public policy, or whether they would do better to adopt the type of non-partisan norms favoured by public accounts committees, which tend to lead to a more informed and genuine debate among committee members.

The MPs who chair these committees will have to ensure that appropriate discipline is observed by members during appearances of public servants. As long as officials are allowed to restrict their comments to the administration of policy, the fears expressed by Wass concerning political exposure of public servants will not be realized. Possibly a code of conduct should be adopted for such committees. If public servants are dragged into politics, ministers will soon curtail the appearances of officials before the committees, and an opportunity for improving relations between the political and administrative arms of government – and for enhancing the influence of MPs over policy – will have been lost.*

Staff Support for Ministers

The second area involving relations between the bureaucracy and the political level of government concerns the issue of staff support to ministers. The analysis in chapter 4 has indicated how complex, and how unmanageable, is the job of the minister. A variety of proposals have been made as to how ministers might be more adequately assisted, ranging from the proposal in Britain's Fulton Report that special policy units be situated in the civil service, with direct reporting relationships to the minister (see appendix 2)[10], to those who would adopt the "spoils system" still practised in the U.S. Administration.

It is sometimes suggested that special advisers or assistants are not very important to ministers, that they are "a minor cosmetic on the great granite face of the body politic: good for appearances ... but not likely to change very much."[11] I disagree. It is perhaps because of views such as this that insufficient attention has been devoted to the quality of appointments to these positions.

Ministers require support in a number of areas which either overlap with, or lie outside the traditional preserve of their departmental staff. These include questions of political strategy and tactics, including the maintenance of relations with their own constituents, the caucus and other members of their party; advice on the political dimensions of relationships with interest groups within their portfolio; assistance of a personal nature in drafting speeches; planning the political dimensions of their agenda and public

---

* Note: a number of recommendations of the McGrath Report seem likely to have a positive impact upon the process of government. However, in one other area touching relations between Parliament and the civil service, I believe the Committee proposals were ill advised, that is, the suggestion with respect to public hearings on the proposed appointments of deputy ministers (chapter 5 of the report). Such a proposal, presumably modelled on the American government (where patronage appointments to the civil service are accepted), would be inconsistent with the concept of a neutral, apolitical public service.

appearances; and questions of public policy outside their own portfolio in which they may become engaged, either through participation in Cabinet meetings, through personal interest or as a result of a special request from the prime minister. In general, much of what the minister deals with will involve a mix of "objective" matters of public policy (where the public service will feel (and often be) best qualified to provide advice), and political or partisan issues where competent political staff can play a very useful role.

Many seasoned public servants, although sometimes diffident about admitting new players into the intimate relationship between departments and ministers, have concluded that personal assistants for ministers are desirable.[12] A Committee of the British House of Commons inquiring into the issue of civil servants' relations with ministers in 1986 concluded that better staff support for ministers was required:

> What we are proposing is . . . an expanded private office [staffed by] . . . a number of special advisers . . . to keep the Minister in touch with his party organization . . . together with a number of career civil servants . . . to keep the Minister in touch with his department . . . and [the Minister's] Private Secretary . . . to keep the Minister in touch with his backbenchers.[13]

A former Secretary to the Cabinet in Canada, Gordon Osbaldeston, has gone so far as to propose a "parallel political bureaucracy" leading to "two strong systems, one bureaucratic and one political, working in harmony."[14]

Special advisers can relieve ministers of a great deal of work. They can help to enhance ministers' political reputations and improve the party's performance at the next election. By careful attention to constituency affairs, they can help them to secure re-election. Depending upon their background and abilities, they may have a not unimportant impact on some policy issues, bringing political intelligence to bear upon the non-partisan analysis brought forward by the civil servants. They can help ministers to maintain effective relations with the prime minister's staff, with important public interest groups, and with key officials in the party.

Conversely, assistants' capacity to inflict damage upon the minister and indeed upon the Government itself can scarcely be underestimated – particularly if they are working in the office of the prime minister. When Prime Minister Brian Mulroney assumed power in Ottawa in 1984, he appointed a group of partisan cronies and political friends to the Prime Minister's Office (PMO). These officials seemed to be somewhat inexperienced in government, unfamiliar with the institutions of the capital, and suspicious of the public service. Over the next two to three years, a number of representatives of the media concluded that these assistants had contributed to a dramatic slide in the PM's personal popularity and in the Conservative Party's standing in public polls. Moreover, relations between the Government and the public service were uneasy, if not hostile, on a number of fronts.

Eventually, the prime minister drafted a public servant from the Department of External Affairs to take over the direction of his office and rethink the organization of the PMO. Most of the old staff were gone within a few months. The standings of the party improved at the polls; the prime minister seemed to run into fewer problems in the House of Commons and with the media. Many observers attributed these developments to the new staff in the PMO and new strategies that had been adopted with respect to the prime minister's priorities.

There has been a good deal of debate over the years as to where ministerial staff should come from: those who helped with the minister's campaign, party workers, or the public service itself. Some ministers like to rely heavily on the public service, believing that promising junior or middle-grade officials seconded to their offices from this milieu will bring established professional credentials and a sound knowledge of the bureaucracy. (One former minister told me, "Throughout my career in politics, I consistently got my best and most knowledgeable assistants right out of the public service."[15] Similarly, Denis Healey, formerly Chancellor of the Exchequer in Britain, set up a personal "cabinet" staffed with "first rate people in mid-career to make sure I asked the right questions and that when decisions were taken I got relevant answers, and then I got the decisions carried out. I found that immensely valuable . . . ."[16])

Other ministers are more comfortable with individuals with whom they have established relationships prior to assuming office, whom they feel able to trust with sensitive assignments. The problem with many of these persons is that they are knowledgeable about the acquisition of power; but they lack the experience, abilities and personal networks necessary to advise the minister on how to exercise it effectively in a complex political and institutional environment. Retaining political power can be a somewhat different challenge from acquiring it.

My own opinion is that where assistants come from is rather less important than their capabilities, experience, personal qualities and temperament. Ministers may well be able to benefit from help in the selection of assistants; Osbaldeston has suggested using former ministerial assistants with proven records to help select new ones.[17] The attributes of effective assistants are unlikely to be found in one person alone. They include:

- a "nose" for political issues and the experience and contacts to be able to advise the minister effectively both on questions of regional or national political consequence which may bear upon his or her mandate, and also on more parochial issues directly connected with the minister's own constituency

- an understanding of the institutions of government; an appreciation of the concept of a neutral public service and the constraints within which public servants must work

- an awareness of the technical and intellectual contributions which public servants can bring to the formulation of policy, and of their ability to provide context and background for most issues that will confront the minister

- the sensitivity and willingness to work collaboratively with the public service (in particular with the department head and his or her office. As Lord Bancroft has observed, "All turns upon whether [special advisers] work too abrasively against the grain of the department, because to work against it to some extent they must.")[18]

- the judgment to know when it is appropriate to invoke the minister's authority and when it is not in relating to the department

- the experience to be able to advise the minister on questions of public relations and communications, and to help to see that the minister is portrayed in circumstances or situations which are politically favourable; the ability to maintain cordial relations with representatives of the media

- a capacity to draft engaging prose for speeches and to save the minister from having to employ some of the more tedious and incomprehensible "bureaucratese" which all government departments seem to produce from time to time

- the ability to anticipate situations which could involve the minister in potential conflict of interest situations, or in situations where the minister (or his or her staff) could be censured for using public resources for partisan ends

- a judicious mixture of humility and self confidence

- the administrative competence, in more senior staff members, to run an efficient office on behalf of the minister.

Improvements in the quality of ministerial staff will not come about of their own accord. An important challenge for public management, which invites a response from both public service and political organizations, is to find ways of assisting ministers in this sphere and to help ensure that the right kinds of individuals are appointed to these sensitive positions.

Tailoring Accountability to Departmental Mandates

Anyone who has studied public administration or worked in government will be well-acquainted with the familiar complaints against central agencies and the cloying regulations with which public servants must so often contend. Every new report on management in government calls for more authority for departments, and for less bureaucracy. Yet little seems to change. Attempts to hack away at the undergrowth of regulations seldom produce enduring results: any clearing established in this way is soon reclaimed by the forest. There is, in my view, a way out of this problem, but it requires a new conception of how the relationship between departments and central agencies should function. As long as old patterns of thinking persist within central agencies, departments are unlikely to achieve any significant improvement in their situations.

As indicated earlier in this book, much early thinking about management was premised on the view that there were universal principles: golden rules which could be used to tell managers how to manage in any situation, and which established the standards of "good management" for every organization. As an outgrowth of this line of thought, management became viewed by some persons as a profession in its own right; a "professional" manager who had mastered the "universal principles" could run anything. We now know that management is a situational discipline. There are few golden rules. As discussed in more detail later in this part of the book, the notion of the professional manager has also been discredited.

The idea that central agencies should relate to departments on the basis of common policies in such areas as personnel, finance and administration arises in large measure from the idea that government is a collectivity. Certainly, if there is to be coordinated control over public expenditures, government finances have to be managed on the basis of principles and practices which are broadly consistent from one department to the next. However, it is by no means clear that the requirement for consistency exists to the same extent in other spheres of administration. The idea that policies must be common in other areas of management may be another example of the "finan-centric" thinking about management which was alluded to in chapter 6. Practices in the sphere of finance do not constitute a model for all other areas of management.

Many central agencies appear still to be mired in pre-1950s ideas about administration. Instead of accepting the fact that considerable variety exists among government departments, and instead of recognizing that contemporary knowledge about management would *demand* discrimination among departments with different mandates and functions, some officials continue to seek to force them all into a Procrustean bed of common policies. The idea that these policies might be formulated on an individual basis for different organizations, or different groups of organizations, conjures up visions of chaos in the minds of such officials. To give up the principle of commonality of policies would be like selling their birthright.

RELATIONSHIPS AND ACCOUNTABILITIES

This is a sphere of public administration where Canada is showing leadership. The IMAA (Increased Ministerial Authority and Accountability) policy alluded to in chapter 7 has opened up the possibility of new relationships between the Treasury Board Secretariat and departments. The management contracts under IMAA contemplate, at least in principle, the possibility of different sorts of accountability frameworks for different sorts of departments.

Experiments with new accountability structures are not confined to IMAA negotiations. Transport Canada, one of the biggest departments of the federal government, is at time of writing working with central agency officials to try to institute a new "public enterprise model" for the country's airport system. The notion underlying this initiative is to determine what needs to be changed within the conventional public service environment in order to provide managers with the latitude to achieve new objectives agreed to for airports by the Cabinet. A more economy-conscious, market-sensitive mode of operation of the airport system is expected to result from this initiative. Other departments in Ottawa are engaged in other experiments along somewhat similar lines.

Instituting this new type of relationship between central agencies and line departments is a major challenge for public management. The challenge has two facets or dimensions. There is, first of all, the conceptual challenge involved in situating central agency-departmental relationships on a new footing. Second, there is the challenge of making the policy work in practice.

It seems likely to me that this second aspect of the challenge may prove a more difficult and enduring problem than the first. Departments like Canada's Treasury Board Secretariat are staffed with many officials who have spent their careers working in the context of common policies. Many central agency officials probably continue to believe that common procedures are the only responsible way to run a government. At time of writing, evidence from departments on the receiving end of the IMAA initiative is that central agency officials responsible for day-to-day contact with departments may be having difficulty understanding the implications of the IMAA philosophy. (It is also likely that a number of departments of government are having difficulty appreciating the kinds of opportunities that might be available to them under the IMAA approach.)

The idea that departments should be handled on an individualized basis is an adjustment of very considerable dimensions to the traditional posture of many central agencies. Its implementation may well necessitate structural alterations within those agencies, to allow for better coordination of relationships with individual departments. It is also likely to call for carefully managed programs of organizational change, to educate officials in the new ways of doing things and reinforce new patterns of behaviour. Unless these requirements are recognized, there is a real danger that the inertia of old methods of thinking will insinuate its way into the relations between central agencies and departments. If this occurs, initiatives such as IMAA will have little long-term impact upon how governments work, and the forest of common policies will grow back as it has in the past.

Alternatives to the Public Service

The closer government organizations lie to the political centre, the more difficult it is to protect them from political influences. The conventions put in place to protect administration from political abuse, and the nature of politics itself, tend to make the process of management tortuous, frustrating and time-consuming in the public service. There are limits to what can be achieved by trying to create within government an environment that is more conducive to effective management.

In considering the role of government in society, perhaps we need to make a clearer distinction between what government *itself* should do and what government should *cause to be done* by other institutions. Government is good at some things, and less good at others: therefore, we should encourage governments to do what they do best, and indeed, what they have to do, namely, set the socio-economic context.[19] Conversely, we should perhaps consider what sorts of functions might better be placed in a context which is less rule-bound and less susceptible to external political or administrative intervention.

RELATIONSHIPS AND ACCOUNTABILITIES

There are several options to be considered in this connection.

Incentives for Business or Not-for-Profit Agencies: The first is to leave the activity entirely in the hands of the private sector, broadly defined to include both business and not-for-profit organizations, and to try to guide the private sector in certain directions through incentives or disincentives (grants, tax "expenditures" or concessions, regulations, legislation, levies, etc.) Obviously, the danger here is that if carried too far, such initiatives may distort both the operation of the market economy and the character of private sector organizations; one may wind up with private sector institutions so overlaid with political goals that they begin to look like part of government.

Sale of Government Assets to the Private Sector (Privatization): Where government is engaged in an activity deemed to be more appropriately carried out by business, the activity may be "returned" to the private sector, or, in the jargon of the 1980s, "privatized" through the sale of the shares in the enterprise to private investors or to corporations. Both Britain and Canada have been engaged in programs of this nature during the 1980s.

New Forms of Contracting: A third option is for governments to contract out activity to the private sector. Historically, governments have tended to contract for the acquisition of products or services for which the productive capacity is known to be already available in the private sector (e.g., manufacturing, construction, other public works, certain forms of research, etc.) Contracting is particularly advantageous where there is no possibility of a monopoly being created, and where a contract price can be determined with reference to the market.

Recently, some governments have been moving toward contracting in service areas conventionally viewed as the prerogative of the public sector. In spheres such as youth employment, social services for children, nursing homes or international development, some governments already provide operational funding or conditional contributions to outside organizations in order to encourage them to carry out defined functions or to pursue objectives consistent with those of the government. Such arrangements constitute a loose sort of contract, and are sometimes also considered to be a form of privatization.

Contracting in the more conventional sense is also being extended into new areas. For example, in the mid-1980s, one Canadian federal government department was reviewing the pros and cons of having nursing services delivered by private contractors rather than nurses on the public service payroll. A provincial department was examining whether certain administrative functions associated with the processing and delivery of welfare cheques could be performed under contract. The U.S. federal government and the Canadian government have both adopted policies to explore the possibilities of contracting for services conventionally viewed as part of government. Contracting for services of this type carries certain risks, in particular, that of creating a monopoly in the private sector in cases where there is no free market for the service in question. However, if these risks can be dealt with, the idea of contracting may become more widely accepted; it may come to be seen as a legitimate alternative to the more conventional model of "government owned and operated" programs.

Unfortunately, almost all the incentives in governments typically run counter to the contracting of established services. Affected employees feel threatened; unions worry about loss of membership; managers of the activities face the prospect of a diminishing work force, which in turn could threaten their job classification and personal incomes. In addition, most managers are disinclined to subject their employees to the personal stresses associated with the transfer of a function to the private sector. Finally, the process of change itself involves disruption and extra work, prospects which most managers are unlikely to welcome. In short, there is little motivation for managers to try out this approach, and there are several reasons to ignore or resist it. Unless incentives are changed and commitment to this option at the political level is strengthened, it seems unlikely that we will witness any widespread adoption of this approach to administration. (There are, in any event, limits upon how many services can realistically be privatized in this way.)

Crown Agencies and Quangos: Crown agencies and corporations offer another alternative to the public service. Department heads frustrated by government red tape are often tempted by the possibility of converting their organizations to this status. Such a change involves the establishment of a new accountability framework characterized by what is sometimes referred to as an "arm's-length relationship" with the government.[20]

From a managerial viewpoint, the Crown agency/quango structure has the great advantage of "liberating" the organization (to a greater or lesser extent, depending upon the length of the arm) from many of the controls and constraints of the public service environment. This accountability framework tends to let managers manage to a much greater degree, and (at least in principle); it is supposed to foster a relationship between the agency and the elected Government where there is somewhat more emphasis upon the results achieved, and fewer controls and checks related to how the agency attains them.

In principle, the Crown corporation model undoubtedly provides a context which is more geared to allowing managers more room for judgment and freedom of manoeuvre than the public service. Unless subjected to political interference, such institutions can have a clearer sense of purpose and a less cluttered mandate than a government department; there can be fewer restrictions upon personnel management, and more options available to motivate and reward staff. Less time will need to be devoted to supporting the responsible minister. Such agencies can also have the advantage of insulating the minister from having to be directly involved in certain types of decisions.

There can, however, be problems with this type of organization. Particularly for ministers who are dirigiste by nature, the Crown agency structure is frustrating. Their authority over such agencies is supposed to be restricted to broader policy issues, and they resent the fact that as elected representatives of the people, they are nonetheless unable to exact the kind of accountability from the management of the agency that they want, or to exercise detailed control over agency decisions.

In general, the Crown agency/quango model works well in cases where the Government is willing to operate on a hands-off basis, where it appoints responsible and effective individuals to the agency's governing council, where there is consistency of philosophy between minister and the agency; and where, directly or indirectly, the Government ensures that sound appointments are made to top executive positions within the agency. Where any of these conditions do not obtain, there can be troubled relations between the Government and the agency and/or problems with the agency's performance and management. Crown agencies are thus not a panacea to the problems of management in the public service, although they can be a viable option in some cases.

Increasing the "Public" Content in Public Policy

The classical view of the public servant as the faceless administrator carrying out ministerial wishes no longer has much credibility. However, the tradition that public servants should be anonymous as well as neutral remains well established. It is also believed in some quarters that it is the job of the minister and elected members of Parliament to read the public pulse and to convey to the public service the mood and wishes of the people.

This is an area of public administration where principle may not have entirely caught up with contemporary reality. Public servants who are urged to be "anonymous" on the one hand (see chapter 5) are on the other encouraged to keep in touch with the public.* The range of issues upon which governments are engaged is so diverse and so complex, it would be quite impossible for members of Parliament to constitute the sole, or even the principal, conduit of information from the public to the policy-making process.

A Canadian deputy minister has argued that public servants at top levels

> should be less averse to taking risks and should actively assume responsibility .... Outreach should be an essential component of almost every important government initiative. Yet, generally, the bureaucracy has not been skilled in communication and consultation. Our traditions

---

* "[P]ublic administrators ... have been brought very much into the traditional role of the politician as arbitrator, conciliator, and definer of the interests to be fostered, placated, rewarded, or penalized through public policy." J.E. Hodgetts, "Government responsiveness to the public interest: has progress been made?", *Canadian Public Administration*, vol. 24 no. 2, (Summer 1981), p. 221.

are rooted in the concept of single-line accountability to the minister, which is inadequate to serve either our ministers or the public effectively.[21]

An American official has stated the argument for external consultation by public servants cogently: "[C]ommunity groups represent your consumers, and they are often right, or at least partly right, in their complaints. If you cannot accept this proposition, you ought to be in another business." (He provides a number of suggestions for relating to such groups effectively.)[22]

My impression is that, perhaps because of the traditional civil servant's concern about not up-staging the minister and perhaps also because of the persistence of a dated view of the "faceless" official, we are not sufficiently forthright in either encouraging our public servants to consult the public or in educating them in how to do it effectively. Likewise, we may not emphasize sufficiently the importance of their responsibilities in this sphere.*

I recently had occasion to interview officials in a cross-section of government departments concerning their experiences in public consultation. Their comments, reinforced by the growing literature on public participation in policy development, made it clear that there is a good deal more to such consultation than may meet the eye. Space precludes any in-depth discussion of consultation techniques here, but a summary of some of the questions associated with consultation indicates the complexities that may be involved:

- How does the public servant determine who has a legitimate voice in the consultative process?

- What type of preparations should be made before engaging in a process of public consultation? How long should such a process last? What techniques might be used to collect information?

---

* While the "Drafter's Guide" for memoranda to Cabinet circulated by the Privy Council Office in Ottawa (undated) requests officials to tell ministers what they think the public's attitudes are to policy issues, there is no requirement for officials to undertake consultations, nor are they even asked to specify what consultations with the public have been undertaken. Departments tend to talk to their "primary clients" if they do consult on policy, and would not necessarily engage other interest groups who are not part of their primary clientele.

- What should be done with respect to groups or individuals who may have a legitimate role but lack the time or resources to participate?

- At what stage in the process should consultations be entered into: prior to the articulation of options, or after?

- In what circumstances might it make sense to turn the actual decision (and perhaps the resources) associated with the resolution of a public policy issue over to interested parties to work out (or divide up) among themselves, rather than having government do it for them?

- When should the minister(s) be involved in the consultative process, and what role should he, she, or they play?

- When should white (or green, or other-coloured) papers be employed?

- How might the process of public consultation be employed to resolve interdepartmental conflicts over policy alternatives?

- To what extent is it legitimate for a public servant to advise members of the public on tactics that might be used to raise the public visibility or political priority of a particular issue?

- Is consultation advisable when dealing with a single interest group whose views on an issue are already known, and who are not receptive to considering alternative positions?

- What responsibilities exist for communicating the results of a consultative process back to those who participated in it? To what extent might such feedback betray confidential advice to ministers?

- When is it advisable to make the process of consultation formal, and when is it preferable to take an informal approach?

- If the time frame available for consultation is constrained, is it better to consult quickly but inadequately or not at all?

- What are the merits of establishing an ongoing advisory committee of representatives from the public to provide input to policy, as opposed to using the "travelling road show" approach?

- Under what circumstances are public hearings appropriate? Upon what basis or set of procedures should such hearings be run?

- How does one consult with the public on issues where the concern is general but diffused (environmental policy might bean example)?

- What is the role of the member of Parliament in public consultations? What if regions of the country are affected where the sitting member is not a member of the Government?

Many public servants have little or no training in how to handle issues of this type. They should have. Public consultation is, very roughly, the public sector analogue of the marketing function in the private sector. Marketing is a recognized discipline in business; it is a field of specialization for students of business administration. How many students of public administration graduate with specializations in public consultation techniques?

We are clearly well beyond the stage where public servants can expect to sit behind their desks and wait for elected politicians to serve as their conduit to the public. Public servants have a responsibility to keep themselves informed on the views of the public on policy issues relevant to their portfolios, and to ensure, as suggested in chapter 5, that they have a first-class "intelligence system". An important practical challenge for public management is to ensure that officials are properly equipped to perform this role; a related challenge at the level of principle is to provide guidance as to how this responsibility should be reconciled with precepts regarding the anonymity of public servants.

Summary

As populations grow and the issues of public policy become more complex and intertwined, the role of the public servant has to evolve to accommodate these developments. No longer can the government official pretend to be uninvolved in the development of policy or disengaged from obligations in the sphere of public consultation.

This chapter has identified several challenges with which public management should, in my view, be wrestling in the years ahead. These are:

- developing conventions and traditions which allow public servants to support the emerging role of parliamentary committees, without becoming caught up in partisan controversy

- improving the quality of staff assistance available to ministers in the execution of their impossible jobs

- defining new, "customized" accountability relationships between central agencies and departments – and implementing these relationships effectively

- determining which types of functions are likely to be best performed by government departments and which might be better suited to alternative accountability arrangements or managerial environments

- ensuring that officials understand, and are trained to execute, their roles in public consultation in the context of policy development.

In the following chapter, we turn to the question of managing people more effectively within the public service: the last and possibly the biggest challenge facing public management today.

Footnotes:

1. As one of the designers of the Canadian system has stated, the PEMS process appears to have "set real and visible limits for Cabinet decision-making . . . . It has . . . [provided] an effective mechanism for reallocating resources in response to changing priorities. Decentralization to committees has allowed Cabinet to handle efficiently the large number of "routine" items brought to it while leaving the Prime Minister and senior ministers time to concentrate on major issues. In sum, it has, I believe, helped the Government stay on top of its affairs in difficult economic circumstances. See Ian Clark, "PEMS and the central agencies," Background notes for a presentation to the North American Society for Corporate Planning, (Ottawa: Privy Council Office) October 27, 1983, p. 15.

2. Gordon Aiken, *The Backbencher, Trials and Tribulations of a Member of Parliament,* (Toronto: McClelland and Stewart, 1974), pp. 95, 182-184.

3. *Report of the Special Committee on Reform of the House of Commons,* (Ottawa: Supply and Services Canada, 1985), p. 1.

4. *Ibid.,* p. 11

5. *Ibid.,* p. 2.

6. Aiken, *op.cit.,* pp. 175 ff.

7. Douglas Wass, "Critical opposition: part of the polity," in *Government and the Governed,* BBC Reith Lectures 1983, (London: Routledge and Kegan Paul, 1984). Reprinted in *The Listener,* 8 December 1983. See also Hugo Young and Anne Sloman, *No, Minister,* (London: British Broadcasting Corporation, 1982), pp. 68-72.

8. Wass, *op. cit.*

9. *Ibid.*

10. Concerning the fate of these proposals, see Peter Kellner and Lord Crowther-Hunt, *The Civil Servants,* (London: Macdonald General Books, 1980), pp. 206-209.

11. Young and Sloman, *op. cit.*, pp. 88-91.

12. See, for example, the views of Lord Bancroft, formerly Head of the Civil Service in Whitehall: "In small numbers, and in a staff not a line capacity, [special advisers] have proved their worth." (Lord Bancroft, "Whitehall: Some Personal Reflections," Suntory-Toyota Lecture, delivered at the London School of Economics, December 1, 1983.) Similarly, Douglas Wass has commented, "[P]olitically committed special advisers have a key role in the help a department gives to its Minister." (Douglas Wass, "The Privileged Adviser," in *Government and the Governed*, BBC Reith Lectures 1983, (London: Routledge and Kegan Paul, 1984). Reprinted in *The Listener*, 8 December 1983.) A former Cabinet secretary in Canada, has stated, "The Minister . . . needs a competent political staff that views advice and programs from a political perspective, as he would do, if he had the time." (Gordon Osbaldeston, "The Public Servant and Politics," *Policy Options*, vol. 8 no. 1 (January 1987), p. 3.

13. *Seventh Report from the Treasury and Civil Service Committee*, Session 1985-86, "Civil Servants and Ministers: Duties and Responsibilities, vol. 1, (London, Her Majesty's Stationery Office, 12 May 1986), p. xxv.

14. Osbaldeston, *loc. cit.*, p. 6.

15. Author's discussion, February, 1988.

16. Young and Sloman, *op. cit.*, p. 91.

17. Gordon Osbaldeston, "Dear Minister, Letter to an Old Friend on Being a Successful Minister," remarks to the Association of Professional Executives, (Ottawa: January 22, 1988).

18. Lord Bancroft, *op. cit.*

19. See Charles Wolf, "Policy Analysis and Public Management," *Journal of Policy Analysis and Public Management*, vol. 1 no. 4, (Summer 1982), pp. 546-551. Wolf, Dean of the Rand Graduate Institute in California has written of how, in every field of public policy, we constantly encounter "a combination of good intentions with perverse outcomes," and has suggested that, beyond a certain size, inefficiencies inevitably set in in government organizations because of "the profound diseconomies of scale to which government is prone." These exist because the

difficulty of defining outputs restrains governments' ability to decentralize or delegate, while conversely, the possibilities for centralization are constrained by the limitations of leaders' judgment and time, span-of-control problems and the difficulties of consultation associated with centralized administration. Wolf proposes that there should be a ceiling to the scale of government operations.

20. Under this arrangement, "those elected – and thus responsible – give direction and set policy and financial boundaries, and select the most senior people to whom to delegate operational responsibility. If necessary, they can replace people in whom they have lost confidence. But the arm's-length principle is in its way an iron law: between ministerial responsibility and program delivery there is an intermediate power [usually, a board of directors or council of some type] over which there is no operational authority . . . . [The principle puts] decision-making in the hands of the qualified and [insulates] the political power from direct access to resource distribution." See Gérard Pelletier, "Canadian Culture and the Arm's-Length Principle," Notes for a Presentation to the Fellow's Luncheon, Canadian Museums Association, Winnipeg, 27 May 1987. Pelletier traces the origins of the principle to the Board of Commissioners established to discharge the Office of the Lord High Admiral in the U.K. and to protect the conduct of naval affairs from the patronage of King Charles II.

21. Bruce Rawson, "The responsibilities of the public servant to the public: accessibility, fairness and efficiency," *Canadian Public Administration*, vol. 27 no. 4, (Winter 1984), pp. 601-610.

22. See Gordon Chase and Elizabeth C. Reveal, *How to Manage in the Public Sector*, (Don Mills: Addison-Wesley, 1983), pp. 130ff.

Chapter Thirteen:
People and Performance

In the last chapter, several challenges confronting management in government were outlined. These were primarily concerned with certain institutional relationships in a parliamentary democracy. In this chapter, we consider the motivational aspects of performance. The discussion is based upon two premises: first, that people are the heart of management, and that getting the "people" aspects of management right is probably more important than any of the others, taken alone; and second, that this issue is not simply a matter of good will. Although treating people in ways that are just, considerate, and humane will be a goal sufficient in itself for many managers, there are always some who pride themselves on being "hard-headed" when it comes to personnel management. These are the managers who take the view that there is no point in doing things for their employees unless it can be demonstrated to improve productivity.

The message in this chapter is that in organizations where there is room for discretionary effort—that is, in organizations where employees have the latitude to make more or less of their jobs, depending upon their own discretion—productivity and motivation are inextricably linked. This includes virtually every organization in the public sector (and most in the private sector as well). If people want to make the place work, they will, in ways that will not only overcome defects in formal systems and procedures, but even make many such systems irrelevant. Conversely, if they feel like the public servant cited previously in the book, ("Why should I stick around? I'm going home"), no amount of cunning in the design of structures or procedures will achieve real improvement in productivity. People have to want to work productively, and if they do not, their organization will not find it possible to perform at full capacity. Ironically, because discretionary effort is intangible, senior management will never even know that it is being withheld.

The evidence cited in chapter 11 suggested that there are serious problems in the way people are managed in public services. This chapter suggests what needs to be done to rectify some of these problems.

Departmental Mandates

Motivation starts with a sense of purpose and with clarity of direction. The need for clarity of intention for departments should send a message to both politicians and central agency officials concerned with designing the machinery of government. Departments with complicated, conflicting mandates and multiple policy interests will be difficult organizations in which to instill any sense of coherent direction. A department structured in this way will be hard to lead effectively.

A good illustration of what not to do to promote productivity and morale is provided by the Canadian government's tinkering with the machinery of economic policy during the 1970s. This episode, described in appendix 1, resulted in the creation of a pastiche of departments and ministries all of whom were partially involved in policy development and none of whom was clearly accountable. The reputation of flagship departments such as Finance declined; the prestige of the economist/statistician occupational category diminished; and day-to-day contact with public servants provided considerable evidence of a general disaffection among those involved in economic policy work.

Elected governments and central agencies which are seriously committed to improving the quality of service to the public and to ensuring value for money in the expenditure of public funds should strive to structure government organizations so that their purposes are clear and they are not encumbered with multiple, or mutually inconsistent mandates. Regrettably, as Lord Bancroft has observed, in politics, whim and fashion seem often to prevail when decisions are being made about the machinery of government.

Vision and Leadership

Sadly lacking in many government departments is any sense of vision. A vision is a view of the future that can give staff a sense of involvement, direction and "the feeling of being at the active centres of the social order."[1] Vision may derive from the political level, or from a deputy minister or permanent secretary who is able to work effectively with a minister receptive to his or her ideas. An organization with visionary leaders has a sort of motivational overdrive relative to one which has none.

A vision may be based around, but is not dependent upon, a well-drafted Cabinet document. It is broad direction communicated to others in ways that inspire confidence and commitment. Managing through vision places confidence in subordinates' ability to find their own way within the framework of general direction.

> When the organization has a clear sense of its purpose, direction, and desired future state and when this image is widely shared, individuals are able to find their own roles both in the organization and in the larger society of which they are a part. This empowers individuals and confers status upon them because they can see themselves as part of a worthwhile enterprise .... A shared vision of the future ... helps individuals distinguish between what's good and what's bad for the organization, and what it's worthwhile to achieve. And most important, it makes it possible to distribute decision making widely.[2]

Vision may serve as one of the organization's most effective management control tools, by providing a framework within which individuals can control themselves.

The practice of rotating ministers clearly militates against the establishment of any consistent vision or direction for departments of government; but at least there is (presumably) some political justification for this practice. The justification for frequently moving department heads from one organization to another is much less easy to defend. Prime ministers who are interested in having their public servants perform for them would be well advised to abandon this kind of practice.

Below the political level, perhaps the most serious problem related to the management of people in government is that the public service culture has not traditionally attached high priority to leadership or the management of people. Intellectual leadership is valued; but in many quarters, the effective direction and motivation of subordinate staff is still not seen as a requirement for promotion. An up-and-coming public servant, adept at reading organizational values, might well conclude that when decisions were being made about promotions, the leadership of people would count rather less than such factors as mental agility, drafting skills, central agency connections and contact with ministers.

Differences between the culture of the civil service and a major business firm have been well described in a penetrating article by a British civil servant, David Howells, who had an opportunity to work with Marks and Spencer (M&S), a respected retail chain with a good reputation for staff relations. Howells' article, written in 1981, foreshadowed the findings of the Zussman/Jabes survey to a remarkable degree.

M&S' high standards do not typify all private firms by any means. However, Howells' comments show what can be attained in a well-managed private company, and the contrast with the situation in Whitehall is vivid.[3] M&S accords great importance to building a sense of cohesion and identity between the company as an institution and its employees. "[T]he company wants staff to identify with M&S, to understand its aims and to feel part of an organization which does worthwhile things. In this it has succeeded to an impressive degree; the outsider cannot fail to be struck by the strong and sometimes fierce loyalty shown by staff at all levels, and the feeling that they work for an organization which is both efficient and socially useful."

Howells paints a contrast between the personal style of M&S and that of the civil service, and highlights the priority accorded to leadership in the private firm. He notes the low importance accorded to the management of people and to making organizations work in the culture of the civil service.

> [T]he subject of leadership [in the civil service] is little stressed. More emphasis is placed on intelligence, tactical judgement and the ability to perform well on paper . . . . [M]ost officials see themselves (in many cases correctly) as the confidential advisers of ministers [rather] than the managers of activities; they look up, not down.

> Jobs which involve the management of activities therefore command comparatively low prestige, even though they may involve control over very large resources. The reward and promotion system accordingly places relatively low emphasis on qualities of leadership and personality which would be much more critical within M&S . . . .

> Partly as a result of all this, the gap between the centre and the field is far wider in the civil service than at M&S. Motivation is probably highest near the top . . . . But elsewhere levels of satisfaction and motivation are much lower, reflecting the changes in composition and outlook which have taken place, especially in departments with large local office networks . . . . Compared to the pre-war period, or even to the 1950s, today's civil service is much younger, less stable and committed, and less motivated by an ethic of public service. Many, if not most, civil servants are not particularly attached to their work or to the civil service as a career but see it just as a job, whose attractiveness is set against alternative jobs in different organizations. They neither meet nor identify with senior officials; nor do they share the same outlook or experience 4

This sounds very similar to the findings of Zussman and Jabes. Howells says that civil service values tend to be "instrumental in character – neutrality, personal integrity, intellectual rigour – and do not bear primarily on end results . . . ."

> [T]hese values . . . are scarcely effective motivators in today's conditions. The same is true of the particular policies of government, which are often complex, conflicting and liable to change; they cannot serve as a source of motivation except in certain circumstances, e.g. where the unit is close to ministers or where it is new and expanding.

The aim of accommodating the minister and getting the government's business through — however logical and right this may appear in the head offices of departments — can have little appeal to staff down the line.[5]

Promotional Practices

Today, it is no longer sufficient for governments to advance officials on the basis of their policy skills alone. Leadership and motivational ability should also be criteria. Promotional decisions are one of the most important ways of communicating organizational priorities and values to staff. They are the tangible manifestation of the norms of the organization, providing unmistakable evidence of what the culture of the institution *really* is, as opposed to what top executives may *say* it is.

[T]he tremendous significance of promotions and appointments is not fully realized ... directives and policy statements and messages to staff ... are nothing compared with promotions. Promotions are the one visible, unmistakable sign of the corporation's standard of values, an irrevocable declaration of the qualities it prizes in its staff, a simultaneous warning and example to everyone who knows the nature of the job and the qualities of its new incumbent.[6]

Studies of both the Canadian and Ontario governments at the end of the 1970s underlined the importance of performance appraisal and noted that this area was not receiving the priority it warranted.[7] Elsewhere, the Canadian government was accused of paying more attention to the mechanical aspects of the selection process and to making sure that a promotional decision was "appeal-proof", rather than ensuring that individuals' pace of advancement was governed by their work history or record of accomplishments.[8]

If more attention is to be given to leadership skills in the staffing of senior positions in government, then questions arise concerning the use of policy departments as a sort of breeding ground for top officials.* The practice of naming officials who have little

---

* In a study of the Government of Ontario, it was noted that many deputies had no experience in the departments to which they were named, and that six ministries tended to act as "feeders" for senior appointments.

demonstrated managerial competence to take over departments with major administrative responsibilities accords too much credibility to policy skills and insufficient priority to leadership ability. Of course, some officials from policy departments may well have the ability to motivate others and to lead big organizations; but policy competence in itself is no guarantee of this.

In addition to leadership ability, an interest in, and aptitude for, the effective management of resources should also be a criterion for advancement to many top posts. The culture of government does not place a high priority on this area. With respect to the U.S. government, Irving Shapiro has commented:

> The people who fill the line offices [in government]... may show outstanding records in a professional or academic setting... but none of this demonstrates an ability to administer a departmental staff and budget. Individuals the private sector would not trust with the management of a large plant are given executive spots in government organizations dealing with public problems of major importance, with responsibility for billions or hundreds of millions of dollars.[9]

The Myth of the Professional Manager

A practice that seems to be common to many public services is that of rotating intermediate officials around government. There is much to be said for broadening the experience of individuals as they move up the management hierarchy; but there is a point at which the systematic enlargement of a person's experience deteriorates into a sort of crazy quilt, devoid of pattern or logic. Job rotation or career development through different postings should be directed to defined goals; in government it often seems to amount to little more than a random collection of unrelated assignments.

The popularity of this practice in government was founded in part upon the notion that the main objective in developing a civil servant was to enhance the individual's policy skills, to create a "generalist". Policy competence is certainly improved through exposure to a variety of experiences and policy fields. This makes an official sensitive to the many different interests at play in government, widens thinking, and provides better insights into the subtleties of the bureaucracy. However, this sensitivity should be combined with a sound knowledge of the substance of one or two specific policy fields, and of the administrative problems associated with running departmental operations.

Such knowledge cannot be acquired by the official who skips from one department to another or who has never worked in an operational or field position. (Consulting studies conducted at the time of the Fulton Report in the U.K. found that in the 1960s, most administrators spent only two years in their jobs before moving on to the next.)[10] As Howells has noted, attitudes in the private sector to operational experience differ from those in government. In M&S, for example, managers are expected to start their careers in the field; executives are required to stay in close contact with in-store activities through regular visits.

> By comparison with M&S, the work of Whitehall is London-bound and desk-bound . . .. Even where the job is managerial or where decisions are involved which bear on local administration, there is no institutionalized pressure as in M&S to observe things at first hand. This is reflected in a willingness to work through hierarchies and to rely on paper-based systems of communication . . . .[11]

The practice of rotating officials around the government was also sustained by a belief which held particular currency in the 1960s and early 1970s to the effect that one could, and should, seek to develop a breed of "professional managers". Such a manager would be a man (or woman) for all seasons, able to cope with any challenge or contingency.

The notion of the professional manager is founded on a misunderstanding of the manager's role. It overlooks the technical dimensions of management. One of the classic *Harvard Business Review* articles on human resource management, written by Robert Katz in 1955, suggested that there are three types of abilities that should form the basis of selection decisions for managers: technical, human and conceptual.* On the specific issue of technical or

---

* "Technical skill implies an understanding of, and proficiency in, a specific kind of activity, particularly one involving methods, processes, procedures or techniques . . . .

substantive skills, Katz's original assessment was that "it has its greatest importance at the lower levels of administration." Significantly, however, in writing a retrospective commentary on this article 20 years later, Katz recanted.

> In the original article I suggested that specific technical skills are unimportant at top management levels. I cited as evidence the many professional managers who move easily from one industry to another without apparent loss of effectiveness. I now believe this mobility is possible only in very large companies, where the chief executive has extensive staff assistance and highly competent, experienced technical operators throughout the organization.[12]

Similar conclusions were reached by John Kotter, author of a landmark study on general managers' jobs in industry, who, in reflecting on his earlier research into senior executives' jobs, observed that he had become skeptical of the term "general manager," and that he increasingly thought of senior managers as specialists in a particular company or industry.[13] Perhaps Katz's professional managers who purportedly moved easily from industry to industry without loss of effectiveness never existed. Governments should be careful not to import myths from the private sector as models for their own policies. Effective managers need to understand the operations under their control; their effectiveness is greatly enhanced by hands-on operational experience and by the personal contacts which they develop through sustained experience in a specific policy field or industry setting.

Building Institutions that Value People

Studies of business suggest that successful CEOs show a strong sense of identity with their corporation. They assume that it is their job to

---

[H]uman skill is the executive's ability to work effectively as a group member and to build cooperative effort within the team he leads.... Conceptual skill...involves the ability to see the enterprise as a whole; it includes recognizing how the various functions of the organization depend on one another, and how changes in any one part affect all the others; and it extends to visualizing the relationship of the individual business to the industry, the community and the political, social, and economic forces of the nation as a whole." (See Katz citation in footnotes to this chapter.)

make their organization the best. They rely on "a consistent internal value system" to tie disparate parts of the organization together and to maintain the integrity of the whole. They see it as their job to build enduring corporations, and to take a vigorous interest in promoting, communicating and reinforcing those organizational values that establish the character of the institution. They also take a strong personal interest in their employees.

> All were aware of the need to touch their own people and made a practice of it.... They were especially affectionate with people close to them, while still maintaining an appropriate distance.... [T]hey were...supportive... compassionate and empathetic. They were sensitive to people's self-esteem and face-saving needs; the lower in the organization, the greater the concern for the person. They did not confront people easily, although they usually did so when required.... They tried to rescue or defend some people at times when perhaps they should not have made that effort.... They went out of their way to extend personal kindnesses.[14]

My own exposure to the public service certainly supports Zussman's findings that business leaders have a more powerful sense of attachment to their organizations than do the top people in many government departments. Certainly most ministers, as birds of passage, have little ongoing commitment to their departments. Deputy ministers appointed to departments where they have little or no background are unlikely to be very sensitive to the history and traditions of the organization. Many civil servants seem to see their deputies as somewhat remote figures. My impression is that many DMs do not identify very strongly with their role as institution builders (this may be less true in the U.K. as permanent secretaries are civil servants and are not rotated as they are in Ottawa. However, Howells' article would seem to suggest that institutional leadership may be a problem here as well.) Other observers have pointed out that it is not easy to nurture an "organizational family" in the public service.[15]

This impression is reinforced by the fact that on institutional matters, the strategic orientation tends to be different in government than in the private sector. In business, the strategic concern of top executives is the health of the institution itself: this is the economic, legal and social entity which has been entrusted to the CEO, and it is his or her job to add value to the organization and to enhance its stature in the business community. By contrast, in government the strategic concern is focused upon the policy field, rather than the institution. The principal interest of top government officials is the "health" of the area of public policy for which their department is responsible. The department as an institution is a secondary and somewhat derivative concern; it is not the object of policy or strategy in the same direct way as it is in business, nor are the people employed within it.

This would help to explain why civil servants seem to have less pride in their organizations than do business managers. There is some question as to whether government leaders consider it important, or even legitimate, to encourage their staff to develop this sense of pride and identity, even though many employees may *want* to be proud of their institution, and would probably feel more positively about their job situation if such a sense of pride were encouraged. The evidence in the Zussman/Jabes survey indicates that Canadian government departments are not perceived by their managers to have a strong orientation toward their employees, and that there are serious problems in the government's performance in this sphere.*

More Authority to Deal with People and Structure

The following case study, based on experience, (although slightly adapted to conceal the identity of the department in question), illustrates the sorts of problems frequently encountered by department heads confronting organizational problems.

A deputy minister decided that to provide efficient service to clients, it was necessary to unite two separate programs into a new, larger entity. To staff the new senior position required, the head had

---

* In business, almost 40 per cent of managers one level below the CEO indicated that they thought the firm was "employee oriented", compared with 18 per cent at a comparable level in government; five levels down from the CEO, 34 per cent of business managers still thought the organization was oriented to staff, as compared with a worrying five per cent in government.

in mind a particular individual who he knew would be competent both to manage the amalgamation of the programs and to operate the unified organization once the restructuring was complete. However, he discovered that, despite the availability of this individual, a number of requirements still had to be met:

(1) A submission to Treasury Board was required, since the proposed new position put the department over the senior management quota accorded by the Board.

(2) Since the job classification for the new position had to include an outline of the organization structure that the position was to supervise, the new manager could not be asked to direct the reorganization — a new provisional structure had to be devised first. Staff in the affected organizations wanted to know why the restructuring was going to occur without the involvement of the new manager.

(3) As there was no one available internally to develop the new organization structure, the deputy minister had to become personally involved in structuring the new unit. To assist him, he decided to hire an outside consultant, but because of a recent cross-government hiring freeze, a special request to the minister for the necessary authority was required.

(4) Once the new position was classified, a competition advertised nation-wide would have to be held in a search for candidates from both public and private sectors, this despite the fact that government salary scales for this type of job were well below comparable private sector rates at the time. The likelihood of attracting a qualified candidate from the private sector was minimal.

In the normal course of events, in the business world, within a matter of weeks, or even days, a president would have appointed the new manager and the reorganization would have been under way. Only a few individuals would have been involved in making the necessary decisions. However, in this department, it became evident that by the time the consultant had been hired, the provisional structure agreed to, the position classified, the complement problem resolved, the competition held, the candidates elected and (if necessary) relocated, somewhere between 12 and 18 months were likely to elapse (this assuming that the request for a supplementary executive level position was approved). Three departments, six Cabinet ministers,* and several dozen civil servants would be involved at one stage or another.

In government, corporate or government-wide policies affect almost every decision related to people. Special objectives may be established in relation to certain groups such as disabled persons or female employees, or to increase language capabilities of the public service, as in the case of Canada's bilingualism program, or to create a "representative" public service. Factors only distantly related to job competence are thereby added to the selection criteria for appointments. Each new objective entrains a cluster of regulations intended to ensure its implementation. Often accompanying these regulations are controls on the complement or establishment of departments. Such controls are inconsistent with the philosophy of managing by "outputs" or results; but they still seem to persist in many jurisdictions.

Many objectives which are served by governments' personnel-related policies and rules — equity, merit, affirmative action, due process, neutrality, bilingualism, etc. — are laudable; but no one states what priority they should enjoy relative to other goals such as speed of response, administrative simplicity, or accountability for program results. Usually, no one in government is in a position to act as an arbiter between the application of these rules and the priorities of line departments. In general, if there is a conflict between personnel objectives and departments' operational goals (e.g., getting a new program under way quickly), the former will prevail, because they are enshrined in legislation and regulations, backed by central agency officials, and treated as conditions of program delivery. When personnel-related regulations are passed in government, their cumulative impact on departments' ability to deliver programs and services is seldom taken into account. Little by little, the arteries permitting rapid action become constricted. Often no one notices the

---

* The request for change in complement had to be approved by Treasury Board, a Cabinet committee of five ministers. The departmental minister had to approve the consultant's contract.

progressive loss of energy until a coronary bypass is required to keep the patient alive.

Many departmental officials believe that they have insufficient control over the critical issues affecting people management. Pay, accommodation, conditions of work, benefits, financial incentives, industrial relations policies all tend to be determined centrally. Officials at the departmental level who might wish to tailor personnel practices to the needs of their own organizations often find their path is blocked by the desire to ensure consistency of practice across the public service. The Zussman/Jabes survey confirms that managers at all levels in the Canadian government feel they have insufficient authority to hire, fire, promote and set salaries.*

Perhaps because of the tendency to assume that financial matters are the crux of management, there has been insufficient recognition of the debilitating effect of government personnel policies and practices upon the practice of management in the public service. We know from private sector experience that successful CEOs make extensive use of their power to build a team of like-minded, effective colleagues, to assert corporate values, to reassign responsibilities where necessary and generally to fashion the organization of the firm in a way that will result in superior performance. However, we hobble top managers in government with regulations and policies that make this almost impossible, unless a manager has the patience of Job.[16]

In order to protect operational programs from excessive delays arising from personnel-related policies, governments might give more attention to setting and enforcing operational performance standards in regard to key personnel actions such as staffing. For example, a standard might be set to the effect that on average, it should take no

---

* Of the respondents from business to the Zussman/Jabes survey one down from the CEO, 14 per cent indicated they felt they had insufficient authority to promote people, compared with 41 per cent in government one level below the DM. Five levels down, 40 per cent of business managers expressed this view compared with 76 per cent in the public sector. With respect to authority for hiring people, only 14 per cent of business executives one level below the CEO thought their authority was insufficient, compared with 34 per cent in government; five levels down, the replies were 36 per cent private and 66 per cent public. As regards authority to fire non-performers, a little over 15 per cent of business managers one down from the top indicated a deficiency of authority compared with almost 60 per cent in government; five levels down, the statistics were about 40 per cent for business and roughly 75 per cent for government.

more than, say, three months to fill a management position (less if the competition was internal to government). Canada's Public Service Commission currently undertakes audits within departments, directed not only at staffing but at other personnel activities. But sluggishness in many personnel matters persists, suggesting that either the standards of performance are too forgiving, or that the audits are narrowly focused on compliance and do not address the question of the impact of regulations on operational ability to perform. Certainly we do not as yet appear to be witnessing the system-wide changes that would be needed to increase the flexibility of line managers. Periodic reviews should relate personnel policies to the achievement of operational goals, and prevent departmental operations from being suffocated by an excess of well-intentioned regulations.

Government managers, particularly those at more senior levels, require adequate authority in personnel and organizational matters if they are to be held accountable for the morale of their departments and the performance of departmental programs.

Coping with Inadequate Performers

It is generally accepted today that ministers cannot be held accountable for every last act of their officials. This move to gradations in the degree of accountability which the political level of government is prepared to accept for problems or errors in judgment raises the question of accountability at lower levels in the hierarchy. The question of official accountability has to be faced. As a British House of Commons committee has noted, "If . . . Ministers are not accountable to Parliament for some actions of their officials, then who is? . . . [W]ho ought to resign or to be penalised if mistakes are made? If it is not Ministers, it can only be officials."[17]

For many years, there has been a strong tradition in many public services that civil servants should be protected from dismissal. I have run across effective senior managers in the Canadian public service who believed that they could not fire employees for incompetence or error. This is in fact, not the case, but the fact that many managers seem to think it is true indicates how widespread the disposition against disciplining non-performers in government may be.

The tradition of neutrality of the public service is a shield designed to protect public servants from arbitrary dismissal upon changes of Government. The merit principle is intended to ensure that people who are well qualified are appointed to positions in government. It would appear, however, that these principles may have somehow expanded into a general disinclination to deal with problems of non-performance.*

Disciplining individuals for failure to perform duties as required is a difficult and unpleasant exercise. However, it is quite widely believed that this is easy in the private sector, and difficult to the point of impossibility in government. Certainly in Canada, this is not the case. Employees in the private sector are protected by a considerable body of legislation and legal precedent from arbitrary or unjust dismissal. These legalities have to be taken into account by any employer who wishes to discipline an employee, and the more senior the employee, the more care has to be taken. Dismissals, whether justified or arbitrary, have to be carefully planned and properly executed. The process often takes time, and, especially in the case of senior employees, it often costs quite a lot of money.

The situation is much the same in government. While the protections available to public servants may be somewhat different than they are in the private sector, and perhaps somewhat better from the employee's perspective, employees can be, and are, removed from government positions when they fail to meet the demands of the job. However, it does appear that this occurs rather less often than it should. Since departments are not subject to the test of profitability, and since for many years it was not difficult to secure more resources to finance the salaries of new employees, the easy route was to siphon marginal performers off into ineffectual staff positions or into known

---

* On this issue, the Lambert Commission made the following observation: "One of the greatest difficulties faced by deputy heads is handling performance problems .... [P]rocedures for dealing with unsatisfactory performance are inadequate .... [L]egislation should be enacted to ensure that personnel whose performance has been evaluated as unsatisfactory can be disciplined or removed." The Report also recommended that deputies should have the authority to dismiss, demote or transfer employees below the level of ADM, and that a placement and counselling service be established in a central agency to assist employees who have been dismissed. See the *Final Report*, pp. 226-227.

backwaters of the public service where they would be unlikely to get in the way of the higher priority work (a piece of organizational choreography not unknown in business, sometimes described as a lateral arabesque).

Organizations which are serious about encouraging a sense of commitment among their employees cannot afford too many lateral arabesques, or too many marginal performers left in positions of power. People who do not perform, particularly if they happen to be in charge of other hapless individuals, have a depressing impact upon morale and motivation. The performance of their own unit suffers; but perhaps more serious, they serve as a living signpost attesting to the fact that senior management is not seriously committed to such values as quality, reliability, good judgment, trustworthiness, or whatever other attributes the person in question is known not to possess. People who are paid less but who know they work harder and better than a non-performer are constantly reminded (by his or her presence) that their employer does not believe in treating employees equitably.

People who do not measure up, and who are allowed to get away with it, are like an acid eating at the innards of an organization. Senior government officials owe it to the public (who pays them) and to their colleagues and subordinates (who look to them for leadership) to deal humanely but effectively with problem employees. How an organization deals with its non-performers sends messages to staff that are almost as powerful as promotions; senior managers should ensure that the right messages about what is valued in the organization are sent to those staff who are committed and who do perform.

Rehabilitating the Personnel Function

Simplifying personnel rules in government may help to rehabilitate the function of personnel management. In many departments, personnel managers have come to be perceived as individuals whose *raison d'être* depends upon these rules: a self-perpetuating bureaucracy. They are often viewed as hurdles rather than helpers in the selection, appraisal and development of employees. (This perception is not confined to government. Peter Townsend's irreverent bestseller, *Up the Organization*, suggested the best personnel policy was, "Fire the whole personnel department.")[18]

Personnel officials in departments occupy an unenviable position. On one side, they face central agencies to whom they are accountable for implementing government-wide policies and systems.* On the other side, they face line managers who want to get on with their jobs without having to fight through a bramble patch of procedures. Personnel officials who side with line managers risk the ire of central agency officials and may see their career prospects dimmed in the government personnel community. Conversely, personnel managers who toe the central agencies' line are likely to be viewed as intransigent and bureaucratic by line colleagues.

Personnel officials in government seem to spend too much of their time policing, implementing and monitoring a vast range of personnel-related regulations. The personnel manual of the Canadian government exceeds 30 volumes of material which is in a state of continual review and update. Many officials who have attained their position by working their way up the personnel hierarchy (and through these reams of regulations) might be forgiven for having a blinkered view of the role of the personnel shop. In fact, the primary responsibility of a personnel unit should be to support the senior executives of the department and provide a strategic perspective to the management of people, linking human resource management initiatives to the overall policies and strategies of the organization. In particular, personnel officials should see that the key human resource management functions — selecting, appraising, rewarding, and developing staff — are effectively executed for the key positions in the organization. Personnel directors surrounded by 30 volumes of manuals can easily lose sight of the strategic dimensions of their job and turn into paper-pushers who add little to the actual performance of the organization.[19]

---

* In Britain, for example, the senior personnel official, known as the Principal Establishment Officer, is appointed by the permanent secretary, but the PEO's job description is written in the Treasury Department, and a reading of this document makes it abundantly clear that resource control, not motivation or service to line managers, is considered the essence of the job. See the U.K. manual, *Government Accounting*, Section C, 10.1-10.14, June 1986 version.

The Importance of Employee Communications

Often overlooked as a factor affecting morale is the importance of communication with employees. Employees who are largely unaware of the reasons for decisions – all too often this includes all employees not directly involved in top management – will seek their own logic for the actions taken by the institution. Where the lack of communication is not rectified, I have known staff to weave a fabric of half-truths and misperceptions that jaundices their entire view of the organization's goals and of the abilities of senior officials.

Good employee communications are not a frill; yet they usually receive low priority in government. In almost every government department with which I have been associated over the years, no member of senior management (other than the deputy minister, who is often too busy) has viewed it as his or her specific responsibility to be concerned with this area. Often employee communications end up being not much more than an occasional memorandum to staff from the department head. Public relations or information officers are usually busy with external communications and support to the minister; personnel officials are caught up with administering central agency regulations, monitoring complement and running personnel systems. As a result, employees are the last to find out the department's intentions. The main channel used to convey important information to staff is that problematic and unreliable vehicle, the office grapevine. This situation contributes to the feeling that employees are of no great importance to the department.

There are, of course, exceptions to these generalizations, and there are signs of change. However, some government departments would do well to look at progressive practices now being used in other organizations – general meetings, videotapes and other audio-visual presentations, bulletins, focus groups, employee "hot lines", newsletters, staff surveys, etc. The goal in employee communications should not just be to disseminate social information (the focus of many employee newsletters), but to facilitate a two-way flow of information on matters of significance in the organization. Departments should strive to keep staff posted on plans and on developments likely to affect their work before changes are instituted, and to build some sense of community. Good employee communications require a focus of accountability, as well as an awareness that this is an ongoing, not a sporadic function.

Performance Pay in Government

Incentive pay, or pay for performance, is one of the instruments frequently associated with improving motivation in the private sector. This technique may be part of the overall solution, but for several reasons I think it is unlikely to occupy a central place in most programs directed at public service morale.

In the private sector, the most effective financial incentive schemes seem to be those where rewards are linked to tangible achievement. For example, at lower levels of the organization, sales people often work on commissions tied directly to sales volume. At senior levels, the formula can get more complicated, but in well-managed enterprises a significant proportion of the total compensation of key executives is often tied in one way or another to enhancement of the share value of the corporation over the longer term. Assessments of individual performance are typically based upon a mixture of objective and subjective information, but to the degree possible, the company's financial results play a key part in the determination of how much key people get paid. In a good year, it would not be unusual for some business persons to supplement their base income by anywhere from 25 to 100 per cent, or even more in selected cases. Bonuses of this size get people's attention.

Bonuses of four or five per cent do not. Government performance pay schemes in Canada and Britain are limited in scope, and, by and large, the possibilities for income supplementation, at time of writing, are not great. The usual constraints on pay levels in the public service tend to hold down the size of performance bonuses – a perennial concern is, how much more can a public servant earn than a member of Parliament to whom he or she is nominally subordinate? Moreover, in times of restraint, civil service pay tends to be held back by the elected Government as evidence of its commitment to fighting inflation or cutting the deficit. This creates tensions in the system as pay falls further and further below comparable private sector salaries. Managers in government, seeing their staff squeezed by this process, are tempted to award "performance" pay or bonuses as a substitute for economic increments, and performance pay programs become progressively devalued.

A final difficulty with performance pay in government is that public sector programs are typically unable to link bonuses to any objective measure of achievement or to an enhancement to the financial value of the organization. Usually performance assessments are primarily based upon qualitative factors; and if an individual fails to achieve his or her goal there are often extenuating circumstances such as ministerial indecision or interference by other departments. These considerations make incentive pay programs in the public sector difficult to administer and vulnerable to manipulation and to outside criticism.[20]

Incentives that Mis-motivate

In chapter 7, a number of incentives "to manage badly" were identified: lapsing funds, inability to retain savings that have been realized, classification systems that accord excessive weight to the number of employees or size of financial resources supervised, over-regulation. There are good reasons why some of these misdirected incentives exist. However, central agencies are, in my experience, often rather less alive to the motivational aspects of regulations and policies which they promulgate than they might be. Lapsing funds, for example, might not be conventionally considered to be an incentive in government. A regulation in this area would be more likely to be viewed as an element of financial policy.

Organizations' characters, and individuals' behaviours, as Chester Barnard pointed out many years ago, reflect the incentives at play. As part of a program to take stock of people management in government, central agencies might want to take a fresh look at certain policies not conventionally viewed as part of the incentive structure. In a well-designed organization, managers who perform appropriately will feel that they are working with the grain of their organization, and in a manner consistent with their own self-interest, not against it. Incentives should not be defined purely in terms of direct financial rewards to employees.

Summary: Productivity through People

Despite the complexity of the issues associated with motivation and morale, there are a few home truths that apply most of the time. By and large, people are more motivated when:

- they understand where the organization is headed, even if only in a general sense; they have confidence in the leadership and identify with the leaders' objectives and values;

- they feel that they know what's going on, and that superiors think of them as if they were part of a team;

- their work is directed by a manager in whom they have confidence, and better yet, whom they admire, who is reasonable but demanding;

- the organization demonstrates by its actions and policies that it is interested in them as people, not just factors of production;

- they know to whom they are accountable (fewer reporting relationships are easier to deal with than many);

- they know what they are accountable for — that is, they understand their job clearly (and the rules don't change unexpectedly);

- they are personally challenged by their work;

- their authority to take decisions is roughly commensurate with their responsibilities;

- they have clear goals to achieve within the context of their job responsibilities;

- they see the results of their work;

- they are rewarded for accomplishment through recognition, praise, attention, status, advancement, a sense of personal achievement and/or in material ways;

- they believe they are being treated fairly in relation to others in the same organization (even if they think persons in other organizations are getting a better deal, this is often a secondary consideration);

- they feel a sense of pride in the organization; belonging to it contributes to their sense of self-worth;

- the organization permits them to realize their work objectives, and does not frustrate them by delaying the taking of decisions, by unreasonably changing course or by failing to follow through on its commitments.

Some organizations have adopted a philosophy of human resource management or a framework of broad principles intended to serve as a credo in relating to their people. (An example of such is shown in Exhibit 13-1.)[21] In some organizations, such statements probably have no operational consequences; managers pay lip service to them, but will not assume the risks associated with their implementation. However, where such statements have been hammered out as an articulation of top management values and policies, they may help to shape the culture of the organization and let subordinate managers know what is expected of them as long as top management's actions prove compatible with their principles. In general, the appearance of such credos may reflect a growing appreciation of the importance of people in improving organizational performance.

The most important reason why issues of people management need to be addressed in government is because if they are not, many of the best people will leave, and others will refuse to join. It is generally accepted that remuneration in government, for more senior positions, is below what is available in the private sector. Nonetheless, people continue to work in the public service because of the intrinsic interest of the work, the influence and the sense of public service. However, if too much of the work in government becomes viewed as frustrating, regulation-bound, and thankless; if politicians treat public servants as if they were disposable assets; if managers feel they have insufficient scope to exercise judgment or imagination, then they will go elsewhere. There is some cause for speculation, in Canada, as to whether this is already occurring to some degree.

If a trend develops along these lines, then it will become harder and harder to attract outstanding individuals to government. The problem may become particularly severe at middle management levels, where the Zussman survey has suggested the morale problems

EXHIBIT 13-1

A Philosophy of Human Resource Management
An Example

People are our most valuable resource. Our objective is to recruit, develop, reward and retain knowledgeable, talented and loyal staff and to create an organization with which staff are proud to be associated.

We shall conduct our business with integrity. Each employee is entitled to know this organization's mission, objectives and priorities. We will communicate this to our staff on a regular basis, and keep them abreast of significant developments which may affect them.

We shall encourage two-way communication on matters affecting the policies and priorities of the organization. Although decision-making is the prerogative of management, following consultation, we will strive to communicate the substance and the reasons for decisions to employees once decisions have been taken.

In order to provide a stimulating and supportive work environment where people may pursue individual goals consistent with those of the organization, we shall undertake to provide a wide range of opportunities for career development and growth for staff.

Good performance should be recognized and rewarded. It is the duty of every manager to ensure that staff are involved in setting objectives related to their work, that staff performance is fairly and routinely reviewed, and that the results of appraisals, and the reasons for these results, are communicated to each employee. It is likewise every manager's responsibility to support the achievement of this organization's objectives in the area of career development. A major component of a manager's own appraisal will depend on his or her success in carrying out the above responsibilities.

Staff should be accountable for their decisions and actions; we shall strive to provide an environment where responsibilities are clearly understood and authority is, to the degree possible, commensurate with responsibility.

We shall encourage innovation and shall be receptive to ideas forwarded by employees, related to the improvement of our operations or policies. We stress collegiality and teamwork and we expect staff to support each other and to share ideas and information.

are more severe. This will result in a gradual erosion of the public service, and it bodes ill for the quality of government in the longer term. Generations are required to build sound government institutions; a decade or two of comparative indifference to people is all it may take to erode them. Rebuilding will be much more difficult, and probably more costly, than preservation.

This chapter has indicated a range of actions which could be taken to improve motivation in government. They include: attempting to ensure that departmental mandates are kept relatively unencumbered by diverse, unconnected functions; more attention to leadership and the motivational aspects of management in promotional decisions; more stability in senior appointments; abandonment of the myth of the professional manager and the according of more importance, in managerial appointments, to incumbents' knowledge of the substance of the work to be supervised; more interest in building institutions that value people; greater delegation of authority to departments and managers in areas related to people and structure; more attention to employee communications; ensuring that personnel managers focus on the strategic rather than the administrative aspects of their jobs; and getting rid, to the degree possible, of "mis-incentives" in government. Change of the scope proposed here will not be easy to implement; it constitutes something close to a change in the culture of government, in terms of how it relates to its public servants. Change on this scale will take commitment and time to institute.

The lack of priority accorded to the management and motivation of people reflects the powerful tradition of policy primacy described in chapter 3. It also reflects the relative disinterest of politicians in issues related to the internal workings of the civil service. Rightly or wrongly, most politicians do not seem to perceive a very close relationship between the way in which people are motivated in the public service and the performance of the elected Government at the polls.

Politicians and the Public Service

Politicians cannot escape a considerable measure of accountability for the state of morale in government organizations. They make the rules. They have not, in general, shown a great deal of interest in the people working for them, and as Lord Bancroft has noted, "The ritual words of praise, forced out through clenched teeth in public . . . deceive no-one if they are accompanied by noisy and obvious cuffs about the ear in semi-private."[22] The British House of Commons Committee cited earlier in this chapter raised the somewhat unusual topic of ministers' responsibilities to the civil service and suggested that the prime minister might promulgate some guidelines on this matter. However, more than this is required—as the Cabinet Secretary observed at the time, there is a strong possibility that such guidelines might turn out to be "an anthology of cliches with no practical application."[23]

Until political attitudes change, efforts to make the government a better place for people to work in will, unfortunately, be swimming against the stream to some extent. Senior officials, particularly those in central agencies, will be called upon to try to enlist more ministerial interest in, and commitment to, resolving the issues raised in this chapter. Leaders in the business community and elsewhere who are interested in better government and who understand the importance of people to performance can contribute to this cause by conveying a similar message to our elected representatives.

The Prospects for Government

Despite the imperfections of government, there is little cause to believe that it is withering. On the contrary, even though in some countries there has been a reduction in the size of government in the 1980s, it seems likely that, subject to the limits of financial capacity, governments will continue to grow over the long term, if only to keep pace with the growth of population and wealth.

Governments will grow because of the many specific interests that constantly call upon them to fix social or economic problems. The "revolution of rising expectations" seems to find expression in new demands upon government; today, individual initiative, which a generation ago might have been channeled toward self-help and private enterprise, often seems directed to finding new ways to tap the public purse. Many interest groups currently in receipt of public funding want further assistance to finance new initiatives. Those not already at the public trough consider themselves unfairly treated and feel they have a "right" to their share of support. No one is interested in giving up resources to someone else's purpose: the solution to new problems is new money, not old money redirected to new uses. Unless there is a basic change in the expectations of government, these pressures will continue and will prove difficult for politicians to resist.

There are other, more sobering trends suggesting that governments may be called upon to play an increasingly obtrusive role in future in order to control forces and interests whose power is on a scale unimagined even fifty years ago.

Political philosophers since Plato and Aristotle have identified the fundamental role of government as the maintenance of the social context, through the enforcement of civil order and the rule of law. The dilemma of political science has been to determine how to foster these conditions while preserving individual rights and freedoms. To some extent this traditional role of government has been obscured by the shift in focus of more recent writings, particularly since the time of Karl Marx, which have tended to concentrate on government's economic functions and its social responsibilities.

For reasons that few people will welcome, the 21st century may witness a renewed recognition of the need for governments to exercise their classic role as context-setters, accompanied by a trend toward increasing, rather than diminishing, government control. A major cause of this will be demographic growth. The world is finite. Current rates of population growth cannot be sustained indefinitely, but plagues and wars, the methods of population control forecast by Thomas Malthus over 150 years ago, are hardly the best solution to this problem. As populations grow, it seems inevitable that governments will find it desirable to establish and if necessary enforce limits to growth. In some countries, this trend is already apparent.

Demographic, economic and technological growth all make the world more complicated. With each passing year, more opportunities for friction and disorder develop within the shrinking boundaries of the global village. Many Third World countries are now impinging on the rest of the world both politically and economically: the resulting changes in international relations are generating a need for more inter-governmental liaison. The greater the number and variety of commercial entities in the world, the more call there will be upon governments to establish rules and systems to govern business, to adjudicate among competing parties and to ensure that the public interest is not damaged through industrial or commercial operations. The greater the number of municipalities, the more friction there will be with agricultural interests. The bigger cities become, the more difficult they will be to administer, and the harder it will be to maintain workable urban support systems and civil order. Governments will be expected to see that these challenges are met.

Of particular concern in the 21st century will be the issue of pollution control and environmental damage. Here too, there are clearly limits to what the world can sustain. As the biosphere is progressively degraded, governments will almost certainly have to assume a stronger hands-on role. The longer it takes to recognize the need for supervision and international co-operation in this area, the more serious the problems will become, and, ultimately, the more intrusive will be the role of governments as environmental policemen.

Perhaps the most troubling issue is the spread of nuclear technology and the progressive dissemination of destructive weapons through the arms trade. Many of these seem to find their way into the hands of terrorist groups and governments with deep mutual distrusts and differences in values. To combat international terrorism, it may be only a matter of time before governments will have to move beyond such measures as security checks at airports to more far-reaching and objectionable control initiatives. "Isolated" military confrontations between Third World governments may become more difficult to contain as local conflicts, as the Iran-Iraq conflict has already shown. Failure to reduce the gaps between the populous poor nations and the wealthier countries of the world will exacerbate international tensions. Nuclear technology will make it increasingly dangerous to leave the conduct of international relations in the hands of independent nation states. As the risks of nuclear confrontation grow and as "local" wars make their effects more widely felt, the need to contain conflict will increase. A resurgence of interest in new forms of international federation, or even world government, may emerge.

In short, ensuring that government institutions are effectively led and well managed will be all the more important in the future. At the same time, there must be appropriate checks upon government authority to ensure responsiveness to public concerns, and to prevent abuse. The need for new approaches to the management of our public institutions is apparent. With good will and commitment, the institutions of government can and must be made good places to work and effective in meeting the requirements of the public they serve.

Footnotes:

1. Warren Bennis and Bert Nanus, *Leaders — The Strategies for Taking Charge*, (New York: Harper & Row, 1985), pp. 82-109.

2. *Ibid.*

3. David Howells, "Marks and Spencer and the Civil Service: A Comparison of Culture and Methods," *Public Administration*, vol. 59, (Autumn 1981), pp. 337-352.

4. *Ibid.*

5. *Ibid.*

6. Antony Jay, *Management and Machiavelli*, (Harmondsworth: Penguin Books, 1970), pp. 172-173.

7. Royal Commission on Financial Management and Accountability, *Final Report*, (Ottawa: Supply and Services Canada, March 1979), pp. 220-221. "What is needed to improve the quality of performance appraisals is not new systems and procedures, but that more deputies assign high priority to this basic management task ...." Price Waterhouse Associates/The Canada Consulting Group, "A Study of Management and Accountability in the Government of Ontario," (Toronto, January 1985), pp. 10-11: "Performance appraisal is a key element in relating the requirements of the system to individual actions .... Our interviews suggested that the kind of dialogue that appraisal requires is too often absent."

8. H.L. Laframboise, "The responsibilities of a senior public servant: organization, profession and career," *Canadian Public Administration*, vol. 27 no. 4, (Winter 1984), pp. 594-600.

9. Irving S. Shapiro, *America's Third Revolution: Public Interest and the Private Role*, (New York: Harper & Row, 1984), p. 123. See also Hugo Young and Anne Sloman, *No, Minister*, (London: British Broadcasting Corporation, 1982), p. 34.

10. Peter Kellner and Lord Crowther-Hunt, *The Civil Servants*, (London: Macdonald General Books, 1980), p. 35.

11. Howells, *op. cit.*

12. Robert L. Katz, "Skills of an effective administrator," *Harvard Business Review*, (January-February 1955); reprinted with an additional "Retrospective Commentary," in *Paths Toward Personal Progress*, (Harvard Business Review, 1983). See p. 34 here. See also Laframboise, *loc. cit.*, p. 595.

13. John P. Kotter, *The General Managers*, (New York: The Free Press, 1982), "Preface to the Paperback Edition," p. xi.

14. Harry Levinson and Stuart Rosenthal, *CEO — Corporate Leadership in Action*, (New York: Basic Books, 1984), p. 72.

15. Laframboise, *loc. cit.*

16. For the Lambert Commission's view on this issue, see Royal Commission on Financial Management and Accountability, *Final Report*, (Ottawa: Supply and Services Canada, March 1979), pp. 222-223.

17. *Seventh Report from the Treasury and Civil Service Committee*, Session 1985-86, "Civil Servants and Ministers: Duties and Responsibilities, vol. 1, (London, Her Majesty's Stationery Office, 12 May 1986), p. xiii.

18. Robert Townsend, *Up the Organization: How to stop the corporation from stifling people and strangling profits*," (Greenwich, Conn.: Fawcett Publications, Inc., 1970), p. 128.

19. See Noel Tichy, Charles J. Fombrun and Mary Anne Devanna, "Strategic Human Resource Management," *Sloan Management Review*, vol. 23 no. 2, (Winter 1982), pp. 47-61.

20. See David Zussman, "Bonuses and Performance in the Public Sector," *Canadian Psychology*, vol. 23 no. 4, (1982), pp. 248-255.

21. For other examples derived from several business corporations, see James Nininger, *Managing Human Resources, A Strategic Perspective*, (Ottawa: The Conference Board in Canada, April 1982), Appendices A to D, pp. 107ff.

22. *Seventh Report from the Treasury and Civil Service Committee*, Session 1985-86, "Civil Servants and Ministers: Duties and Responsibilities, vol. 1, (London, Her Majesty's Stationery Office, 12 May 1986), p. xiii.

23. "Civil Servants and Ministers: Duties and Responsibilities," *op. cit.*, p. xii.

Appendix One:
Systems and Sisyphus:

Three Decades of Management Change in Ottawa

Improving Management: An Uphill Battle

During the past 25 years or so, in Canada, Britain and numerous other jurisdictions, there has been a growing awareness of the need for better methods of management in the public sector. Government is a different institution than it was 40 or 50 years ago. Changes in its size and responsibilities have occurred in response to significant alterations in public expectations of it. Now, parliamentary democracy is adapting to the era of big government. The adaptation has not been easy, nor has it been welcomed by many public servants. Some top officials have embraced the need for better management while others have viewed the incursions of management theory into the bastions of the public service somewhat as the Romans viewed the attacks of the Gauls.

Some public servants seem to believe that management is just a fad, a passing fashion, after which the government will return to its classical values and methods of operation. Such beliefs are fueled by the knowledge that better management is seldom an abiding political priority, and that ministers are, by and large, uninterested in administration. One British official observed,

Permanent secretaries are wily old birds and they have spent a lifetime learning to sniff every changing political wind. Some may genuinely understand what this thing called management is all about, and may be personally committed to it. But for others, this may simply be the latest political enthusiasm, to be endorsed politely until it goes away and is replaced by something else.[1]

The resistance which many officials have shown to the efforts to improve management has not arisen simply from pig-headedness. A number of initiatives undertaken in the name of "management improvement" have considerably increased stress on line officials, and some have added to overheads at a time when resources have become scarcer. Experience with such initiatives have jaundiced many officials, causing them to associate attempts at management improvement with busywork, budget cuts and battles with central agency officials. To some public servants, "management" does not involve getting the job done, but is synonymous with the rules and procedures that stand in the way of efficiency. Other officials are cynical about the degree to which good management is a serious priority in government. Some factors contributing to these attitudes are:

- inconsistent or superficial commitment from politicians to reducing deficits or to facilitating the task of administration in government;

- central agencies' periodic practice of introducing initiatives necessitating a lot of work in departments, only to change to different and apparently inconsistent initiatives a few years later;

- the introduction by central agencies of rafts of new administrative procedures or management policies without seemingly assessing their cumulative impact on the workload of departments;

- lack of co-ordination among central agencies, leading to inconsistent levels of delegation to departments, to a plethora of unconnected demands for "improved management" emanating from different sources, and to the installation of systems unco-ordinated at the centre, each of which makes different demands on departments;

410

- misunderstanding of the concept of management, causing senior departmental officials to abdicate important management responsibilities;

- the institution by central agency officials of administrative policies that treat departments as if they were all the same, instead of allowing for variations in their character and mandates;

- the introduction of private-sector methods of management not necessarily suited to all public-sector organizations, (such as some of the flirtations with management by objectives, cybernetics and corporate planning in Canada during the 1970s;

- confusion of the concept of accountability with the concept of control.

Surrounded by such difficulties, many departmental officials must at times feel like the mythical King Sisyphus, condemned forever to roll a huge rock up a hill, only to have it roll down again. No matter how many times they try to move the rock of better management to the top of the slope, no matter how many new systems and procedures are developed in the department, there is always something more to do. Yesterday's management priority passes out of fashion, to be replaced with some new technique requiring more paper and more management time.

This appendix provides an overview of the efforts of the federal government in Ottawa to improve management over the last 25 years. The purpose here is not to provide a definitive history but to illustrate the type of problems with which the government was grappling. (A similar review of British experience appears in appendix 2.)

The 1960s

According to Hubert Laframboise, a former senior public servant in Ottawa, during the period from about 1945 to 1960,

> [T]he rate of management change was exceedingly low and eminently digestible. [However, during the 1970s,] four decisions . . . spelled the doom of this tidy little world. In a short span of years it was decided (a) to establish a Royal

Commission on Government Organization [the Glassco
Commission] and to implement its recommendations; (b) to
introduce collective bargaining for federal employees; (c) to
bilingualize the federal public service; (d) to establish the
Treasury Board Secretariat as the "general manager" of the
public service, and as "the employer" as required for
collective bargaining.

Taken one at a time, the merits of these decisions are
defensible or at least arguable. Taken in their totality ...
they have resulted in such an increase in the internal
administrative work-load that only huge increases in staff
numbers and unprecedented demands on available
managerial work-time have made their imperfect implementation possible."[2]

During the last half of the 1960s, the federal government also
was subjected to the implementation of a program planning and
budgeting system (generally known by the acronym PPBS), imported
from the United States and implanted in Ottawa just as certain
aspects of the system were falling into disrepute in many American
jurisdictions. PPBS (see chapter 9) called for major changes to the
way budgets were prepared, and added substantially to the workload
of both financial officials and line managers. It also called for the
creation of new staff units charged with analyzing all spending
programs.[3]

According to Laframboise, whose views were shared by many
other managers in the public service, there was increasing doubt
about the cumulative merit of this plethora of changes. Resistance
grew to the burgeoning administrative overhead being added to the
service in the name of good management, and, in Laframboise's
evocative phrase, a "saturation psychosis" developed among harried
departmental officials. (However, his lament apparently had little
impact among the central agency officials of the day.)

The 1962 Glassco Report had rightly recognized that critical to
management in government is the relationship between central
agencies and departments. Glassco made so many proposals that
would have led to greater delegation to departments that his Report's
philosophy became summarized in the phrase, "Let the managers
manage!" Nonetheless, progress toward decentralization was slow
and problematic. Ten years after the Report was published, a

retrospective article in *Canadian Public Administration* based on interviews with about 40 top public servants stated that control by central agencies was a continuing concern among officials responsible for operating departments. The biggest complaint, according to one frustrated deputy minister, was Treasury Board's continuing control over the structure and organization of departments and the classification of senior officers. "The number of persons working for him too often is the criterion for determining a supervisor's classification and pay. The man at the top can only reward merit by joining in the game, creating phony jobs to satisfy the phony criteria imposed by the system."4

Deputy ministers suggested that departments should be allowed to set salaries subject to limits on the number of persons they could hire and subject to the constraints of collective agreements. Central agency officials, however, pointed out that when they had extended certain types of staffing authority to a few departments, the result has been 'over-classification' of some personnel and 'raiding' between departments. Treasury Board officials argued further that it took time to unravel "the accumulation of forty years of controls", and that "the freedom to manage or mismanage must await the development of effective tools to audit the performance of individuals and departments." They further emphasized the importance of maintaining a "rough equality" within the public service and the need to respect the principle of Cabinet responsibility by allowing the Board to evaluate the effectiveness of departmental performance.5

The problem of securing a balance of authority between central agencies and departments in Canada was not made any easier by the philosophy of the top official of the Treasury Board at the time, A.W. Johnson. One of the suggestions advanced to the Board, for instance, was that departments should have more power to allocate money from lower to higher priority projects within their own sphere of responsibility. Johnson saw the Board as the representative of the collectivity of ministers, whose responsibilities could not be usurped by departments. In his view, greater delegation was antithetical to the very fabric of Cabinet government.

> [T]he reconciliation of the principles of modern management and the principles of cabinet government is not an easy task . . . . It has been suggested to me by at least a few

> very knowledgeable people in government that ... depart-
> ments concerned should be allowed to decide how to allocate
> funds between alternative projects and programs I
> disagree: in my view the collectivity [of ministers] is nearly
> always going to make these decisions ... given the nature of
> cabinet government.[6]

Johnson's articulation of this position provides an interesting insight into how principles of public administration, if pressed too far, can conflict with sane management practices and with simple common sense. His view, almost certainly shared by many central agency officials both before and since, was that only on a very exceptional basis could priorities be set on other than a cross-governmental basis (i.e., by Treasury Board) even if the amounts involved were modest. However, the demands on ministerial time are such that it strains one's imagination to believe that Treasury Board ministers were able to perform this role adequately. At the time this issue arose, Treasury Board ministers were supervising a federal budget of more than $13 billion administered by about 50 departments and several dozen organizations and agencies. How could they manage this portfolio effectively and, at the same time, make informed decisions about every one or two million dollars? It is doubtful that Treasury Board, as a small committee of Cabinet, truly represented the views of the collectivity of ministers. If Treasury Board ministers were indeed dealing with decisions at this level of detail, it seems inevitable that they must have become lost in the trees of individual decisions, and lost sight of the forest of their larger responsibilities for public expenditure management. (Indeed, during the 1970s, the deficit of the Canadian government grew dramatically.)

In 1986, Treasury Board finally reversed its position, adopting a policy known as IMAA – increased ministerial authority and account-ability – which specifically authorized ministers to make decisions concerning modest reallocations of expenditures within their own portfolios.[7] This development, discussed at greater length in the main text of this book (see especially chapter 12), was the logical culmination of the envelope system adopted in the 1970s. However, more than 15 years passed before central agency officials were prepared to recognize the need for arrangements of this type.

APPENDIX ONE

Beyond Glassco: The Age of Reason

Despite pleas that federal public servants be allowed some time to digest the many administrative reforms of the 1960s, efforts to improve management practices in Ottawa continued unabated during the 1970s. The election of the Government of Prime Minister Pierre Trudeau in 1968 brought a group of new senior officials into high places who were fascinated with the possibilities of more rational approaches to the direction of government. Regional desks were established in the Prime Minister's office (PMO) to monitor public opinion, a development that left some members of Parliament wondering what their job was. Systems experts were hired to apply project management and industrial engineering techniques to the development of public policy.

Efforts were made in the Privy Council Office to develop a Cabinet planning system to co-ordinate policy development in government. Meanwhile, to the confusion of public servants removed from the machinations among competing central agencies, other systems were developed in the Department of Finance and in Treasury Board which were also designed to facilitate planning and co-ordination, but which were not linked to the PCO system. Each new system carried with it demands for departments to prepare briefs, reorganize information into new formats, or adjust to new planning schedules. According to one insider, during this period, "[E]laborate charts intended to capture and interrelate the government's many planning exercises provided an often bizarre iconography for the corridors of power."8

This was the heyday in Ottawa of delphi studies, environmental scanning, technology forecasting, planning systems, cost-benefit analysis and futurology. A new, high-powered Planning Branch was set up in Treasury Board whose purpose was to "rationalize" the public expenditure management process, to conduct special evaluations (often in areas that departments considered their own territory), and to press for the greater use of analytic techniques in policy formation in government. Largely in response to Treasury Board's encomiums about the need for better planning and clearer objectives, departmental planning and co-ordination units sprang up like weeds. The number of civil servants in what was then known as the SX (senior executive) category increased so fast that the Treasury

Board Secretariat, dismayed at the sorcerer's apprentice it had let loose in the bureaucracy, had to freeze staffing of SX officials. A centralized "temporary assignment pool" of top civil servants allowed high-priced talent to be moved from one department to another as projects drew to a close; it also helped to check the flow of senior appointments which had swelled to such worrying proportions.

Ottawa became fascinated with co-ordination and with systematization. New central agencies were established, first to co-ordinate federal policy in urban affairs and then later in the field of science and technology and still later, in economic policy and social policy. Departments were required to integrate new financial management systems with new approaches to corporate planning. Reorganizations turned many officials who had been hired as policy analysts in the days of PPBS into the operators of departmental planning systems. In 1974, Treasury Board invited departments to implement a complex "operational performance measurement system" (OPMS) which, officials were assured, would permit "realistic performance targets to be established and the necessary resource requirements to be determined."* OPMS carried the jargon of evaluation to such a level of complexity, few officials could even remember, let alone apply, the terminology to their operations. Concurrently, the falling cost and increasing power of electronic data processing was leading to large-scale attempts to construct computerized management systems within departments, attempts that also required substantial organizational changes and that involved major adjustments to operating procedures. Public servants were being buffetted from all sides: by initiatives deriving from the political level of government, by a growing number of central agencies competing for turf, and by technological advances entirely outside the sphere of government.

---

* OPMS required managers to understand four different "proxy levels" for measurement and to distinguish among such terms as operational efficiency, program efficiency, operational effectiveness, program cost-effectiveness and contributions to well-being. Although the basic concepts of OPMS were sound, the system was over-complicated. Its terminology passed into richly deserved obscurity within a few years (a number of the basic concepts survived and have now become part of the federal government's standard evaluation methodology). See Treasury Board, "Operational Performance Measurement: vol. 1 – A Managerial Overview," (January 1974).

Were this not enough, another development, which may have seemed innocent enough to those outside the public service, was to have significant consequences for managers within the federal government. This was the report, published in 1975, of an independent committee of inquiry into the role of the federal auditor general, inviting the auditor general to investigate what became known as "value-for-money" issues.[9] Informed observers were concerned, first, that no real standards existed for the conduct of such inquiries, at least not in the guise of "audits" as these were conventionally understood, and second, that such an enlargement of the Auditor's mandate might engulf his office in damaging political controversy.

Nevertheless, as soon as the new auditor general's Act was passed in 1977, representatives of the Auditor General set off into the forests of the public service to hunt down the beasts of waste and inefficiency. The budget and the staff of the Audit Office swelled to such an extent that, according to one reliable source, soon after the new act was proclaimed there were more officials working for the auditor general, either on contract or on full-time basis, being paid at the level of a deputy minister than there were deputy ministers in the entire public service. Many public servants felt that these audits were little more than fishing expeditions on which auditors cast about hopefully until they hooked an issue worthy of the taxidermists who stuffed the auditor general's annual report with examples of government mismanagement. Predictably, early reports of the Office, conducted under the acronym SPICE (Studies in Procedures in Cost Effectiveness) were heavily criticized within the public service for their lack of professionalism and for their limited scope. One outside observer, who perhaps had a more objective viewpoint, condemned the initial crop of value-for-money reports as poorly planned and poorly executed, and suggested that they were verging on intellectual dishonesty.[10] Nonetheless, the audits continued apace and indeed swelled in volume and scope as the Office consolidated its mandate.

Accountability and its Consequences

The activities of the auditor general during the late 1970s, the growing concern over government spending and the discovery that several Crown corporations had been engaging in questionable business practices, led to a new demand in Ottawa for "strengthening accountability". Accountability, a concept usually of greater interest to auditors than to managers, became the preoccupation of central agency officials and, to some extent, of ministers who would normally have little time for such administrative concerns. A perception arose, fueled by the media and by inflammatory reporting by the then auditor general, James Macdonnell, that government spending was "out of control". The solution urged upon the government was to reinforce the "accountability of the public service". Under this banner a host of changes was instituted.

An important institutional innovation was the establishment, in 1978, of a new organization *within* the public service (unlike the Office of the Auditor General, which is outside it) to promote good management practices. Just what the relationship of this new organization, called the Office of the Comptroller General, was to be to the Treasury Board Secretariat (which already had a mandate for management in the public service) was clear to few other than the auditor general (who had recommended this course of action to a reluctant government). Nonetheless, the office was constituted, and now, close on the heels of the auditors from the Office of the *Auditor* General, came the experts from the Office of the *Comptroller* General, fanning out across the government in an exercise known as IMPAC — Improvement in Management Practices and Control. The IMPAC teams were in fact able to identify many useful managerial improvements within departments, and to highlight issues that might otherwise have lain dormant. The action programs arising from their reports were negotiated with DMs and ultimately endorsed by them in many departments. However, from the perspective of many harried departmental managers, the OCG teams were just another wave of outside interference analyzing existing practices, developing recommendations for improvement and getting in the way of the day-to-day work.

At about this time, another development occurred: the promulgation of a new Treasury Board policy requiring departments to execute evaluations of all their programs on a revolving, five-year cycle. This involved not only the establishment of another layer of administrative overhead in departments, but the creation of another brand of assessor of departmental activities: the program evaluator. The evaluator was not so much concerned with the efficiency of delivery of the program as with its fundamental impact. Evaluators headed into the public service concurrently with the auditors from the auditor general and the IMPAC teams from the OCG: one more group of reviewers, checker-uppers and examiners who were wearing down carpets in federal offices.

In addition, departmental managers had also to contend with auditors from the Public Service Commission who visited departments to assess their compliance with staffing policies. Reviewers from the Treasury Board Secretariat came by to examine the application of legislation and regulations with regard to the use of Canada's two official languages in the bureaucracy. Other examiners, also from the Treasury Board Secretariat, conducted audits to determine whether departments were adhering to proper classification procedures or grading of positions. Still, other visitors included departments' own internal auditors conducting reviews on behalf of management, or consultants hired from outside the organization to assist with special studies, such as the installation of new computer systems or the improvement of financial controls that might have been recommended in an earlier study by the auditor general. (The more studies completed by the auditor general, the more recommendations there were to contend with, usually leading to further studies directed toward the implementation of recommendations.)

By the latter part of the 1970s, Ottawa was awash in auditors, assessors and evaluators, mostly operating in the name of "enhanced accountability" — which was generally viewed as synonymous with control. From the bureaucracy one increasingly heard the wistful plea, "Why can't they leave us alone and let us get on with our jobs?"

Toward the end of the 1970s, the prime minister, again largely because of criticism in the auditor general's reports, established a Royal Commission on Financial Management and Accountability. The report of this Commission (the Lambert Report), tabled in 1979, contained major recommendations for management change. The commissioners produced a report that took the broadest possible interpretation of their mandate, covering such issues as the role of central agencies, strategic planning, the reporting relationships and performance appraisals of deputy ministers, the management of

Crown corporations and personnel management. Implementation of the Report's proposals, mostly on a piecemeal basis, provided another spurt of management change during the early 1980s.

Yet another chapter in the saga of enhanced accountability was provided by the roundup of Crown corporations during the 1970s. Ministerial and central agency attention began to focus on the many different agencies that surrounded the core of departments at the centre of government. The imprudence of a few commercial Crown corporations in their business dealings encouraged the Auditor General to conduct a series of audits of major corporations, leading to further cries for tighter controls over these agencies. Difficulties encountered by the government in stating exactly how many of these corporations existed, gave the impression to the taxpayer that corporations were multiplying indiscriminately. If the government couldn't count them, how could it control them?*

During the 1970s, officials in central agencies began to draft legislation to herd these unruly organizations into a corral where they would be subject to more consistent controls. The Lambert Report provided an extensive analysis of the relationship between Crown corporations and government, which finally resulted in Bill C-24, a piece of legislation passed by Parliament in 1984,[11] supplanting the old Financial Administration Act that had previously governed Crown corporations. Among the clauses of the new act were provisions regarding the roles and duties of directors, the presentation and approval of capital and operating budgets, the power of the government to issue directives and the appointment of auditors.

Another administrative change during this period was the effort to improve the public reporting by departments and agencies. The major initiative here was the adoption of a new form of the financial Estimates, tabled by the Government in the House of Commons early

---

* Counting quangos or Crown corporations involves both conceptual and pragmatic difficulties (see chapter 2). Government organizations are created in various ways – by legislation, by regulation, by order-in-council – and in addition, agencies could (and did in the 1970s in Canada) create subsidiaries. Further, government departments sometimes delegate authority to citizen groups to such an extent that a quasi-independent corporate entity may come into being. Governments may also own shares in some corporations. In general, classifying and keeping track of all the entities attached to government in one way or another is not easy.

in each new calendar year, as the official record of the government's spending intentions. The Estimates of a government are (or ought to be) tied to a document called the Public Accounts, which records what actually happened to those expenditures. During the 1970s, there was growing criticism of Canada's documents as inadequate, obscure and confusing. In response, the government made numerous changes in format and presentation and added "Part Three" to the Estimates, which contained information that went well beyond the traditional financial statements. Still evolving at time of writing, Part Three attempts to display quantitative information concerning the performance of government programs; it is supposed to include not only descriptions of the programs and their costs, but also data on their efficiency and effectiveness over time.

In principle, the decision to prepare this type of information and make it available to Parliament represented a major advance in public administration. It is certainly consistent with the tenets of good management which hold that substantive reports on progress should be prepared periodically in any organization. In practice, however, despite the very substantial effort that has been put into the preparation of these data in some departments, the reaction of Parliament has been virtually inaudible. And there is concern that, if parliamentarians do show any interest, it may be more to mount partisan attacks on the elected Government, not to engage in fair-minded examination of departments' performance. Not surprisingly, some senior officials in Ottawa have begun to wonder whether the effort involved in preparing the data is warranted. Preliminary experience with Part Three illustrates that in the absence of institutional and/or behavioural change at the political level, there is a limit to how far reform can proceed if it is confined to the public service alone.*

Two other developments should be mentioned. One was the creation by the Public Service Commission in 1981 of a "management category" designed to bring the top four to five thousand public

---

* Changes to the committee structure of the Canadian Parliament instituted in 1986 by the Government of Prime Minister Brian Mulroney may provide the opportunity for MPs to play a more active role in reviewing departmental performance and may increase the utility of Part Three. (See chapter 12.)

servants with administrative responsibilities into a common occupational framework. To make the public service more attractive than it was in comparison to the private sector, improvements were made in the remuneration and benefits for this group, a modest bonus plan was instituted for those whose work was considered exceptional, and special management training programs were set up. (Subsequently, a number of serious problems developed in connection with administration of the management category, but the difficulties appear to have more to do with the implementation of the idea and with resource shortages than with the basic concept.)[12] The other development, which had more far-reaching implications, was the institution in 1979 of a new Policy and Expenditure Management System (PEMS). By the late 1970s, it was clear that a full-blown Program Planning and Budgeting System (PPBS) was not what Ottawa wanted or required. PEMS represented both a modification of PPBS and a set of new procedures designed to facilitate the overall control of government spending. The most important feature of PEMS was the creation of envelopes of government expenditure that were managed by committees of Cabinet with sectoral responsibilities: economic policy, social policy, external affairs and defence, and general government operations. New procedures for the preparation of departmental plans and budgets were proclaimed. In addition, as noted above, two new ministries, the Ministry of State for Economic Development and the Ministry of State for Social Development, were set up to co-ordinate policy in these sectors, and "mirror committees" of deputy ministers were formed to assist with the co-ordination of policy at the official level.

While the establishment of envelopes has proven to be a reform of lasting value, the institution of these ministries and committees was less successful. It was one of those machinery-of-government decisions that doubtless looked good on paper but in practice it created a labyrinth of institutions and procedures within an already highly bureaucratic system. Indeed, there was some irony in the establishment of the new ministries in an era when accountability was a governing priority. So many co-ordinating agencies were being set up, knowledgeable commentators were baffled as to who was in charge of important areas of government policy. In the critical field of economic policy, for instance, accountability which had previously been focused in the Department of Finance was progressively diluted and diffused among four central agencies: PCO, Finance, the Ministry of State for Economic Development and the Treasury Board Secretariat.13 Ultimately, both the ministries and the committees of deputies were disbanded.

Although the envelope system undoubtedly sharpened accountability at the ministerial level, for officials at the working levels in departments, all this making and unmaking of agencies and committees must have raised some concerns as to whether the responsible central agencies really knew what they were doing at the time.

Summary

From the early 1960s to the mid 1980s, the Canadian federal bureaucracy was deluged with initiatives in the name of improved management and better accountability. Some have been false starts, and some created rather more smoke than light. Others have been more constructive. These initiatives have included:

- the Glassco Report

- collective bargaining

- adoption of program budgeting

- development and abandonment of the Cabinet Planning System

- passage of the new Auditor General's Act

- adoption of the policy on program evaluation

- creation of the Office of the Comptroller General

- establishment, and subsequent disbanding of the Treasury Board Planning Branch, the Ministry of State for Urban Affairs, the Ministry of State for Economic Development, the Ministry of State for Social Development, and the mirror committees of deputy ministers;

- passage of the new Crown corporations act

- the establishment of the management category in the public service

- adoption of PEMS and the envelope system

- implementation of the IMAA policy providing for the possibility of greater delegation of authority to ministers.

These changes originated from several different institutional sources: the Auditor General, Comptroller General, Treasury Board Secretariat, Privy Council Office and the Public Service Commission. Lack of co-ordination on some matters created a situation where departmental managers had both to contend with an ever increasing flow of auditors and examiners, and to sort out for themselves differences in terminology, in approach, and even in basic philosophy underlying directives that emanated from the centre. No one at the centre of government seemed to be monitoring the cumulative impact of these changes on the prosaic issue of running the government's day-to-day operations.

Despite the problems and the false starts in some areas requiring subsequent back-tracking, there is no doubt that the federal government has made progress in trying to improve management. Before the mid-1960s, management was almost a foreign concept in the federal government; this does not mean that the government was poorly managed then, but it was a smaller, less complicated organism with less need for the application of sophisticated techniques or formal systems.

However, the times and the needs of the public service have changed. The envelope system is perhaps one of the major achievements of the last several years (see chapter 12); others include the improvement in financial controls, the better reporting by departments, and the establishment of the management category. In the area of bilingualism, not discussed at any length above, there has certainly been (at very considerable cost and disruption) a quantum increase in the use of French within the bureaucracy, a change that was long overdue. The policy regarding improved accountability to ministers — IMAA — cannot be assessed as yet, but it might prove to be another important advance.

These advances have been almost entirely in systems and procedures. There is virtually nothing on the human and motivational front that stands out as a signal achievement during this period. Indeed, as discussed in part three of this book, here the federal government has made little progress, and it may even have regressed over the period. Management improvement efforts in Ottawa have been dominated by the financial types and the systems people.

Ottawa was not alone. The same is true of most of the initiatives directed at management improvement in Whitehall during the same period (see appendix 2).

Footnotes:

1. Author's interview, June 1986.

2. H.L. Laframboise, "Administrative reform in the federal public service: signs of saturation psychosis," *Canadian Public Administration*, 20th anniversary ed. (1978), pp. 112-113. Originally published in *CPA*, vol. 14 no. 3, (Fall 1971).

3. See Michael J. Prince and John A. Chenier, "The rise and fall of policy planning and research units: an organizational perspective," *Canadian Public Administration*, vol. 23 no. 4, (Winter, 1980), esp. pp. 525ff.

4. Michael Hicks, "The Treasury Board of Canada and its clients: five years of change and administrative reform 1966-71," *Canadian Public Administration*, vol. 16 no. 2, (Summer 1973), p. 199.

5. *Ibid.*

6. A.W. Johnson, "Management Theory and Cabinet Government," *Canadian Public Administration*, 20th anniversary ed. (1978), pp. 54-62. (Originally published in 1971 edition of *CPA*.)

7. Treasury Board of Canada, Minute No. TB 800978/79/80 of Meeting of 20 February 1986, "Increased Authority and Accountability for Ministers and Departments," (30 June 1986).

8. For an interesting description of the turmoil and inter-agency competition of this period, see Richard D. French, *How Ottawa Decides*. (Toronto: James Lorimer and Company/The Canadian Institute for Economic Policy, 1980), pp. 22ff.

9. *Report of the Independent Review Committee on the Office of the Auditor General of Canada*, (Ottawa: Information Canada, March 1975).

10. See Michael Pitfield, former Secretary to the Cabinet, as cited in Robert D. Carman, "Accountability of senior public servants to Parliament and its committees," *Canadian Public Administration*, vol. 27 no. 4, (Winter 1984), pp. 546-548; also Sharon Sutherland, "On the audit trail of the Auditor General: Parliament's servant, 1973-1980," *Canadian Public Administration*, vol. 23 no. 4, (Winter 1980), pp. 616-644.

11. S.C. 1984, c.31.

12. See the Auditor General of Canada, *Annual Report, 1986-87.*

13. Rod Dobell, "How Ottawa Decides Economic Policy," *Policy Options*, vol. 1 no. 3., (Sept./Oct. 1980), p. 15. See also Ian D. Clark, "Recent changes in the cabinet decision-making system in Ottawa," *Canadian Public Administration*, vol. 28 no. 2, (Summer 1985), pp. 185-201.

Appendix Two:
Improving Management
in Whitehall

Traditions and Perceptions

In the British civil service, at least up to the late 1970s, management was still regarded in many quarters with a mixture of puzzlement, impatience and even contempt. Puzzlement, because (with significant exceptions) management was often not well understood among senior public servants educated in the classical quadrangles of Oxbridge rather than at Harvard, Stanford or MIT. Impatience, sometimes tempered with contempt, because of the strong tradition that the job of the senior public servant is policy pure and simple; management (as understood in the culture of Whitehall) was considered to be concerned with the implementation of policy and in a somewhat separate sphere. Policy analysts proposed, ministers decided, and subordinate managers disposed once the decisions had been taken. Management was a little below the salt, faintly unintellectual, the sort of thing done by junior officials, technicians, businessmen and Americans, but not by senior civil servants.

The following observations are those of an experienced British official who had worked in both policy and regulatory responsibilities in a major department, and who then was appointed to a senior post in a "trading fund" — an organization that operates nominally within the interdepartmental milieu, but on a charging-for-services basis that affords considerable freedom from the usual controls. He tells how upon assuming his trading fund responsibilities, he came to realize that management had a rather different meaning from what he had previously understood.

> The essence of the managerial situation [in the trading fund environment] is that you are effectively your own master . . . . You actually perform, achieve, effect significant economies, improve productivity, do all these satisfying things; whereas in the upper echelons in Whitehall, generally, . . . you are a creature of the minister. If a decision is worth taking at the top, the minister takes it, by definition. If a minister is good, and they nearly all are good, . . . he is very much in charge and you spend your life submitting recommendations to him which are very cautiously received, which are kicked around in an endless process of consultation. Ministers are by no means their own masters — there's this endless round of Cabinet committees, and it goes on and on and on. . . . A lot depends on one's temperament — a lot of senior people don't like taking responsibility or taking decisions — they are happy to lean on the minister. It's part of the culture or code that they are there to provide him with everything he wants and that's the end of their role . . . .

Reflecting on Whitehall as he had known it, he added,

> One of the tragedies is that most permanent heads of departments aren't in the slightest interested in the management of the departments . . . .[1]

A parliamentary committee inquiring into management in the civil service in 1981-1982 stated,

> So far as management skills are concerned, we do not think that, in the past, the most senior civil servants have given the consistent attention to their management role that its importance justifies. Nor have all of them the necessary experience or training to equip them to manage the vast resources which they are expected to control.[2]

Although some officials believe that change has taken hold at the top of the British civil service and that there is now a real commitment to improving management at the highest levels, others are less sure.[3] A former permanent secretary of defence, Sir Frank Cooper, reported in 1983,

> Frankly, I doubt whether the management culture of the civil service has changed all that much at the higher levels of the service. In the main they still see their task as being responsive to Ministers' political aims and policies and they are insufficiently armed with those technical skills which are required for efficient management . . . . There is still too strong a belief that the way to the top lies exclusively along the policy road. There is still a gentlemen-players view, in which the former make policy and the latter implement it. These attitudes are wrong in themselves . . . .[4]

The British attitude toward administration has pervaded generations of Whitehall officials, and indeed it has extended well beyond Whitehall to influence attitudes in former colonies and dominions, including Canada.[5]

The Advent of PESC

There were two major developments which had a bearing upon the practice of management in British government in the late 1960s. The first of these was the institution of a new system for controlling public expenditure, which became known as PESC (see below). The second was the publication of an important report primarily concerned with personnel management practices, known as the Fulton Report (see following section).

The PESC system in the U.K. was created to facilitate the management of public expenditure in aggregate, in lieu of a fragmented, ad hoc methodology that had been in place prior to 1960.[6] It arose out of the work of a committee known as the Plowden Committee, chaired by Sir Edwin Plowden, whose mandate was to report on the theory and practice of expenditure control as it existed in the late 1950s.

The committee's 1961 report introduced major changes in the way in which the bureaucratic process of government interacted with the political level. The key elements of these changes were as follows. First, budgetary estimates in future were to be presented, at the aggregate level, according to functional "programs". This approach, which later became one of the cornerstones of the program planning and budgeting system (PPBS) introduced in the U.S. and then in Canada, allowed all expenditures related to a particular function of government, such as education, defence or criminal justice, to be examined together as a single "program", even though in practice the expenditures in question might be administered by several different departments or agencies of government.

A second change was the decision to present budgetary proposals for several years (initially five, later reduced), not just for the forthcoming year. In addition, the estimates for later years were to be presented in constant prices – that is, there was to be no allowance for inflation in projecting future needs. The idea was to introduce a longer term element into the planning of government programs, and to encourage departments and ministers to think about the cost of programs and services in real terms, rather than dealing with projections that were distorted due to the effect of inflation. (This latter feature of PESC was dropped in 1981, in part because it was found to be too difficult to correlate assumptions about inflation with the actual rate of economic growth, and there was a persistent tendency to overestimate the rate at which the economy would grow. The practical impact of this was to create a growing gap between the uninflated numbers used to prepare budgets and the actual performance of the economy. This greatly complicated the job of financial management.)[7]

The system also introduced the concept that Cabinet should establish aggregated expenditure guidelines which would constitute a framework within which proposals for new spending would have to be situated. These proposals, instead of being considered on a case-by-case basis, as in the past, would be looked at collectively. This was to be done through an interdepartmental survey of requirements conducted under the auspices of a newly created Public Expenditure Survey Committee (whose acronym PESC became a shorthand method of referring to the overall public expenditure management process).

In short, PESC was designed to introduce into Whitehall a comprehensive, medium term planning apparatus. It was hoped that the system would help to bring public expenditure under control, and that it would force both ministers and civil servants to consider intentions in the light of available resources. PESC had a very substantial impact upon the way in which budgets were to be prepared, and it led to a huge increase in the amount of work associated with budget preparation. It anticipated a number of features of PPBS, and was undoubtedly the first effort to implant what might be called modern methods of expenditure management within the British civil service in the post-1960 era. Although it brought more discipline to financial management in the U.K., it did not, regretably, succeed in holding back a surge in public expenditures in Britain during the next two decades.[8] (An analysis of the reasons why PESC did not achieve this goal lies beyond the scope of this discussion; suffice it to say that the failure to restrain expenditures arose from a combination of political and economic forces. While the PESC system suffered from certain defects (and has been engaged in a continuous process of modification since 1961), there is little evidence to suggest that any budgetary system, however well-defined, will of itself be sufficient to hold the lid on expenditure growth in government.[9])

The Fulton Report

In 1966, a committee of Parliament under the chairmanship of Lord Fulton was set up to inquire into the Home Civil Service. Its report, published in 1968, opened by asserting that the civil service was "still fundamentally the product of the nineteenth-century philosophy of the Northcote-Trevelyan Report [whereas] the tasks it faces are those of the second half of the twentieth century."[10] It stated that the service was still based too much on the concept of the "amateur, generalist or all-rounder." "Too few civil servants are skilled managers." The system of classes in the service hindered its work and many competent persons, particularly those with scientific and technical education, were being needlessly excluded from positions of responsibility.

The committee felt there was insufficient contact between the service and the public. Furthermore, it said, "personnel planning and career planning are inadequate." It presented a variety of proposals, including the establishment of a Civil Service Department, a Civil Service College, the devotion of more resources to career management and training, greater mobility between the service and other employments, the application of the principles of "accountable management" in departments, and the establishment of new Planning Units in departments headed by a new position, that of senior policy advisor to the minister.

Unfortunately, much of value in the Report was obscured by weaknesses in its presentation and by a few highly contentious proposals that reduced some debate on its merits to emotional posturing. One was the labelling of civil servants as "amateurs" in a service that prided itself on its professionalism. The Committee's denigration of the generalist was almost certainly seen by many civil servants as an attack on the carefully nurtured tradition of dispassionate neutrality and dissociation from special interests (see chapter 3).

The second especially controversial suggestion was that ministers should have their own senior policy advisors who would head up the Planning Units inside the service and hence be privy to its internal policy discussions. The suggestion that the cherished role of the civil service in providing policy advice to ministers should be shared with a new group of policy advisors who would not report through the permanent secretary offended the Report's own principle of accountable management (by splitting responsibility). By proposing to excise, even partially, the most valued role of the civil service from the department's traditional responsibilities, the Report more or less guaranteed itself a hostile response from the civil service.

The furore created by Fulton was remarkable. Passions ran high. One commentator proclaimed,

> I would far rather be ruled by men who were familiar with the tragedies of Sophocles, who had a grounding in the wisdom of Socrates and Plato and then topped it up by a wide reading of Shakespeare, Hobbes, Locke and Stuart Mill, than by one who was an expert electronics engineer or a first-class nuclear physicist. By acquiring all this expertise in the most modern of sciences, a man is bound to cut himself off from the wisdom of the ages.[11]

In a retrospective on Fulton, John Garrett, a former member of the "management consultancy group" that had provided advice on management to Fulton, allowed as how

> [T]he Fulton Committee ... did ... present its analysis and its proposals for change in a self-defeating way. If implementation was to succeed it had to have some support among the administrators in command at the time, yet its tone and style alienated them from the outset .... [Fulton] did, however, spot most of the cracks, pressure points and distortions which appeared in the management systems of the Civil Service and it gave the initial impetus to a number of overdue reforms ....
>
> The Fulton Committee set the scene for the adoption of some useful management practices in central government .... [12]

A decade after the Fulton Report was issued, one pair of observers, journalist Peter Kellner and former Committee member Lord Crowther-Hunt, published a cutting denunciation of the process of implementation. They argued that the senior bureaucracy had sandbagged Fulton, providing the appearance of action while in fact doing little by way of concrete response to what was a declared priority of the then Prime Minister, Harold Wilson. (Credence is lent to this accusation by the fact that 14 years after the Report's publication, the civil service was still appointing individuals with no professional financial training to the position of chief financial officer[13] — the top financial job in departments that spend billions of pounds annually.)

On the other hand, it appears that many civil servants felt that the Fulton Report was superficial, unbalanced and ultimately unfair. However, when civil servants come under attack their ability to respond is hampered by the requirement of anonymity (see chapter 3). Their cause must generally be championed by a politician or some other public figure. Politicians will, from time to time, proclaim the virtues of the public service, but such professions of confidence are relatively infrequent and tend to be unspecific and unconvincing. Whatever the merits of the Fulton allegations, there was little effective counter-criticism of the Report by the civil service itself, and no political champion emerged at the time who was willing or able to discredit the Report. As a result, almost 20 years after publication, discussions of Fulton can still generate anger and frustration among some Whitehall mandarins.

The 1970s

The Fulton Committee may have introduced the issue of management to centre stage, but during the 1970s there was not a great deal of action on the set. There was no major thrust to carry Fulton's work forward on an ongoing basis, no grand attempts to implement system-wide changes in management of the type that characterized the Canadian public service during the same period.

One exception was a little-known program of management reviews of individual departments, carried out under the auspices of the Civil Service Department which, in the wake of Fulton, was accorded a partial mandate for "management" in the civil service (financial aspects of management remained under Treasury's jurisdiction). This initiative improved administrative practices on a department-by-department basis, but it was hampered by a lack of a strong political commitment and the absence of an agreed set of principles or standards as to what constituted good management.[14] The political problem diminished its impact, and the conceptual problem led to disagreements with some departments that dulled its effectiveness. The program was also impeded by certain limited ideas about the scope of management, about which more is said in chapter 5. Ultimately, it lapsed into obscurity in about 1979.

Another, higher-profile initiative during the tenure of Prime Minister Edward Heath in the 1970s was PAR (Program Analysis and Review), a program of reviews of major areas of government expenditure nominally under the direction of ministers, with heavy participation from central agencies. Although a number of PAR reviews were conducted during the 1970s, PAR was not really directed at resolving systemic difficulties in management in the civil service; rather it was a series of one-shot attempts to address the spending levels in discrete areas of government activity. Despite high hopes associated with its establishment, its ultimate impact was not great. Toward the late 1970s it too lost momentum and disappeared from view.

The uncertain response to Fulton during the 1970s had both good and bad consequences. On the positive side, since it was not clear that all Fulton's proposals were workable, the British civil service was mostly spared the "two steps forward, one step back" dance to which the Canadian public service was subjected during the 1970s. In addition, the pace of management change was perhaps less frantic — an uncharitable observer might say that in some departments it was positively somnolent — as the political interest in management improvement waned, and the senior civil service returned to its classical preoccupation with policy matters. Structural turmoil in Whitehall during the 1970s derived mostly from what Lord Bancroft, former Permanent Secretary of the Civil Service Department and head of the Home Civil Service in Britain, has since called a propensity to dicker with organization without sufficient attention to the disruptive consequences of such changes.[15]

While other governments were attempting to make officials more conscious of their responsibilities as managers by building improved management information systems and by linking budgets to responsibility centres, Britain resisted these innovations despite the fact that Fulton had made a major plea for the adoption of "accountable management" in departments. In addition, (following precedents hotly criticized by Fulton in 1968) Britain continued its practice of appointing people whom Fulton would have called amateurs to the position of principal finance officers in departments — incumbents who were not burdened with previous training or experience in financial management. It decided not to follow the fashion of other jurisdictions in adopting the concept of program planning and budgeting (see chapter 9), except at very aggregate levels of expenditure, and there was no system-wide emphasis on objective-setting or upon clarifying the expected impacts of government activity. By and large, changes in management approach in Whitehall during the 1970s occurred on a piecemeal, department-by-department basis. Some legitimate reforms proposed by Fulton which could have had an important positive impact — particularly some aspects of his recommendations in favour of more accountable management — fell on stony ground.

This era of comparative peace ended in 1979 soon after the new Conservative Government of Margaret Thatcher came to power in

May. Mrs. Thatcher took the unusual step of making management improvement a political priority and keeping it there throughout her first term in office and into her second. The winds of change began to sweep the placid landscape of the civil service.

Thatcher and Management

The Thatcher Government decided to confront management issues in the civil service for a number of reasons. One was undoubtedly the personality of the prime minister herself, and her interest in seeing things done efficiently. Another factor was the feeling that government, especially during the 1960s, had grown in an uncontrolled fashion, with too many quangos popping up on its fringes. There was the right-wing philosophy of the Conservative Party, given new vitality under the leadership of the 'Iron Lady', that favoured the private sector over the public sector. Two other factors were noted by a senior Whitehall official:

> In the '70s ... there developed a concern about ministerial patronage – a large number of people who were owing their keep to the government. As far as I know, there was no particular event that gave rise to this.... Probably more significant was a growing feeling in the '70s among MPs that government had got too powerful, that Parliament was no longer exerting the right sort of checks on the executive that it had in the past.[16]

An early step in the energetic program to address these concerns was the appointment of Derek (later Lord) Rayner, who subsequently became Chairman of the well-known and well-regarded Marks and Spencer chain of retail stores, as personal Efficiency Adviser to the Prime Minister. This was followed by a barrage of developments during the next five years: a major reduction in the size of the civil service through widespread personnel cuts; a program of quango reduction and of privatization; the launching of "Rayner scrutinies", a series of efficiency studies in departments; an attack on obsolete methods of financial management and unclear accountability under the banner of what became known as FMI (Financial Management Initiative); a blooming interest in improved management information systems initiated, surprisingly, by a minister who became frustrated with his department's inability to brief him effectively on what it was doing; and a variety of related initiatives in such areas as training and succession planning. These enterprises derived further momentum from a decision by a committee of the House of Commons to launch an inquiry into efficiency and effectiveness in the civil service.

Reducing the Size of Government

A key element in the Thatcher Government policy on the civil service was a determination to reduce its size. In May 1979, there were 732,000 people employed by government in a wide variety of departments and agencies (In 1854, the Northcote-Trevelyan Report on the civil service had counted 16,000!)[17] By October of 1983 the figure had fallen dramatically, to 636,000, and the projections of the Government were that by 1988, the number would fall to 593,000.[18] A variety of means were used to accomplish these goals, including reductions in the staff of existing institutions, the abolition of certain functions altogether, and the transfer of other functions to the private sector.

An important component of this program was a systematic quango hunt, whereby Leo Pliatzky, a respected former second permanent secretary at the Treasury, was commissioned to stalk "the whole range of non-Departmental bodies with a view to eliminating any which had outlived their usefulness or which could not be justified in the context of the Government's objectives of reducing public expenditure and the size of the public sector." The review also examined arrangements for control and accountability for these bodies. The hunt bagged 30 out of a population of 489 executive quangos, proposing "winding up, rationalisation or withdrawal of support"; it wrought further devastation among the 1,561 advisory bodies by identifying 211 for extinction. The Government decided that "Pliatzky reviews" should be conducted on a regular, cyclical basis of each quango in future. (New policies in areas such as accountability, audits and board membership were also defined.) As a result of these later reviews, another 200 quangos were eliminated, with savings of a further 106 million pounds.[19] Perhaps in the spirit of the hunt, the Cabinet Office took to publishing slightly grisly press releases tallying up the latest body counts: "A further drop in the numbers of quangos is shown in 'Public Bodies 1984,' released today . . . by the Cabinet Office (MPO). The quango population has fallen to 1,681 – a reduction of nearly 500 . . . ."[20]

As the population in the game park fell, however, it became increasingly clear that insofar as quango hunting was directed to cost reduction – its principal purpose was to reduce patronage – it had limited potential. Remaining quangos were less easily flushed and more likely to raise an outcry if attacked. The Government decided to redirect its fire on internal management practices within quangos, and in November 1984 it launched a "Financial Management Initiative for Non-Departmental Public Bodies". The purpose was to bring to bear on the residual quango population a somewhat similar type of "FMI" review to those that had already been visited on many departments of government.

Throughout the campaign against quangos, a continuing theme was the need to reduce the size of the civil service, a goal which, as discussed elsewhere in this book, is not necessarily consonant with improving internal management in government organizations.

Reforming the Centre of Government

While quangos were an important part of the reform agenda, an even more intensive program of management improvement was directed at departments. One element of this comprised Lord Rayner's internal reviews of departmental activities. Rayner sought to keep his scrutinies lean and unbureaucratic: "Do not create a bureaucracy to defeat a bureaucracy. All past attempts to achieve progress in this way have failed."[21] Rayner believed that lasting change had to involve those who would have to implement the new procedures – line managers, not committees or staff groups. He created a small seven-person unit attached to the prime minister's office to establish policies, to act as a catalyst for the execution of scrutinies and to ensure that certain standards were observed. The work itself was conducted by promising younger officers in departments who, for purposes of the scrutinies, reported directly to the minister, and who were instructed to work within a limited timetable, usually under three months. Reports were usually published.

Scrutinies were focused and specific. They addressed such diverse subjects as the enforcement of grading regulations for eggs, inquiries from the public at Customs and Excise, defence building projects, the administration of teachers' pensions, various statistical services, arrangements for withdrawing national savings certificates, procedures for identifying internal talent in departments and the administration of juries in the Lord Chancellor's Department.[22] By April of 1983, (shortly after Lord Rayner was replaced by industrialist Robin Ibbs), about 140 scrutinies had been completed. Government statistics on the scrutinies maintained that savings of 56 million pounds "once and for all" had been made, plus a further 400 million realized in "potential savings and extra income".

Looking back on his experiences over the previous four years, Rayner noted that the reviews had been received with an enthusiasm that was less than total. The frequent reaction: "Reform like chastity is a fine and splendid thing, but let it begin elsewhere." Rayner's overall assessment was as follows.

> It is ironic that despite the talent [of so many public servants] the quality of so much Whitehall management should be so low; and that leadership has too often in the past fallen into the hands of those who know nothing of management and despise those who do . . . .

> [T]oo many of the early scrutinies demonstrated a staggering double flaw in Civil Service management — first, an inability to identify the true cost centres and services being provided through want of systems or through many functions, activities and services being provided without charge, and secondly, a widespread obscurity about who was responsible to whom and for what; one Permanent Secretary rightly described this in his own Ministry as a prevalent "fuzziness" of accountability.

> As a whole, the Service was content with a "gentleman's agreement" form of accountability which has served us well in the past, and secured a high degree of integrity but was not enough in the last quarter of the twentieth century. Too often there was not delegation but abdication.[23]

While Rayner's scrutinies were going on, the House of Commons' Treasury and Civil Service Committee was conducting its own investigation into efficiency in the government. In 1982 it produced a report containing 26 recommendations for improving management, starting with ministerial accountability and moving on to address the preparation of departmental estimates, program management and review, the role of central agencies and of the Comptroller and Auditor General, and matters related to personnel policy. It noted that "morale in the Civil Service is in a precarious state" and, although it was relatively silent on issues related to people, it looked hopefully for a "fortifying of good traditions and a restoration of morale."[24]

An interesting feature of the Committee's review was its endorsement of a system known as MINIS devised under the direction of the then Minister of the Environment, Michael Heseltine. MINIS was a form of management control system intended to attribute costs to clearly defined responsibility centres in the department and to establish measures of performance for those centres. It also involved regular review meetings attended by Heseltine himself at which officials explained what they were doing and planning to do and at which they received direction from the minister on priorities. The acronym stood for Management Information System for Ministers, a somewhat misleading designation since the system was in fact more a general planning and control system (see chapter 9) than a management information system. (It was a too-detailed instrument of management for use by most ministers on other than an exceptional basis, since most ministers have neither the time nor inclination to manage their departments. Heseltine was atypical in this respect.)

MINIS represented an admixture of sensible and, on the whole, well-known managerial techniques of planning and control embodying many features of program budgeting. Similar systems of one sort or another had been in use in North America in many jurisdictions for well over a decade. A London Business School professor judged it to be a major contribution to government accounting practices but noted, "[T]he reaction of other departments has been decidedly cool. They have not rushed to apply it . . . ."[25] Its arrival in Whitehall was greeted with a measure of quizzical fascination in the civil service which had previously tended to reject the need for anything so radical as an accounting system that related resources to results or to responsibility centres.[26] Doubts about its utility and transferability to other departments were expressed during the Committee's hearings by both Lord Bancroft and also by Robert Armstrong, head of the Cabinet Office. Nevertheless, the Committee's decision to endorse Heseltine's approach apparently had the effect of causing the government to review Treasury's historical disinterest in management accounting, and in due course MINIS clones and mutations began to spring up in many other departments.[27]

In May 1982 the British government launched its most sweeping attack on management practices with the "financial management initiative," a review of management in departments that, like the Lambert Royal Commission in Canada, took a very broad view of the term "financial." The FMI, as it became called, amounted to a general review of objective-setting, accountability, management information and financial procedures. Somewhat in the manner of the IMPAC studies in Canada, each department was called upon to establish a plan by the end of the year setting forth the improvements it considered necessary, under the guiding eye of a new joint Treasury-MPO division known as the FMI Unit. The FMI was the government's general response to the proposals of the Treasury and Civil Service Committee. It announced a variety of initiatives with respect to the estimates process, program evaluation, the role of parliamentary committees in reviewing departmental expenditures, the role of central agencies, the appointment of permanent secretaries and several related subjects.[28] Concurrently, it gave MINIS the official system-wide blessing it had hitherto been lacking.

A final interesting development in the U.K. at time of writing is a move toward what Treasury calls "running costs limits" — a potentially significant change to the accountability regime between departments and the Treasury. The general intent is to push responsibility for operating (non-program) resources down the line, an approach similar in some respects to Canada's program for increased ministerial authority (IMAA), though less comprehensive. Specifically, it moves detailed control over individual expenditure items from Treasury to departments, giving them more authority to transfer approved resources between line items — that is, from one type of expenditure, such as office services, to another, such as accommodation — without having to secure central agency approval.

Under this system, departments are to be "required to ensure that all their administrative costs for current expenditure are met from within their running costs limits.... By concentrating on the total cost to each department, [the new arrangements] provide departmental managers with the flexibility to decide how they can most effectively use the resources available to meet their objectives."[29] Starting in 1983-84, Treasury also relaxed certain provisions related to year-end capital spending by departments, allowing some carry-forward to the following year.

Treasury officials were predictably concerned lest the transition to the new regime proceed too rapidly, citing "a lot of weak management and a lack of contingency planning and commitment scheduling in departments.... It will take a long time before the arrangement is mature."[30] So far, the arrangement applies only to running costs or operating costs; pay and related staff costs are not included. In the longer term, subject to experience with this initiative, Treasury has undertaken to review the need for manpower controls. This could lead to a quite significant development, since manpower costs are the largest element in running costs, and the historical preoccupation of politicians and central agencies with staffing levels has been a significant source of frustration to departmental managers. A move away from specific control over staffing levels might give departments an important new dimension of managerial flexibility.

Summary

Improving management in Britain has followed a somewhat different path than it has in Canada. Since 1960, we have witnessed:

- the advent of PESC in 1961, followed by an ongoing program of modifications and elaborations;

- the well-intentioned, but largely ineffectual Fulton Report in 1968 dealing with personnel management issues;

- a few discrete initiatives aimed at reviewing and improving various bits and pieces of the government's programs and administrative structures during the 1970s, such as PAR, which ran into the sand after a few years, and the Civil Service

Department's low-profile program of management reviews, which likewise appeared before the end of the decade;

- the greatly increased priority accorded to management after 1979, in the wake of the election of Prime Minister Thatcher's Government, leading to Rayner scrutinies, the FMI, Pliatzky reviews and quango hunts, cutbacks in the civil service; and a variety of other initiatives undertaken by the Cabinet Office (MPO) or by the Treasury;

- a new interest in Parliament in management issues, resulting in examinations of administrative matters by the Treasury and Civil Service Committee in the early 1980s;

- some limited experimentation by Treasury with new policies related to running costs controls and other aspects of its relationship with departments.

Despite the differences between the British and the Canadian approaches, it is clear that both governments have been wrestling with similar issues. These include the management of public expenditure and the design of planning and budgeting systems; the type of the accountability relationship that should prevail between central agencies and departments in an era of "big government;" the improvement of management information relative to government programs and the general problem of monitoring performance; and the issue of the size of the public service and the types of activities that should be positioned in departments as opposed to quangos, Crown corporations, or the private sector. The problems are complex, and the search for solutions (if indeed there are clear solutions to problems of this nature) seems likely to continue for many years.

Footnotes

1. Author's interview, May 1985.

2. *Third Report from the Treasury and Civil Service Committee,* Session 1981-1982, "Efficiency and Effectiveness in the Civil Service," vol. 1, HC 236, (London: Her Majesty's Stationery Office, 8 March 1982), p. xxxv, para. 88.

3. Author's interviews, May 1985 and June 1986.

4. Sir Frank Cooper, "Freedom to Manage in Government," Lecture in Royal Institute of Public Administration Winter Series, 19 April 1983.

5. Robert Boase, a management consultant who has worked in Nigeria and Jamaica, advises that such attitudes are much in evidence in these countries. Conversation with the author, February, 1986.

6. For a more thorough description and appraisal of the PESC system and of efforts to get public expenditures under control in the U.K. from 1960 to 1980, see Leo Pliatzky, *Getting and Spending: Public Expenditure, Employment and Inflation,* rev. ed., (Oxford: Basil Blackwell, 1982). See also Peter Mountfield, "Recent Developments in the Control of Public Expenditure in the United Kingdom," *International Budgeting and Finance,* vol. 3, no. 3 (Autumn, 1983), pp. 109-130.

7. Pliatzky, *op. cit.,* pp. 202ff.

8. See Pliatzky, *op. cit.,* esp. pp. 52ff, 81, 89, 136, and 179-180.

9. This discussion is pursued in more depth in an unpublished report by the author entitled, "Government Budgeting Systems," written in 1985 on behalf of the Government of Alberta.

10. *Report of the Committee on the Civil Service, 1966-68,* (Fulton Report), vol. 1, Cmnd. 3638, (London: Her Majesty's Stationery Office, June 1968), pp. 104-107. The Northcote-Trevelyan Report of 1854 introduced to the U.K. the concept of a professional civil service appointed on merit through periodic, centrally administered, competitive examinations. See Appendix B to the Fulton Report, pp. 108ff.

11. Wilfrid Sendall, in the *Daily Express*, 1 July 1968. Quoted in John Garrett, *The Management of Government*, (Harmondsworth: Penguin, 1972), pp. 48-49.

12. John Garrett, *Management in Government*, (Harmondsworth: Penguin, 1972), pp. 52-57.

13. Peter Kellner and Lord Crowther-Hunt, *The Civil Servants*, (London: Macdonald General Books, 1980); *Third Report from the Treasury and Civil Service Committee*, Session 1981-1982, "Efficiency and Effectiveness in the Civil Service," *op. cit.*, p. xii para. 14.

14. Author's interview, May 1985.

15. Lord Bancroft, "Whitehall: Some Personal Reflections," Suntory-Toyota Lecture, delivered at the London School of Economics, 1 December 1983. Available from the library, Royal Institute of Public Administration, London.

16. Author's interview, May 1985.

17. Fulton Report, *op. cit.*, Appendix B, p. 10.

18. Briefing papers supplied by Cabinet Office/MPO, 1985.

19. *Report on Non Departmental Public Bodies*, Cmnd 7797, (London: Her Majesty's Stationery Office, January 1980), p. 4. Commonly referred to as the Pliatzky Report. While the number of organizations affected was quite impressive, the actual savings were less so. Although total expenditures by both executive and advisory quangos at the time were approximately £5,837 million (capital and operating), immediate savings were just under £12 million. See also *Non Departmental Public Bodies: A Guide for Departments*, (London: Her Majesty's Stationery Office, 1982). Under revision at time of writing.

20. Press release MPO (84)1. 18 December 1984.

21. Lord Rayner, "The Unfinished Agenda," University of London, Stamp Memorial Lecture, 1984.

22. From documents supplied by the Efficiency Unit, 70 Whitehall, London SW1 2AS. For details on the conduct of a major review, see Norman Warner, "Raynerism in Practice: Anatomy of a

Rayner Scrutiny," *Public Administration,* 62, (Spring 1984), pp. 1-22.

23. Rayner, *op. cit.*

24. *Third Report from the Treasury and Civil Service Committee,* Session 1981-1982, "Efficiency and Effectiveness in the Civil Service," *op. cit.*

25. Andrew Likierman, "Management information for Ministers: the MINIS system in the Department of the Environment," *Public Administration,* 60, (Summer 1982), pp. 127-142.

26. See Mountfield, *loc. cit.,* and Pliatzky, *op. cit.,* pp. 98-99.

27. *Financial Management in Government Departments,* Cmnd. 9056, (London: Her Majesty's Stationery Office, September 1983).

28. *Efficiency and Effectiveness in the Civil Service - Government Observations on the Third Report from the Treasury and Civil Service Committee,* Cmnd. 8616, (London: Her Majesty's Stationery Office, September 1982).

29. See *Supply Estimates 1986-87: Summary and Guides,* Cmnd. 9742, (London: Her Majesty's Stationery Office, March 1986), p. 15; also *The Management of Public Spending,* (London: H.M. Treasury, May 1986), paras. 55-70.

30. Author's interview with Treasury officials, June 1986.

Appendix Three:
A Brief History of Management

The Origins of Management

Compared with other professional disciplines taught at universities and colleges today – law, engineering, medicine, for example – management is a mere stripling. Even in relation to economics, which itself has a heritage of only a couple of centuries, management is a young field of inquiry. Some trace its earliest roots to the work of Frederick Taylor, an American preoccupied with how to increase the productivity of industrial workers. Taylor's book, *Scientific Management*, published in 1912, introduced the notion that, through systematic observation and analysis, it was possible to formulate rules or principles to improve performance on the job.

In fact, Taylor's concept of productivity improvement through rationalization of the workplace was not entirely new. Early economists, notably Adam Smith in the opening of his 1776 classic, *The Wealth of Nations*, discussed the division of labour.[1] He suggested that in the manufacture of large numbers of similar items such as pins, the work could be divided among workers possessing different skills and abilities; productivity would thereby be enhanced. However, with the industrial revolution's fascination with the possibilities of engineering solutions to problems of production, Taylor moved the discussion of productivity improvement from the realm of hypothesis to that of scientific investigation.

He studied how the better workers did mechanical tasks (for example, in handling pig-iron, shoveling or bricklaying), timed their movements with stopwatches, and then analyzed how the amount of energy and time required could be reduced. Taylor's techniques of objective analysis of routine work gave birth to "time-and-motion" experts. Even today, three generations later, this label is often attached to students of management and to management consultants, despite the fact that most modern management "experts" are concerned with problems very different from those that occupied Taylor.

There were four "principles" involved in scientific management as Taylor defined it. First, managers were expected to "gather in" knowledge formerly in workers' heads, tabulate it, and reduce it to "laws, rules, and even mathematical formulae" for the conduct of work that would supplant the old rule-of-thumb methods of the workers. Second, workers were to be selected according to their character, performance and potential, and then trained for advancement wherever suitable. The third principle was, in Taylor's words, the "bringing together" of the rules and the workers, a process that today might be called organizational change; the fourth was the notion of the transfer of certain responsibilities (those that involved planning and organizing work) from workers to managers. "[U]nder this new type of management there is hardly a single act or piece of work done by any workman in the shop which is not preceded and followed by some act on the part of one of the men in management."[2]

During the early years of management theory, clear general precepts akin to those that had been evolved by Taylor for mechanical tasks were propounded for other types of managerial work, leading to the development of what is sometimes called the classical school of management. The teachings of this school were full of "simple-minded injunctions to plan ahead, keep records, write down policies, specialize, be decisive, and keep your span of control to about six people."[3] And, for certain purposes and in certain contexts, they worked.

Two of the best-known authors of the classical school are Colonel Lyndall Urwick and the French industrialist, Henri Fayol. Urwick's efforts to provide a scientific codification of universally applicable principles of management drew heavily on his experience in both military and industrial settings.[4] These principles stated that in any organization, authority and responsibility should be co-terminous (principle of correspondence); that superiors should be responsible for the acts of their subordinates (principle of responsibility); that there should be a clear line of authority running from the top to the bottom of the organization (scalar principle); that no superior can supervise directly the work of more than five or six subordinates (principle of the span of control); that a person's work should as far as possible be confined to one leading function (principle of specialization); that work has to be smoothly co-ordinated (principle of co-ordination), and that every position in the organization should be clearly described in writing (principle of definition). While Urwick later called these principles "flexible guidelines," some disciples regard them as stone tablets. Some contemporary management studies and audit reports suggest that a few "management experts" and, more recently, value-for-money auditors, may not have carried their studies of management much beyond the precepts of the Colonel — who, incidentally, published his major works before 1950.

Fayol's *General and Industrial Management* was another seminal work in the evolution of management thinking. Originally written in French and published in 1916, Fayol's work only found its way into the English literature with the publication of an initial translation in 1929, and a later, somewhat better one, in 1949. Fayol introduced the notion that the job of management involved five basic functions — planning, organizing, co-ordinating, commanding and controlling. Restated in various ways (another author, Luther Gulick, preferred POSDCORB — planning, organizing, staffing, directing, co-ordinating, reporting and budgeting), these functions continue to be the basis of many curricula for management study courses, for the writing of job descriptions, for the evaluation of managerial performance, and for the review of organizational practices (even though they were formulated as descriptions of the jobs of individual managers and *not* of general organizational functions).

Fayol's statement of responsibilities is not, in fact, very useful as a basis for assisting managers in their work or for analyzing what they do, but the terminology has become so embedded in managerial thinking that managers themselves, asked to describe their work, will often use his words. Henry Mintzberg, a professor of management at McGill University, argues that this language is too general to be revealing:

> These four words [planning, organizing, coordinating, controlling] do not, in fact, describe the actual work of managers at all. They describe certain vague objectives of managerial work . . . . [T]he writings of the classical school have served to label our areas of ignorance, and may have fulfilled the need of telling managers what they should be doing (even if it did not tell them what they did). But the classical school has for too long served to block our search for a deeper understanding of the work of the manager.[5]

Another author from the non-English speaking world who has heavily influenced management thinking is Max Weber. At about the same time that Taylor was formulating his views on industrial productivity, Weber wanted to abolish patronage and nepotism, practices that were rife in his native Germany, by establishing more objective, or professional, concepts pertaining to the exercise of authority in organizations.

For Weber, bureaucracy was not a pejorative concept, but an alternative to distasteful traditional practices that stood in the way of effective management. Bureaucracy had to be created in order to establish standards, to abolish cronyism and favouritism, and to make employees accountable for their performance. It was characterized by the subjection of officials to strict discipline and control, by division of labour, hierarchy, examinations for positions based on technical competence or merit, and promotion based on seniority, achievement, or both. Officials had to earn their positions, and could not 'own' them.[6] Weber's work made an important contribution to the notion of a professional, apolitical bureaucracy. As chapter 3 observes, this concept continues to be a core principle for the operation of public services in many parliamentary democracies.

It is interesting to note how many "principles" of management, still finding popular acceptance today, arose from the studies of men writing about managerial problems in particular situations, three or four generations ago. One of the reasons for this is the relatively simple and straightforward approach of the classical school. Managers are busy people. Simple solutions may be band-aids for complex problems, but they may be all that can be applied in the time available, and perhaps they can prevent a serious hemorrhage. Therefore, managers tend to grasp at maxims that are easy to understand and to use. Ideas such as Urwick's principles or the plan-organize-co-ordinate-control recipe seemed to make the job of management understandable without imbuing it with too much complexity. However, there are many types of organizations where some doctrines of the classical school are not helpful. Indeed, there are circumstances where certain classical precepts are downright wrong. The shortcomings of the classical school became more evident as the sphere of interest of management expanded.

The Widening Scope of Management Concerns

If, somewhat arbitrarily, one were to take Taylor's industrial shop floor as a point of departure for the activities with which management is concerned, one can think of it spreading through the industrial organization and beyond. Starting in the production department, it has moved to address all the other functions of the business enterprise: finance, marketing, sales and more recently, such corporate functions as strategic planning, public relations, corporate affairs, government relations and, perhaps most recently of all, information management. Both white- and blue-collar employees have become the objects of management's search for methods to improve productivity.

Taylor's original preoccupation was mainly with deploying productive effort in the most efficient manner. He was not much worried about issues such as worker co-operation because his approach tied increases in wages to increases in output; he was convinced that if his methods were properly applied, workers would perceive the advantages to themselves and willingly join in. However, later students of management found that workers do not always embrace ideas for productivity improvement wholeheartedly.

It began to emerge that employees' attitudes toward their work powerfully affected their motivation and thus their behaviour on the job; and it became apparent that attitudes were affected by a host of influences, not all of which were related to the job itself. Pay, for example, was only one of the factors affecting workers, and in many instances it had less effect on motivation than other rather intangible considerations such as recognition, advancement, the degree of responsibility and authority accorded to employees, or their sense of achievement. Performance was affected in subtle ways, through leadership, group norms and peer pressure, as well as through general organizational policies in such areas as employee communications.

It also emerged that generalizing about employees was dangerous: different employees responded differently to different management styles and approaches. For example, some liked more challenging work, others seemed less interested in challenge or job enrichment; some responded positively to well-defined policies and structures of the kind advocated by Weber, and some reacted poorly to working in an environment of this type. In recognition of the complexity of all these issues, there has evolved within the study of management a substantial subsector of inquiry called "human resource management" concerned with motivation, morale and the management of people generally.

As the sphere of management moved to new functions beyond the shop floor, it became evident that organizations were more complex than Urwick's original principles had suggested. Early models upon which organization theory drew were those of the Catholic Church and the military, neither of which is reputed for its adaptability to external pressures, its innovative capacities or its responsiveness to employee concerns. It emerged that what worked in the context of either the religious or the military cloisters would not always work in organizations that had to respond rapidly to changes in their environments, or where top-down direction was less readily accepted. There was no single model for success, no one best way of dealing with different organizations and situations. Formal procedures and policies of the type advocated by Weber were not always the answer; in fact, sometimes organizations worked well *in spite* of formal structures rather than because of them.

Other changes in management thinking related to decision-making and decentralization. As technology and society generally became more complicated, many managers realized that not all the important decisions could be taken at the top of the organization. People who were directly involved in day-to-day relations with clients, or in technical aspects of work were often better placed to decide how to resolve many operational issues than senior managers who were removed from the firing line. Moreover, top managers had less time to run the operations: as the pace of social change increased, more executive time had to be spent managing the relationship of the organization with its environment and new stakeholders such as local governments.

Changing attitudes toward employment made it clear that workers were no longer prepared to let their lives be ruled by impersonal bosses whom they never saw. Employees demanded a growing role in decision-making. Methods had to be found to allow for pooling the practical experience of those who actually did the day-to-day work of the organization with the broader perspective of those in higher positions. This led to the development of theories regarding participative management and decision-making processes linking the two perspectives.

With respect to the structure of organizations, it became apparent that Urwick's principle of the span of control was not correct: there was no single "right" formula, such as one boss to six workers, even for organizations in apparently related lines of work such as manufacturing. Joan Woodward, for example, discovered that how an organization should be structured depended on the technology it was employing, technology being broadly defined as "the kind of work being done". What worked in one setting, such as a continuous-flow oil refinery, was not necessarily suited to another, such as the manufacture of a customized product (e.g., a piece of industrial machinery). Contrary to Urwick, Woodward concluded that different kinds of work *demanded* different organization structures.[7]

Still other research revealed that in designing and managing an organization, two other factors had to be considered: the stage of development of the organization, and the people. For example, in the early stages of a business enterprise, when there are relatively few managers, the firm needs entrepreneurial skills, and often a centralized structure. As the size, sophistication and managerial complement of the enterprise develop, new requirements assert themselves. Managers are now needed with skills in integrating diverse functions, and in the development of administrative and productive systems.

Experience and research also showed that the overall performance of an organization was directly affected by the people, particularly those in top executive positions. Different types of leadership behaviour – directive, supportive, achievement-oriented, participative – were suited to different sorts of tasks and situations; different styles of leadership – delegating, telling, selling – were shown to be more successful with different types of employees. Managers were challenged to take a more thoughtful approach to their employees in deciding how to manage most effectively.

The concerns of management as a discipline did not stop at the margins of the organization but extended to include the interaction between the organization and its environment. Like biological organisms, business organizations consumed certain goods and services sold by other business entities, then processed and produced their own products or services which were in turn acquired by still other corporations. The analogy with living creatures trying to achieve harmonious interaction with their own environment seemed instructive. The business which was able to monitor its markets and anticipate trends would prosper; the firm which misread the demand for its goods or which neglected other important external forces, such as exchange rate fluctuations or government regulations, would fail.

As management moved into these new areas, it began to address such questions as: What techniques could be devised to monitor what was going on outside the organization? What structures and decision-making processes would allow the organization to assimilate this information? How could the organization plan effectively so that it would not be caught by surprise by external developments? Whose responsibility was it to plan the future of the organization – the line manager, a staff group or some combination of the two?

No longer concerned solely with "doing" or "executing," management was moving beyond "how" to address "what" and "why" – beyond implementation into the sphere of strategic planning and policy development. New tools and techniques were emerging that could be used to develop organizational plans and strategies, many (but not all) of them geared to solving business problems, under a confusing array of labels such as strategic planning, corporate planning systems, decision analysis, cybernetics, competitive analysis, portfolio management, scenarios, market research, business policy, futures research and environmental scanning.

Summary: Management Today

Management now has insights to offer concerning virtually any function or relationship bearing upon the effective performance of organizations, over both the short and the longer term. Its concerns are internal and external. It deals with the traditional (such as production), and the emerging (such as information management), with the co-ordination of these functions and with the problems of linking activity at the bottom and the top of the organization. It is interested in the intangible aspects of organizational performance – the norms, values and traditions affecting employees' behaviour and attitudes, and the incentives that motivate them. Further, it is interested in the complex and difficult issues having to do with the relationship between the organization and its milieu, and with the development of strategies designed to ensure survival and effective performance well into the future. It is interested not only in business enterprises, but in all types of organizations, and it recognizes that what is suitable for one type of institution or situation will not necessarily be appropriate for others.

Footnotes:

1. Adam Smith, *The Wealth of Nations*, Edwin Cannan, ed., (London: Methuen & Co., 1925), book I, ch. 1, p. 5.

2. F.W. Taylor, "Scientific Management," in D.S. Pugh, ed., *Organization Theory – Selected Readings*, 2nd ed., (Harmondsworth: Penguin, 1984), pp. 157ff.

3. See Charles Perrow, "The Short and Glorious History of Organizational Theory," in James L. Gibson, John M. Ivancevich and James H. Donnelly, eds., *Readings in Organizations*, 4th ed., (Plano, Texas: Business Publications Inc., 1982), pp. 32-44.

4. See John Garrett, *Management in Government*, (Harmondsworth: Penguin, 1972), pp. 58-67.

5. Henry Mintzberg, *The Nature of Managerial Work*, (New York: Harper and Row, 1973), pp. 9-11.

6. See Garrett, *op. cit.*, also M. Weber, "Legitimate Authority and Bureaucracy," in D.S. Pugh, *op. cit.*, pp. 15-27.

7. Joan Woodward, *Industrial Organization: Theory and Practice*, (London: Oxford University Press, 1965).

Members of the Institute

MEMBERS OF THE INSTITUTE

James S. Cowan, Q.C.
Partner, Stewart, MacKeen & Covert, Halifax
V. Edward Daughney
President, First City Trust Company, Vancouver
Dr. H.E. Duckworth, O.C.
Chancellor, University of Manitoba, Winnipeg
Dr. Stefan Dupré, O.C.
Department of Political Science, University of Toronto
Marc Eliesen
Chairperson and Executive Director, Manitoba Energy Authority, Winnipeg
Emery Fanjoy
Secretary, Council of Maritime Premiers, Halifax
Maureen Farrow
C.D. Howe Institute, Toronto
Dr. James D. Fleck
Faculty of Management Studies, University of Toronto
Dr. Allan K. Gillmore
Executive Director, Association of Universities and Colleges of Canada, Ottawa
Margaret C. Harris
Past President, The National Council of Women of Canada, Saskatoon
Michael Hicks
Principal, Centre for Executive Development, Ottawa
Dr. David Hopper
Washington, D.C.
Richard W. Johnston
President, Spencer Stuart & Associates, Toronto
Dr. Leon Katz, O.C.
Saskatoon
Dr. David Leighton
Director, National Centre for Management Research and Development
University of Western Ontario, London
Terrence Mactaggart
Managing Director, Sound Linked Data Inc., Mississauga
Judith Maxwell
Chairman, Economic Council of Canada, Vanier
Milan Nastich
Canadian General Investments Ltd., Toronto
Professor William A. W. Neilson
Dean, Faculty of Law, University of Victoria
Roderick C. Nolan, P.Eng.
President, Neill & Gunter Limited, Fredericton
Robert J. Olivero
United Nations Secretariat, New York
Gordon F. Osbaldeston, O.C.
Senior Fellow, School of Business Administration, University of Western Ontario, London
Garnet T. Page, O.C.
Calgary
Jean-Guy Paquet
Vice-président exécutif, La Laurentienne, mutuelle d'Assurance, Québec
Professor Marilyn L. Pilkington
Osgoode Hall Law School, Toronto
Eldon D. Thompson
President, Telesat, Vanier
Dr. Israel Unger
Dean of Science, University of New Brunswick, Fredericton

Dr. Norman Wagner
  President and Vice-Chancellor, University of Calgary
Ida Wasacase, C.M.
  Winnipeg
Dr. R. Sherman Weaver
  Director, Alberta Environmental Centre, Vegreville
Dr. Blossom Wigdor
  Director, Program in Gerontology, University of Toronto

Government Representatives

Roger Burke, Prince Edward Island
Joseph H. Clarke, Nova Scotia
Hershell Ezrin, Ontario
Allan Filmer, British Columbia
George Ford, Manitoba
Ron Hewitt, Saskatchewan
Barry Mellon, Alberta
Geoffrey Norquay, Canada
Eloise Spitzer, Yukon
H.H. Stanley, Newfoundland
Barry Toole, New Brunswick
Gérard Veilleux, Canada
Louise Vertes, Northwest Territories

Institute Management

Rod Dobell	President
Peter Dobell	Vice-President and Secretary-Treasurer
Yvon Gasse	Director, Small & Medium-Sized Business Program
Barry Lesser	Director, Information Society Studies Program
Jim MacNeill	Director, Environment & Sustainable Development Program
Shirley Seward	Director, Studies in Social Policy
Murray Smith	Director, International Economics Program
Jeffrey Holmes	Director, Communications
Parker Staples	Director, Financial Services
Tom Kent	Editor, *Policy Options Politiques*

Fellows- and Scholars-in-Residence:

Edgar Gallant	Fellow-in-Residence
Tom Kent	Fellow-in-Residence
Eric Kierans	Fellow-in-Residence
Jean-Luc Pepin	Fellow-in-Residence
Gordon Robertson	Fellow-in-Residence
Alan Maslove	Scholar-in-Residence
James Taylor	Scholar-in-Residence
David Cameron	Scholar-in-Residence
Dennis Protti	Scholar-in-Residence
Eugene M. Nesmith	Executive-in-Residence

Related Publications Available

Order Address

The Institute for Research on Public Policy
P.O. Box 3670 South
Halifax, Nova Scotia
B3J 3K6

David K. Foot (ed.)

Public Employment and Compensation in Canada: Myths and Realities. 1978 $10.95

Meyer W. Bucovetsky (ed.)

Studies in Public Employment and Compensation in Canada. 1979 $14.95

G. Bruce Doern &
Allan M. Maslove (eds.)

The Public Evaluation of Government Spending. 1979 $10.95

Richard M. Bird

The Growth of Public Employment in Canada. 1979 $12.95

Peter Aucoin (ed.)

The Politics and Management of Restraint in Government. 1981 $17.95

Nicole S. Morgan

Nowhere to Go? Possible Consequences of the Demographic Imbalance in Decision-Making Groups of the Federal Public Service. 1981 $8.95

Nicole S. Morgan

Où aller? Les conséquences prévisibles des déséquilibres démographiques chez les groupes de décision de la fonction publique fédérale. 1981 $8.95

BEYOND THE BOTTOM LINE

Jacob Finkelman &
Shirley B. Goldenberg

*Collective Bargaining in the Public Service:
The Federal Experience in Canada.* 2 vols. 1983
$29.95 (set)

Mark Thompson &
Gene Swimmer

*Conflict or Compromise: The Future of Public
Sector Industrial Relations.* 1984 $15.00

Nicole Morgan

*Implosion: An Analysis of the Growth of the Federal
Public Service in Canada (1945-1985).* 1986
$20.00

Nicole Morgan

*Implosion: analyse de la croissance de la Fonction
publique fédérale canadienne (1945-1985).* 1986
$20.00

John W. Langford and
K. Lorne Brownsey (eds.)

*The Changing Shape of Government in the Asia-
Pacific Region.* 1988. $22.00

Index

INDEX

INDEX